Contents

About the editors

Dr Tim French is a 33-year-old house officer at the Countess of Chester Hospital. Prior to taking the plunge into a medical career at the precipitous age of 27, he studied Experimental Psychology at Balliol College, Oxford University, graduating with a first-class honours degree. He then taught sound engineering and production in London, working as a freelance production engineer in his spare time. While studying medicine at Liverpool University he became interested in the idea of publishing a series of books to complement the new problem-based learning courses. After learning hard lessons about not working on important projects with close friends, he eventually found a kindred and industrious spirit in the unlikely guise of his lexical former academic sub-dean.

Professor Terry Wardle: the 'prof' will be fondly remembered by all of those he has taught, chastised, and ritually humiliated (only joking, Tim). Another late starter to medicine, the former joiner is currently the Professor of Clinical Science at Chester University, and Clinical Sub-Dean at Liverpool Medical School. He has considerable experience in the theory and practice of teaching, and has contributed to the development of many aspects of undergraduate and postgraduate medical education including the internationally acclaimed MedicALS course. Aside from these duties, he is a jobbing consultant gastroenterologist/hepatologist at the Countess of Chester Hospital, and resorts to Thai boxing to 'unwind' in the evenings (when I'm not on-call, Terry).

List of contributors

Dr Libby Artingstall MB/ChB(Hons)
House Officer, Royal Liverpool Hospital
Co-author, scenario 3

Mr Alex Blackmore MB/ChB MRCS
Senior House Officer in Surgery, Christie's
Hospital Manchester
Co-author, scenarios 8, 9, 11

Dr Rob Cooper MB/ChB(Hons)
House Officer, Countess of Chester Hospital
Author, scenario 18

Dr Andy Cunnane MB/ChB
Senior House Officer in Anaesthetics, Aintree
Hospital
Co-author, scenario 6

Professor James Elder MD (Commendation) FRCS
(Ed Eng Glas)
Professor of Surgery (Retired), Keele
University
Co-author, scenarios 3, 8, 9, 11

Mr Mike French MB/ChB MD(Cambs) MD FRCS
Consultant Urologist (retired), North
Staffordshire University Hospital
Author, scenarios 4, 8, 12, 14

Dr Tim French BA(Hons) MA (Oxon) MB/ChB(Hons)
House Officer, Countess of Chester Hospital
Author, scenarios 1, 3, 15, 16, 20, 23, 26, 28,
30

Dr Alan Highcock MB/ChB(Hons)
House Officer, Arrowe Park Hospital
Author, scenarios 6, 10

Dr Clint Jones BSc(Hons) MB/ChB(Hons)
House Officer, Arrowe Park Hospital
Author, scenarios 2, 25, 27

Dr Toni Jordan MB/ChB(Hons) MRCP
Specialist Registrar in Respiratory Medicine,
Aintree Hospital
Author, scenarios 5, 22

Dr Josep Macmillan BSc MB/ChB(Hons)
Senior House Officer in Anaesthetics, Aintree
Hospital
Author, scenarios 7, 29

Dr Stephen Newton MB/ChB
Senior House Officer in Accident and
Emergency Medicine, Glan Clwyd Hospital
Co-author, scenario 25

Dr Jon Rosser MB/ChB(Hons)
House Officer, Arrowe Park Hospital
Co-author, scenarios 4, 12, 14

Mr Azi Samsudin MB/ChB MRCS
Specialist Registrar in Urology, Countess of
Chester Hospital
Co-author, scenarios 4, 12, 14

Dr Sameer K Sharma MB/ChB
Clinical Fellow and Anatomy Demonstrator,
Addenbrookes Hospital
Author, scenarios 13, 19

Mr John Taylor ChM BSc FRCS (Gen Surg)
Specialist Registrar in Vascular Surgery,
Countess of Chester Hospital
Co-author, scenario 8

Dr John Tsang MB/ChB MRCP
Specialist Registrar in Geriatric Medicine
Co-author, scenario 25

Professor Terry Wardle MB/BS(Hons)
BMedSci(Hons) DM FRCP
Professor of Clinical Sciences, Chester
University
Consultant Gastroenterologist, Countess of
Chester Hospital
Co-author, scenarios 15, 17, 18, 26, 28
Author, scenarios 17, 21, 24

Dedication

This book is dedicated to my late grandfather Dr EB French.

Acknowledgements

We would like to thank all of the contributors to this book for their help and support. Particular thanks should go to Mr Mike French and Professor James Elder for making the most of their retirement years. Their unending enthusiasm dragged us forwards by making a significant contribution to the surgical scenarios in this book. Furthermore, we would like to thank Dr Guy Sissons for his valuable help with the radiology elements in the scenarios, and his clear-thinking, concise commentary. All the staff in the ECG department of the Countess of Chester Hospital are to be thanked for remembering to get our ECGs. We would also like to thank our publisher Radcliffe, and in particular the managing director, Andrew Bax, for his patience and trust in the concept we presented him with many months ago. He smiled his way through a progression of missed deadlines, and gently persuaded us to hurry up. Lastly, but by no means least, Tim would like to thank his girlfriend Charlotte for her sufferance in the face of what has been a very long year; she considered surgery to maintain her smile after many thousands of hours of discussing 'the book'.

Should we have written this book? We feel the answer is 'yes', and we hope it proves useful for most medical students. However we welcome your views and comments.

Abbreviations

ABCD	airway, breathing, circulation, disability	cpm	contractions per minute
ABCDE	airway, breathing, circulation, disability, environment	CPP	cerebral perfusion pressure
		CPR	cardiopulmonary resuscitation
ABG	arterial blood gases	CRF	corticotrophin-releasing factor
ABPI	ankle brachial pressure index	CRP	C-reactive protein
AC	adenocarcinoma	CSF	cerebrospinal fluid
ACE	angiotensin-converting enzyme	CT	computed tomography
ACE-I	angiotensin-converting enzyme inhibitor	CTPA	CT pulmonary angiography
ACR	albumin creatinine ratio	CVP	central venous pressure
ACS	acute coronary syndrome/American College of Surgeons	CXR	chest X-ray
		DBP	diastolic blood pressure
ACTH	adrenocorticotrophic hormone	DCIS	ductal carcinoma *in situ*
ADH	antidiuretic hormone	DEXA	dual emission X-ray absorbtiometry
A&E	accident and emergency	DHS	dynamic hip screw
AF	atrial fibrillation	DKA	diabetic ketoacidosis
AFB	acid-fast bacilli	DNAR	do not attempt resuscitation
AIDS	acquired immunodeficiency syndrome	DT	delirium tremens
ALL	acute lymphoblastic leukaemia	DVT	deep vein thrombosis
ALP	alkaline phosphatase	ECG	electrocardiogram
ALS	advanced life support	ECHO	echocardiography
ALT	alanine transaminase	EEG	electroencephalogram
AMA	antimitochondrial antibodies	EMA	endomysial antibody
AML	acute myeloid leukaemia	ENS	enteric nervous system
AMT	abbreviated mental test	ERCP	endoscopic retrograde cholangiopancreatography
ANA	antinuclear antibodies		
APTT	activated partial thromboplastin time	ESBL	extended-spectrum beta lactamase
ARDS	acute respiratory distress syndrome	ESR	erythrocyte sedimentation rate
ASD	atrioseptal defect	ESWL	extracorporeal shock wave lithotripsy
5-ASA	5-aminosalicylic acid	EUS	endoscopic ultrasound
AST	aspartate transaminase	EVM	eyes, voice and motor
ATLS	advanced trauma life support	FBC	full blood count
AUA	American Urological Association	FBD	functional bowel disorder
AVPU	Alert, responds to Voice, responds to Pain, Unresponsive	FEV_1	forced expiratory volume in 1 s
		FiO_2	fraction of inspired oxygen
BCG	bacillus of Calmette and Guérin	FNA	fine needle aspiration
BGS	British Geriatrics Society	FNAC	fine needle aspiration cytology
BLS	basic life support	α-FP	alpha fetoprotein
BM	Boeringher Mannheim (test)	FVC	forced vital capacity
BMD	bone mineral density	GABA	γ-aminobutyric acid
BMI	body mass index	GCS	Glasgow coma scale/score
BP	blood pressure	GFR	glomerular filtration rate
BPH	benign prostatic hypertrophy	GGT	gamma-glutamyl transpeptidase
BTS	British Thoracic Society	GKI	glucose, potassium and insulin
CBD	common bile duct	GI	gastrointestinal
CCF	congestive cardiac failure	GMC	General Medical Council
CDSC	Communicable Disease Surveillance Centre	GP	general practitioner
		Hb	haemoglobin
COCP	combined oral contraceptive pill	HbA_{1c}	glycosylated haemoglobin
COPD	chonic obstructive pulmonary disease	HDU	high-dependency unit

HLA	human leucocyte antigen	NSF	National Service Framework
HRT	hormone replacement therapy	NSTEMI	non-ST elevation myocardial infarction
IBD	inflammatory bowel disease	OCP	oral contraceptive pill
IBS	irritable bowel syndrome	OGD	oesophagogastroduodenoscopy
ICU	intensive care unit	OGTT	oral glucose tolerance test
IFG	impaired fasting glycaemia	od	once daily
Ig	immunoglobulin	PaCO$_2$	partial pressure of arterial carbon dioxide
IGT	impaired glucose tolerance		
i.m.	intramuscular	PACS	partial anterior circulation syndrome
INR	international normalised ratio	PaO$_2$	partial pressure of arterial oxygen
IPPV	invasive positive pressure ventilation	p-ANCA	peripheral antineutrophil cytoplasmic antibodies
IPSS	International Prostate Symptom Score		
ISH	isolated systolic hypertension	PBL	problem-based learning
ITU	intensive therapy unit	PCI	percutaneous coronary intervention
i.v.	intravenous	PE	pulmonary embolism
IVU	intravenous urography	PEA	pulseless electrical activity
JCVI	Joint Committee on Vaccination and Immunisation	PEG	percutaneous endoscopic gastrostomy
		PEFR	peak expiratory flow rate
JVP	jugular venous pressure	PND	paroxysmal nocturnal dyspnoea
IVU	intravenous urogram	PIOPED	Prospective Investigation of Pulmonary Embolism Diagnosis (study)
KUB	kidneys/ureters/bladder		
LACS	lacunar stroke	POCS	posterior circulation stroke
LDH	lactate dehydrogenase	PPAR	peroxisome proliferator-activated receptor-gamma
LDL	low-density lipoprotein		
LFT	liver function tests	PPI	proton pump inhibitor
LHRH	luteinising hormone-releasing hormone	PR	*per rectum*
LIF	left iliac fossa	PSA	prostate-specific antigen
LKM	anti-liver–kidney microsomal antibodies	PT	prothrombin time
LMWH	low-molecular weight heparin	PTCA	percutaneous transluminal coronary angioplasty
LREC	local research and ethics committee		
LRTI	lower respiratory tract infection	PTFE	polytetrafluoroethylene
LVF	left ventricular failure	PTH	parathyroid hormone
LVH	left ventricular hypertrophy	PTHrP	parathyroid hormone-related peptide
MAU	medical assessment unit	PVD	peripheral vascular disease
MCH	mean cell haemoglobin	qds	four times a day
MCV	mean corpuscular volume	QoL	quality of life
MDR TB	multi-drug-resistant TB	RIF	right iliac fossa
MDS	myelodysplasia	RNIB	Royal National Institute for the Blind
MDT	multidisciplinary team	RTA	road traffic accident
MI	myocardial infarction	RV	residual volume
MMSE	mini-mental state examination	RVF	right ventricular failure
6-MP	6-mercaptopurine	SALT	speech and language therapy
MRCP	magnetic resonance cholangiopancreatography	SAU	surgical admissions unit
		SBP	systolic blood pressure
MRI	magnetic resonance imaging	SCC	squamous cell carcinoma
MRSA	methicillin-resistant *Staphylococcus aureus*	SHO	senior house officer
		SIADH	syndrome of inappropriate ADH secretion
MSU	midstream urine		
NCEPOD	National Confidential Enquiry into Patient Outcome and Death	SIGN	Scottish Intercollegiate Guidelines Network
NICE	National Institute for Health and Clinical Excellence	SIRS	systemic inflammatory response syndrome
NIPPV	non-invasive positive pressure ventilation	SMA	antismooth muscle antibodies
		SpO$_2$	oxygen saturation measured by pulse oximetry
NG	nasogastric		
NOF	neck of femur	SSRI	selective serotonin reuptake inhibitor
NSAID	non-steroidal anti-inflammatory drug	STEMI	ST elevation myocardial infarction

T_3	triiodothyronine	TPO	thyroid peroxidase
T_4	thyroxine	TRUS	trans-rectal ultrasound
TACS	total anterior circulation syndrome/ stroke	TSH	thyroid-stimulating hormone
		TURP	transurethral resection prostate
TB	tuberculosis	UC	ulcerative colitis
TBG	thyroid-binding globulin	UDPGT	UDP-glucuronyl transferase
TCC	transitional cell carcinoma	U&E	urea and electrolytes
tds	three times a day	U/S	ultrasound
TED	thromboembolism-deterrent (stockings)	UTI	urinary tract infection
TFT	thyroid function tests	vCJD	variant Creuzfeldt–Jakob disease
TGA	transglutaminase antibody	VUJ	vesicoureteric junction
TIA	transient ischaemic attack	WBC	white blood cell
TNF	tumour necrosis factor	WCC	white cell count
TNM	tumour, node, metastases	WHO	World Health Organization
t-PA	tissue plasminogen activator		

Introduction

Historically, medical teaching was didactic. However, this was at a time when diagnosis depended almost entirely on clinical acumen, and little effective treatment was available. Before all this changed, life expectancy in Britain did increase, but this was largely through public health measures such as adequate sanitation, clean water and reducing transmission of disease by decreasing overcrowding.

The past century has seen an extraordinary development in techniques for investigation, treatment and prevention of disease. This has been the main reason for a further increase in life expectancy. It also means that there has been a major change in the content of the undergraduate medical curriculum. The teaching of medicine has now caught up with this rapid and continuing evolution in medical practice with the introduction of problem-based learning (PBL). This could be thought of as getting medical students to *learn how to learn about medicine*, in the knowledge that they are going to have to continue to learn, and thus adapt their practice of medicine until the day they retire.

In keeping with this, the General Medical Council has stated that it is more important for future medical practitioners to have instilled into them the ability and desire for lifelong learning, rather than to acquire a large volume of factual knowledge. 'We should seek to light fires rather than to fill vessels', is their rather odd slogan. There is still a role for didactic teaching and, for students, the straighforward process of memorising facts. Gross anatomy changes little, if at all. The need to know how to avoid cross-infection will never go away. It is said that medical students double their vocabulary during their training. There is also a continuing need to regard a proportion of both undergraduate and postgraduate training as learning a craft from experienced craftsmen. This applies particularly to the use of technic-ally demanding procedures, all of which would be an assault unless performed by someone qualified on someone who consents.

However PBL is different. It is the process of exploring a medical problem, and deciding on the issues that need further exploration. In short, it is the process of becoming efficient at finding the solution to a medical problem. This situation is at its most acute on the first day as a medical student. However, after successfully completing the medical course, the doctor should be proficient as a well-motivated, resourceful, self-directed learner, equipped with the relevant skills to facilitate lifelong learning.

So why this book?

In this book, scenarios will enable medical students, either alone, or in groups to learn about:

- selected clinical problems
- self-directed learning
- what resources are available.

It is not comprehensive, thus having worked through it, you will not know all you need to know, either to pass your final exams or, perhaps more importantly, to become a safe junior doctor. What it does set out to do is to guide you by the use of selected cases and asking you questions as you go through the case. We have tried to encourage and direct you to appropriate answers. You can check your answers against information in the 'teaching notes' where the rationale for 'our answers' is given, and further information provided to expand your knowledge.

We strongly urge you to resist the temptation of either 'a quick look, just to ensure you're on the right track' or just to read the teaching notes. You will derive more benefit by working through the scenarios.

Our intention is to help you to gain *some* new insights. However, we also hope that further insights will be gained by returning to the cases later in your training, when you have actually seen the key cases several times.

Traditional short answer question books tend to focus on differential diagnosis, investigations, pathology, and management. While including these concepts, our book aims to expand the scope of questions, making them relevant to today's PBL courses. Thus, scenarios include the psychological aspects of disease, ethical issues surrounding patient care, and multidisciplinary management, including community and social care.

The scenarios are based on real patients. They have been written by consultants, registrars, house officers and medical students, to demonstrate the range of issues that students need to be familiar with to evolve into competent medical practitioners. We have included investigations from these cases following the protocols of anonymity and consent. It is impossible to fit all of the issues into each case. A book of this nature will encourage you to think about the issues, see more patients, think of the issues that relate to these patients, and reflect on these further. This process could be thought of as writing your own book!

Layout and content

The major components of this book include:

- a list of 'key cases' that students should be familiar with to use the book effectively
- 30 scenarios with associated questions
- answers and teaching notes sections for each of the scenarios
- cross-referencing to aid the development of differential diagnosis skills
- web resources for each of the scenarios
- suggested further reading from commonly used undergraduate/postgraduate textbooks and journals
- index of symptoms, key cases and a general index.

It is important to realise that this book is intended to act as an adjunct to learning. We have presented a series of cases that demonstrate important problems that we have faced in our training. The book in no way constitutes a syllabus, since it is impossible to draw boundaries around the knowledge required to become a competent doctor.

We have deliberately omitted a mark scheme from the questions, since we would encourage you to be able to think around most of the possible answers and justify them. In this way we have 'bulleted' what we consider the most important key points that you should have thought of in response to a question.

If you can justify further answers then that is a good start. The number of key points you can identify should be dependent on your experience. For example, a second-year medical student should be able to work out the signs of dehydration, but might not be able to give the technical details for administration of a fluid challenge in a patient at danger of developing cardiac failure. Similarly, students earlier on in their studies should know that diabetic ketoacidosis (DKA) is treated with insulin, fluid and electrolyte replacement, but might not need to know about the use of glucose, potassium, and insulin infusions to correct the acidosis that may persist after glucose levels have returned to normal.

However, we would make the point that students at all levels should use the opportunity to think about why the sensible answers presented are correct.

Our answers contain brief teaching notes on disease processes. Rather than try to be 'all inclusive' we have included further 'PBL boxes' encouraging you to be aware of further issues in the scenarios. The suggested resources can be used to answer these further questions. We would encourage you to use these 'PBL boxes' to further your knowledge, and to formulate your own learning objectives from each case. Additionally we would encourage you to compare the scenarios with your own clinical experience.

Using this book

This book will help any student on a PBL course in three particular ways: identification of key features, formulation of learning objectives, and self-assessment.

Your first step is to read the scenario and identify the key features. Without these you will not be able to answer the subsequent questions. In some scenarios, the diagnosis will be immediately apparent; however knowing the diagnosis is only the start of your learning journey. Other scenarios contain multiple presenting symptoms and signs, and it is more important to be able to choose between alternatives to answer the subsequent questions. Each question has a different emphasis, with some focusing on community care or psychosocial aspects of disease, and others towards clinical presentation and decision making.

We have deliberately included scenarios that may initially seem similar, such as patients presenting with abdominal pain and vomiting, diarrhoea or breathlessness. That is because these are common presenting symptoms with multiple causes.

An index of symptoms is included in the book, and this is a valuable component of this learning aid. We would encourage students to look at the other scenarios which present with similar symptoms. In this way, students can build up their own clinical decision-making skills based on key feature identification.

An index of 'key cases' or diseases is also included. As an example, diabetes may appear in five different scenarios. Reading these scenarios and answering the questions will help to build a picture of the multiple presentations of diabetes, which can be used as the basis for integrating further knowledge.

When using this book you should ask the following questions:

● why is the problem an important one?
● what do you know about the subject?
● what don't you know about the subject?
● what don't you understand about the subject, and what needs explaining to help you understand?

Clinical PBL learning

When learning during clinical attachments it is vital to take a strategic approach. Every patient presents with a somewhat unique set of problems that require different approaches to management. The scenarios from this book have been developed from a structured, problem-based approach to learning in the clinical setting.

To get the most out of learning in the clinical setting you should:

● introduce yourself to the staff who are working in the clinical environment. Proactively offer to do any jobs that you can, and show staff that you can be useful

● ask staff if there are any patients that they think you should see
● ensure your thorough history and focused examination concentrates on positives and significant negatives
● identify the key features
● think about your management plan for each patient. Write down a problem list if necessary
● clerk the patient, not the notes
● compare your findings with those in the patient's notes. Are there features that you have missed? Why have you missed them?
● present the patient to a more senior colleague
● revisit patients to find out how their condition has evolved. Explore their thoughts and feelings regarding their care
● as the patient's condition improves, think about planning their discharge
● follow up patients. Find out if they have a clinic appointment and ask if you can go
● visit patients at home with a GP.

By following this approach, you will develop insight into some of the elements that will help you to become a competent doctor.

Examinations

PBL encourages you to think about the broader elements of medicine when formulating learning objectives from a scenario. However, exams require a different approach. It is essential to prioritise your thoughts, and marks are given for the important facts.

Although we have presented key facts as 'suggested answers', it is important to realise that this book is not intended as an examination crammer. Case history questions are used in assessments by certain medical schools, however the style and content of questioning in this book are not indicative of any particular examination format.

Self-assessment

The scenarios presented have been designed to bring out important problems and issues, and to aid in the process of self-assessment. Self-assessment is an ongoing process throughout both student and professional life, involving critical self-appraisal and the formulation of learning objectives to enhance knowledge.

Finally . . .

We have set out a framework for using this book, and this can be tailored to your needs. Whatever approach you adopt, the aim should be to understand the principles, rather than rote learning of lists.

Key cases index

The scenarios

1 A student with a 'hangover'

Catherine is 17 years old. She presents to the A&E department at 4 pm complaining of vomiting all night, and has associated severe abdominal pain. She says that she was out with friends from college the night before and drank too much alcohol. She felt hung over this morning and didn't go to college, choosing instead to try and sleep it off. The vomiting and abdominal pain persisted, and now she feels acutely unwell. She has had type 1 diabetes mellitus since the age of 4 years old, and was transferred from the care of paediatric to adult diabetic services 6 months ago. She had not attended her scheduled annual appointment 3 months ago.

(a) What further questions would you want to ask?

....

....

....

While in the A&E department she deteriorates rapidly and starts to show signs of a reduced conscious level.

(b) Which physical signs would support your working diagnosis?

....

....

....

The results of the initial blood tests are shown in (c) below.

(c) Fill in the blank cells with ↑ ↓ or ↔ for increased, decreased or normal.

Plasma glucose	28 mmol/l
Urinary ketones	+++
Urea and electrolytes	
Na$^+$	
K$^+$	5.2 mmol/l
Urea	
Creatinine	100 µmol/l
Arterial blood gases	
pH	6.9
PaO$_2$	13.2 kPa
PaCO$_2$	
HCO$_3^-$	
Anion gap	

(d) Describe your initial management.

....

....

....

(e) What complications might arise during treatment?

....

....

....

She is started on treatment in A&E, and subsequently is transferred to the medical assessment unit. On reviewing the blood test results, the registrar comments that her white cell count is elevated at 36 × 10^9/l and that her serum amylase level is 763 iu/l.

(f) Does this have any implications for management?

....

....

....

Later she is transferred to a general medical ward and appears to have made a good recovery. She is eating and drinking, and has been restarted on her normal insulin regime. The consultant endocrinologist comments that teenage years can be particularly difficult for young people with diabetes, and that he needs to discuss certain issues with Catherine. Additionally he suggests that she see the diabetic specialist nurse whilst still an inpatient to discuss 'sick day rules'.

(g) What would the consultant want to discuss?

....

....

....

(h) What would the diabetic specialist nurse discuss with Catherine regarding 'sick day rules'?

....

....

....

(i) Which healthcare professionals will be involved in her future care?

....

....

....

Key cases

- Type 1 diabetes mellitus
- Diabetic ketoacidosis

Clinical context

Vomiting and abdominal pain are common presenting symptoms in patients who are acutely ill. Such individuals may be referred to physicians, surgeons, and even gynaecologists, as there are so many causes of vomiting and abdominal pain. A pregnancy test is mandatory in all women of reproductive age, diabetic or not! This case illustrates the need for an accurate history to help discriminate between the various conditions; and how clinical examination is of paramount importance in assessing the severity of an illness and monitoring the response to treatment.

Diabetic ketoacidosis (DKA)

DKA should be considered in any unwell diabetic patient, particularly those who are short of breath but not hypoxaemic.

DKA results from either insulin deficiency or an excess of stress hormones with anti-insulin activity. Insulin deficiency results in increased gluconeogenesis in the liver, decreased peripheral glucose uptake and increased lipolysis in adipose tissue. The net result is severe dehydration from a rapid glucose-driven osmotic diuresis, and metabolic acidosis from the eventual accumulation of keto acids produced by fatty acid metabolism.

The symptoms and signs follow from the pathophysiological processes. Thus, DKA presents with nausea, vomiting and abdominal pain (a central effect of ketosis); signs of dehydration (from the vomiting and osmotic diuresis); hyperventilation (an attempt to remove CO_2 to compensate for the metabolic acidosis).

Additionally if the DKA has been caused by serious illness, the patient may present with the symptoms relating to that condition (e.g. myocardial infarction, pneumonia, sepsis). Such symptoms and the associated signs may mask those associated with ketoacidosis. This is particularly true of renal and cardiac causes, which, if volume-retaining, can counteract the usual volume depletion.

The usual causes of DKA are:

- undiagnosed type 1 diabetes mellitus
- missed insulin doses due to illness or poor education
- illness, causing an increase in stress hormones with anti-insulin actions (e.g. glucocorticoids, adrenaline, glucagon).

Other causes include acute pancreatitis and binge drinking of alcohol.

> You must be aware of the spectrum of clinical presentations of diabetes. Diabetes may present asymptomatically, insidiously, with multi-system pathology or as an emergency. Can you think of patients you have seen with these presentations?

(a) History

It is essential to be able to obtain a clear history in a young patient with known diabetes. The history should focus on finding out the cause for the ketoacidosis, whether it is missed insulin doses, intercurrent illness, alcohol, or drugs. Therefore key points in the history must include:

- further symptoms of DKA including polydipsia, polyuria, rapid breathing
- last insulin dose and any insulin doses missed
- recent home BM tests
- food intake
- drug and alcohol history
- symptoms of infection (pyrexia, cough, sputum, dysuria, urinary frequency)
- symptoms of other illness, e.g. pancreatitis (steatorrhoea, abdominal pain radiating to back) or in older patients myocardial infarction (chest pain, shortness of breath, or may be painless in either the elderly or diabetic patient)
- last menstrual period, contraception used, the risk of pregnancy, and any unprotected sex.

> You should be familiar with the pathogenesis of autoimmune diabetes. What are the immunological, genetic and pathological principles involved? What are the current theories of HLA-mediated susceptibility to autoimmune disease? Which immune cells drive pancreatic β-cell destruction? Which other autoimmune conditions are associated with diabetes mellitus?

(b) Physical examination

The clinical features of DKA can be conveniently separated into those of severe volume depletion, and those produced by the combination of acidosis and ketosis.

Signs of dehydration

- Tachypnoea
- Tachycardia
- Hypotension
- Reduced jugular venous pressure
- Dry mucous membranes and skin
- Reduced skin turgor
- Reduced urine output (however in DKA this may be masked by the osmotic diuresis)

Signs of acidosis/ketosis

- Hyperventilation
- Smell of acetone on the breath
- Hypothermia due to acidosis induced peripheral vasodilation (may be masked by dehydration)

> Use this opportunity to revise the signs of volume depletion. How does progressive volume depletion affect the venous and arterial compartments? How does this relate to the early and late signs of dehydration? (*see* p. 105)

(c) Biochemistry

DKA is demonstrated by the presence of hyperglycaemia, ketosis and metabolic acidosis. The biochemical consequences follow from the pathophysiology:

Plasma glucose	28 mmol/l
Urinary ketones	+++
Urea and electrolytes	
Na^+	↓
K^+	5.2 mmol/l
Urea	↑
Creatinine	100 μmol/l
Arterial blood gases	
$_pH$	6.9
PaO_2	13.2 kPa
$PaCO_2$	↓
HCO_3^-	↓
Anion gap	↑

- Hyperglycaemia and plasma hyperosmolality lead to cellular dehydration.

- Hyperglycaemia has a variable effect on sodium concentration, usually the raised osmolality of the plasma pulls water out of the cells, diluting the plasma sodium. Additionally glycosuria leads to impaired tubular reabsorbtion of sodium.
- Hypovolaemia results in uraemia due to a fall in glomerular filtration rate.
- Hypovolaemia worsens the metabolic acidosis by impairing renal perfusion, leading to a relative inability to excrete H^+ ions and ketones.
- Hyperventilation leads to a fall in $PaCO_2$.
- Metabolic acidosis leads to a low HCO_3^- as the excess acid is buffered.
- Anion gap increases since ketones are negatively charged.

> Use this opportunity to revise the control of glucose metabolism. You should be familiar with the effects of insulin, glucagon, corticosteroids and catecholamines on different tissues. Which hormones are affected by stress and illness?

(d) Management of DKA

The principles of management are simple. Rehydration and correction of hyperglycaemia, acidosis and electrolyte disturbance are the priorities. It must also be remembered that there is often a precipitant for DKA. If so, this must be found and treated as promptly as possible.

Most hospitals have a protocol for managing DKA. When managing patients with DKA it is important to follow the protocol and to involve senior doctors as quickly as possible.

The principles of management are:

- *O_2 via facemask*
- *intravenous fluids*: hydration with 0.9% saline (1 l immediately, then 1 l bags sequentially over 1 h, 2 h and 4 h). This is modified according to local protocols and clinical response
- *insulin*: fast-acting insulin should be used (e.g. Actrapid), added to a solution containing 0.9% saline and run at 6 u/h. The infusion should be kept running until the acidosis has been corrected ($HCO_3^- > 20$ mmol/l), this may involve changing the fluids to 5% or even 10% glucose to prevent hypoglycaemia. Alternatively patients can be put on a glucose, potassium, and insulin (GKI) infusion once the serum glucose level is low enough (approximately 11 mmol/l)
- *K^+ replacement*: K^+ is usually added when the serum glucose level falls to 15 mmol/l if the patient is not hyperkalaemic. It is important to

remember that all patients are depleted of total body potassium
- *nasogastric tube*: patients often have gastric distension and a nasogastric tube is needed to remove gastric contents, and to prevent aspiration
- *catheter*: to monitor urine output. Hourly monitoring should be recorded
- *prophylactic anticoagulation*: in severe dehydration there is a significant risk of hypercoagulability.

Obviously it is also important to treat any cause for the DKA such as an infection or MI.

> In the patient with DKA, why is it important to give supplemental oxygen even if they appear to have normal oxygen saturation? Use this opportunity to revise the oxyhaemoglobin dissociation curve.

Monitoring
- Clinical observation. All patients should be watched carefully regarding their fluid balance (respiratory rate, pulse, blood pressure, urine output/signs of fluid overload etc).
- Check blood gases, U&E and laboratory glucose at 1 h and every 1–2 h for the first few hours. Potassium levels might fall rapidly once insulin is started. Some protocols rely on venous bircarbonate measurement after the initial arterial blood gas sample; this is less traumatic for the patient unless there is an arterial line *in situ*.

Patients should be managed in a high-dependency setting. Cardiac monitoring to detect ECG abnormalities, and urinary catheterisation to detect impending acute renal failure are essential. Additionally, patients can become tired after periods of prolonged hyperventilation, developing respiratory failure that may require intubation, ventilation, and management in intensive care.

> Use this opportunity to revise the physiology of fluid and electrolyte balance in different body compartments. Why might a patient with DKA present with hyper- or hypokalaemia? Why are they always depleted of total body potassium?

(e) Complications during treatment
Complications may develop as a result of either over- or undertreatment. Close monitoring should help correct any complications as they develop.

Over-treatment
- Cerebral or pulmonary oedema may result from over-aggressive rehydration causing fluid shifts. Conscious level and SpO_2 should be checked as part of the routine assessment of vital signs.
- Hypoglycaemia may result from insulin infusion. It is vital to check glucose, urinary or plasma ketones and arterial blood gases (ABG)/venous bicarbonate when tailoring therapy, since some patients may show a rapid fall in blood glucose whilst still manifestly acidotic/ketotic. Sometimes many hours of insulin infusion will be required to correct the acidosis/ketosis (*see* above).
- Hypokalaemia is common due to insulin-induced K^+ cotransport into cells, and loss of K^+ in the urine. This is why hourly U&E measurement and K^+ replacement are critical. Cardiac monitoring may also help detect any arrhythmias.

Under-treatment
- Hypovolaemia impairs renal perfusion and hence may cause acute tubular necrosis. If the systolic blood pressure falls below about 90 mmHg then plasma expanders should be given and a central venous pressure (CVP) line considered.
- Hyperkalaemia may cause cardiac arrest. Hourly U&E measurements are important to guide K^+ replacement. Additionally supplementary calcium (i.e. calcium gluconate 10%) may be used to protect cardiac muscle.
- Hypothermia is caused by acidosis-induced peripheral vasodilation and hyperventilation. A core temperature should be taken if hypothermia is suspected.

> Other important aspects to the management of DKA include the changeover to oral carbohydrate and normal daily insulin. When should this be attempted?

(f) Other blood test results
There are several misleading false-positive results in DKA. These include amylase, which may be raised, and the white cell count, which is invariably raised. This is due to the actions of increased stress hormones, and impaired margination of white cells in the hypovolaemic state.

Differentiating between acute pancreatitis and DKA can therefore be difficult on the basis of both symptoms and biochemistry, and on occasion they can co-exist. The abdominal pain in DKA can be so severe that it may be confused with the surgical acute abdomen (*see* p. 67). A diagnosis of acute pancreatitis is unlikely unless the amylase level is extremely elevated (>1000 iu/l) (*see* p. 123). Additionally, the amylase level in DKA responds rapidly to treatment; if it rapidly reduces with fluids and insulin, acute pancreatitis is unlikely. If in doubt a surgical opinion should be sought.

If infection is suspected elicit relevant symptoms and signs such as pyrexia, cough, sputum production, dysuria, urinary frequency, and signs of an obvious focus of infection. C-reactive protein may be of use and, if indicated, a septic screen can be performed (e.g. chest X-ray, midstream specimen of urine for microscopy, culture and sensitivity, blood cultures etc).

(g) Young diabetic patients

Young diabetic patients confront all the normal pressures of physical, psychological and social development. Insulin doses need to be regularly adjusted during periods of peak growth. Strict glycaemic control is needed to ensure normal physical and intellectual development, and to try to avoid the acute and/or chronic complications of diabetes.

Social, cultural and sexual behavioural changes combined with pressure to conform with peers often hampers a teenager's ability to manage his or her diabetes. Teenagers are not renowned for eating a healthy diet and it is a time when experimentation with alcohol and drugs is common. These factors combined with the stresses of college/work, sports activities and socialising often result in poor glycaemic control.

Only the most dedicated teenagers will check their blood sugar regularly enough, and as a result DKA, hypoglycaemic crises and death are much more common.

At the age of 16 teenagers transfer from the care of paediatric to adult diabetes services and non-attendance rates at adult diabetes clinics are high. (NSF Diabetes, Department of Health, 2001)

> You should be able to develop a framework for describing and assessing the psychological impact of suffering from diabetes as a chronic incurable disease.

Every attempt should be made to educate young diabetic patients. In the case outlined above specific importance should be paid to:

- patient education about the importance of regular attendance at diabetic review, reinforcing the importance of good glycaemic control to avoid acute problems, and to minimise long-term complications
- practical diabetes management, including home glucose testing (BM checks), 'sick day rules' and the provision of ketone dipsticks for urine testing

- alcohol and drug advice. Alcoholic drinks often have high carbohydrate content; and in excess, alcohol causes dehydration
- contraception advice
- if pregnancy is planned, it is important to explain that optimal glycaemic control is essential to avoid serious maternal and foetal complications.

The National Service Framework (NSF) for diabetes (2001) suggests that this can be achieved in several ways:

- 'the planned transfer of the care of young people with diabetes from paediatric diabetes services to adult diabetes services'
- 'small group interventions for young people without their parents that address practical diabetes management issues and provide a forum for support and guidance. Evidence suggests that this can lead to improvements in the knowledge of diabetes management, self-care and blood glucose control.'

> What are the social, occupational and legal consequences of suffering from diabetes? How are driving, job opportunities and insurance affected?

(h) Sick day rules

The stress of illness often increases insulin requirement. It is important that patients are properly educated to avoid serious complications. The principles should be explained in person, and supplemented by written information.

Patients should regularly check their finger-prick glucose levels (BMs), and check for ketones in their urine. Fluid intake nearly always needs to be increased, and normal meals can be replaced with sugary drinks if necessary. Insulin doses may need to be increased or decreased according to blood glucose levels.

A discussion with the patient should include the following points:

- patients always need insulin
- be prepared (e.g. having short-acting insulin, ketone dipsticks, and appropriate information to hand)
- check the urine for ketones and blood glucose more often – about four times a day, or more if necessary
- drink plenty of clear fluids
- replace normal meals with carbohydrate-containing drinks if necessary
- seek medical help as quickly as possible if there is

a persistently high BM despite increased insulin, urinary ketones or vomiting.

The diabetes services within individual trusts often produce information regarding the use of supplemental insulin for patients with intercurrent illness and high blood glucose. Increasing the dose of insulin can avoid progression to DKA, however patients have different basal insulin requirements and ideally should have an individualised schedule.

> Use this opportunity to familiarise yourself with your local diabetes service's information on 'sick day rules'. What is their policy on supplemental insulin? Do they suggest incremental doses in units or as a percentage of basal requirements?

(i) Subsequent care

It is important to know about general patterns of care for people with diabetes mellitus. Insulin replacement is lifelong, and vigilance is essential to avoid the debilitating consequences of the disease.

Diabetes management is a true example of a multidisciplinary team approach. Care is often shared between primary and secondary care. Healthcare professionals who may be involved include:

- GPs
- consultant endocrinologists
- diabetes specialist nurses
- practice nurses
- dieticians
- chiropodists
- optometrists
- ophthalmologists
- vascular surgeons.

Review can be in primary and/or secondary care. Most GP-led diabetes clinics and hospital diabetes clinics will have an agreed protocol for 'shared' care and proforma for annual assessment (*see* p. 149 for the format of a normal diabetic review).

Web resources
- Management of diabetic complications: www.prodigy.nhs.uk
- Management of DKA: www.nice.org.uk
- NSF for diabetes: www.dh.gov.uk

Further reading
- Kitabchi AE, Umpierrez GE, Murphy MB *et al.* (2003) Hyperglycemic crises in patients with diabetes mellitus. *Diabetes Care.* **26** Suppl 1: S109.
- Longmore M, Wilkinson I, Rajagopalan S (eds) (2004) *Oxford Handbook of Clinical Medicine* (6e). Oxford University Press, Oxford, pp. 292–300; pp. 818–19.
- Pickup J and Williams G (eds) (2002). *Textbook of Diabetes* (3e). Blackwell Science, Oxford.
- Rose BD and Post TW (2001). *Clinical Physiology of Acid–Base and Electrolyte Disorders* (5e). McGraw-Hill, New York, pp. 809–15.

dysphasia

A 71-year-old lady is brought into the A&E department by paramedics. Approximately 45 minutes before assessment she was found by her husband at home, slumped in an armchair, confused, and talking gibberish. Examination from the bottom of the bed reveals that she is drowsy, with fluid coming from the corner of her mouth, and has right-sided facial weakness. There is spontaneous movement of only the left arm and leg.

drooling (LM)

Initial baseline observations reveal an oxygen saturation of 93% on air, a pulse rate of 78 beats/min, BP 168/96 mmHg, and a temperature of 36.8°C.

The working diagnosis is stroke.

(a) What other differential diagnoses should be considered in this patient?

- hypoglycaemia
- Seizures
- acute metabolic addison

The husband gives a vague history of his wife having a productive cough for two days, but says that otherwise she has been well.

(b) On further history or examination of the patient, what symptoms or signs might you look for to suggest underlying cardiovascular disease?

chest pain
- SOB

During further questioning the husband informs you that his wife recently started new medication and presents a repeat prescription showing the following:

- simvastatin 40 mg once daily
- ramipril 2.5 mg once daily
- warfarin 2–3 mg daily according to INR
- digoxin 125 µg once daily.

(c) Name four cardiovascular risk factors for stroke that the above medication may be used to treat.

- hypercholesterol   - CHF
- hypertension   - AF
- Past MI (IHD)

(d) Which cardiovascular risk factors should be assessed in all stroke patients?

Following full examination of the patient, the SHO in A&E classifies this stroke as a total anterior circulation syndrome (TACS).

(e) When examining the patient, which criteria need to be fulfilled to classify a stroke as TACS?

- htp homonymous homonopre

(f) What initial management steps should be taken for this patient?

Pt airway

NIB PR until formal assessment

– CT scan rule out HS

☞ Below are some results from the initial investigations taken in the A&E department.

WCC	$16.6 \times 10^9/l$
Neutrophil	$13.7 \times 10^9/l$
Hb	9.4 g/dl
MCV	92 fl
Glucose	6.6 mmol/l
Cholesterol	5.4 mmol/l
CRP	197 mg/l
Urea	5.3 mmol/l
Creatinine	86 μmol/l
Sodium	146 mmol/l
Potassium	4.2 mmol/l
INR	1.6
ECG	Atrial fibrillation (ventricular rate 80–95 beats/min) Voltage criteria for LVH (*see* p. 222)
CXR	Right middle lobe consolidation

(g) What likely conclusions can you make from these results?

Ischaemic stroke $2°$ AFB

(h) What is your further management for this patient?

– Thrombolysis + tPa
+ tPa

☞ The following morning the patient has a CT brain scan, sections of which are shown in Figure 2.1.

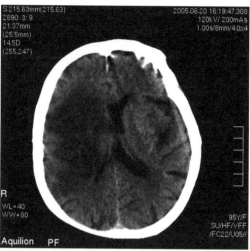

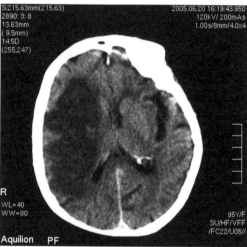

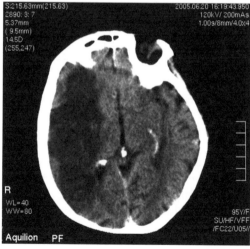

Figure 2.1 CT brain images.

(i) What does the CT scan show?

hypodensity RML

(j) What management is needed after the CT result?

- aspirin 300mg

Prophylactic PPI

☞ The patient is transferred to a multi-disciplinary stroke unit for rehabilitation.

(k) Which healthcare professionals (other than doctors) are in a multidisciplinary stroke team?

SLT - Pharmacist
- Physio - OT
- Nurse - SW

(l) What common complications can patients suffer after a stroke?

aspiration pneumonia

V TE

Key cases

- Stroke
- Hypoglycaemia
- Epilepsy
- Dysrhythmia

Clinical context

Many patients presenting as 'medical emergencies' have acute neurological symptoms and signs. These can be either a primary problem or secondary to many disease processes. You should take 5 minutes and list some of these conditions. If you were allowed one test, what would you request? Your answer should be glucose, as hypoglycaemia has many neurological manifestations and these are reversible, provided the hypoglycaemia is identified and treated immediately.

Stroke is defined as a sudden onset of focal (sometimes global) neurological deficit in a known vascular territory, of vascular origin, that lasts longer than 24 hours, or causes death. It is the third most common cause of death in most developed countries, accounting for approximately 4.5 million deaths each year worldwide. Within the first 30 days of having a stroke, approximately 10% of patients will die, and at 6 months the death rate is at 25%. The risk of severe disability is high for those who survive. Approximately 50% of stroke patients experience some level of disability after 6 months.

This scenario explores the differential diagnosis surrounding stroke, looks at the treatment of acute stroke, and the importance of managing treatable risk factors, going on to discuss the medical, social, and psychological consequences that a patient may suffer following a stroke.

(a) Differential diagnosis

Despite the high probability of stroke in this patient, the following differential diagnoses should be considered:

- *hypoglycaemia*: always assess glucose levels in patients with neurological symptoms and signs. Patients' thresholds may vary, but a glucose level <2.5 mmol/l is enough to make most patients symptomatic. These patients may become sweaty with tremors and feel hungry (autonomic features). Some may be drowsy, agitated, have seizures, or present with focal neurological symptoms such as weakness in an arm or a leg. Hypoglycaemia may exacerbate old symptoms and

signs of a previous stroke. These generally resolve quickly once the glucose level is corrected
- *transient ischaemic attack* (TIA): a sudden-onset focal neurological deficit in a known vascular territory, of vascular origin, that resolves within 24 hours. TIAs are often shorter lasting, resolving over less than 30 minutes. For example a patient may describe 'a sudden loss of vision in one eye that resolved spontaneously after 10 minutes' (amaurosis fugax)
- *subdural haemorrhage*: usually insidious in onset. Monitor for altered or fluctuating level of consciousness, personality changes, sleepiness and headaches. It is an important diagnosis to consider, as neurosurgical intervention is the definitive treatment. Patients at high risk are those with a history of either recent trauma (especially alcoholics)/those on long-term anticoagulation/ or with chronic liver disease (due to coagulation defects; *see* p. 61)
- *tumour*: again the presenting symptoms and signs are usually insidious in onset, and can be similar to a subdural haemorrhage, varying according to the site of the lesion. However patients may present suddenly following haemorrhage into the tumour (*see* p. 127)
- *cerebral abscess*: patients may have symptoms and signs of ongoing infection, e.g. fever, they may be confused or even have a history of meningism. Occasionally the presentation of a cerebral abscess can be sudden due to a bleed into the abscess capsule or alternatively into the surrounding brain tissue.

> Use this opportunity to explore each differential diagnosis. It is important to develop a working understanding of the history, symptoms, signs, appropriate investigations, and treatment.

(b) Symptoms and signs of underlying cardiovascular disease

A stroke can be the first manifestation of cardiovascular disease (e.g. atheroma, atrial fibrillation, or silent myocardial infarction with mural thrombus) in a patient. The following common symptoms and signs may indicate chronic underlying cardiovascular disease:

History:

- *'funny dos'*: possible previous TIA
- *claudication*: peripheral vascular disease
- *angina*: ischaemic heart disease
- *palpitations*: arrhythmia, e.g. paroxysmal atrial fibrillation
- *reduced exercise tolerance*: ischaemic heart disease, heart failure
- *weight loss, polydipsia, polyuria, and lethargy*: diabetes mellitus
- *family history*
- *drugs*.

Examination:

- *carotid bruit*: large-vessel atherosclerosis
- *absent or reduced peripheral pulses*
- *hypertension*
- *apex beat*: prominent in left ventricular hypertrophy – secondary to long-standing hypertension
- *hypertensive retinopathy*
- *irregularly irregular pulse*: atrial fibrillation
- *tendon xanthomas, corneal arcus, xanthelasma*: hyperlipidaemia
- *cardiac murmurs*.

(c) Common cardiovascular medication

Knowledge of common drugs can often help when assessing both the patient's clinical risk factors and the underlying disease. The following risk factors (**bold**) may correspond to this patient taking:

- *simvastatin*: a reversible inhibitor of the rate-limiting enzyme HMG CoA reductase used in the production of cholesterol. It is used in the management of **hypercholesterolaemia and mixed hyperlipidaemia**
- *ramipril*: an angiotensin-converting enzyme inhibitor (ACEI) that reduces the production of angiotensin II. Used in the management of **hypertension, ischaemic heart disease (post MI), heart failure** and diabetic nephropathy (unlikely in this patient as she is not on any other diabetic medication)
- *warfarin*: an antagonist of vitamin K, the essential cofactor for the production of clotting factors II, VII, IX and X, and proteins C and S. Reduces the risk of thromboembolism, e.g. in patients with **atrial fibrillation, metal heart valves, and/or a high risk of DVT or PE**
- *digoxin*: a cardiac glycoside that inhibits the Na^+/K^+ ATPase pump in the heart. It increases the force of myocardial contraction (positive inotrope) and slows the heart rate (negative chronotrope). As a result it is used to control the heart rate in patients with **supraventricular dysrrhyth**-

mias (most often **atrial fibrillation**) and occasionally in **heart failure**.

> Use this opportunity to revise the pharmacology of *common* drugs used in the management of cardiovascular disease. A description of other common antihypertensives can be found on p. 223.

(d) Risk factors for stroke

Strokes can occur at any age, yet more than half of all strokes occur in people over 70 years old. The commonest type of stroke is ischaemic (80%), secondary to thrombotic or embolic occlusion of a cerebral artery; the remainder are mainly caused by intracerebral haemorrhage.

Associated with these common causes of stroke are the following cardiovascular risk factors that promote either atheroma (large and small vessel disease), emboli formation, or both. They should be assessed in all patients:

- hypertension
- diabetes mellitus
- smoking
- excess alcohol intake
- hyperlipidaemia
- atrial fibrillation
- recent MI (< 3/12: associated with a high risk of mural thrombus)
- poor left ventricular function (high risk of thrombus).

There are other rare causes of stroke (e.g. dissection of carotid and vertebral arteries, cerebral venous thrombosis, and vasculitis); however these are generally more common in the younger population (<50 years).

> Assessment of stroke in younger patients can require further investigations and treatment of a rare cause. Study the different causes of stroke in younger patients (e.g. patent foramen ovale, antiphospholipid syndrome, thrombocythaemia and polycythaemia), the additional investigations required for diagnosis and appropriate treatment.

(e) Classification of stroke

There are many classifications of stroke, usually according to the distribution of either individual arteries, or groups of arteries. One such system (Bamford, 1991) categorises patients according to their symptoms and signs into one of the following four groups:

I total anterior circulation stroke (TACS)
II partial anterior circulation stroke (PACS)
III posterior circulation stroke (POCS)
IV lacunar stroke (LACS).

Associated with each classification are differences in pathogenesis, treatment and prognosis.

For the classification of TACS a patient must have symptoms or signs in three of the following categories:

- motor and/or sensory loss affecting the face, arm and/or leg
- higher cerebral dysfunction (dysphasia, perceptual and/or cognitive abnormalities)
- hemianopia.

> Understand the specific criteria for each stroke classification and the associated common causative vascular lesions. What are the effects of occlusion of specific arterial territories supplying the brain?

(f) Initial management of stroke

The initial management of stroke patients involves the management of ABCDE, including the following:

Airway

1 Maintain a patent airway.
2 Keep 'nil by mouth' until swallowing has been assessed (reduced risk of aspiration pneumonia).

Breathing

3 Prevent hypoxaemia.

Circulation

4 Ensure adequate hydration with intravenous access and fluids.
5 Reduce risk of venous thromboembolism by using TED stockings.
6 Reduce BP, if sustained above 230/130 mmHg (there is often a transient rise in BP that settles within 24–48 h).

Disability

7 Correct hypo- or hyperglycaemia (target blood sugar 4–11). Note: all diabetic patients who are nil by mouth should be commenced on a glucose/potassium/insulin (GKI) regime.

Environment

8 Treat pyrexia. Tissue metabolism is higher at higher temperatures. Thus, neural damage is increased in patients with a fever.

In addition

9 Maintain regular turning and keep dry to prevent pressure sores. Some patients may need catheterising to keep them dry (e.g. if they have infected or necrotic pressure sores). Note: catheterisation is not without risks of infection and should not be done routinely.
10 Prevent malnutrition. Be positive and aim for early nutrition assessment with a dietician (see below).

Undernutrition in stroke patients has a direct effect on mortality and functional status at 6 months. Hence it is an important issue to address immediately following admission. This may be complicated by the high prevalence of dysphagia in stroke patients (estimated to be between 22% and 65%).

The largest randomised controlled trial to assess nutrition found that early tube feeding reduced case fatality, but this was at the expense of an increased number of patients with a poor outcome. The other arm of this trial revealed PEG to have no significant clinical benefit over NG feeding. An absolute difference in death and poor outcome was found to be in favour of NG feeding. In conclusion, early enteral tube feeding should be offered to dysphagic stroke patients to reduce the risk of mortality (unless there are strong indications to delay) within the first few days of admission, and NG feeding should be used as first-line therapy (unless there are strong practical reasons to choose a PEG) (Dennis et al., FOOD Trial Collaboration, 2005).

> PEG placement and feeding is not without risks. What are the issues surrounding PEG feeding?

Note: This patient's warfarin should be stopped. Despite the risk of further emboli from atrial fibrillation, anticoagulation in the acute phase of an ischaemic stroke has shown no short- or long-term benefits. It is associated with a significant increase of intracranial and extracranial haemorrhages. Further accurate assessment of the risks for embolic versus haemorrhagic stroke needs to done before anticoagulation can be restarted.

(g) Initial investigations

The results from initial investigations reveal the following significant findings:

- right middle lobe pneumonia
- normocytic anaemia
- rate-controlled atrial fibrillation
- LVH probably secondary to long-standing hypertension
- normoglycaemia
- normal renal function (well hydrated, reduced risk of digoxin toxicity)

- INR below therapeutic range (possibly due to poor compliance).

(h) Management in this case

- Start intravenous antibiotics (the patient has not had a swallowing assessment).
- Note: allergy to penicillin.

(i) CT scan result

The CT brain scan shows a broad reduction in density in the right cerebral hemisphere in the middle cerebral artery territory. There is no evidence of intracerebral haemorrhage.

(j) Further management

- Asprin 300 mg (rectally if nil by mouth).
- Proton pump inhibitor (PPI, e.g. 40 mg omeprazole i.v.).

Early aspirin in the acute treatment of ischaemic stroke (300 mg orally or by suppository within 48 hours of stroke onset) has been shown to have major benefits in reducing patients' risk of death, recurrent stroke and dependency post-stroke (International Stroke Trial Collaborative Group, 1997). In the elderly there is an increased risk of upper GI haemorrhage, therefore a prophylactic PPI should be given.

(k) Multidisciplinary stroke care

The multidisciplinary team on a stroke unit should consist of:

- nursing staff
- medical staff
- physiotherapists
- occupational therapists
- speech and language therapists
- social workers.

However other healthcare professionals can often be found in these teams, e.g. clinical psychologists, psychiatrists, and dieticians.

Organised stroke care saves lives, and has been shown to reduce the risk of death and institutionalisation. With every 33 patients treated there is one extra survivor; for every 20 patients, one extra patient is discharged back to their own home, and another patient becomes fully independent. Admitting patients to stroke units ensures constant focused care by competent healthcare professionals devoted to achieving three important goals of stroke care:

1 general medical management
2 early organised rehabilitation
3 prevention and management of complications.

Multidisciplinary stroke rehabilitation aims to maximise a patient's activity participation (socially and occupationally) and quality of life, and to address carers' concerns. To help accomplish these aims the International Classification of Functioning, Disability and Health (ICF) suggests that the following areas of function are assessed, and input is provided where needed:

- learning and application of knowledge
- performance of general tasks and demands
- communication
- mobility
- self-care
- domestic life
- interpersonal interactions and relationships
- community, social and civil life.

(SIGN Guideline 64, *Management of Patients with Stroke*, 2002)

This patient has suffered dysphasia, hemianopia and hemiparesis as a consequence of her stroke, and therefore requires specific intervention. Speech and language therapy (SALT), an ophthalmological referral and physiotherapy would be of benefit.

(l) Complications of stroke

There are many barriers to recovering from a stroke. A list of common problems is presented below – it is important to prevent as many of these as possible by the provision of optimal care:

- residual neurological deficits (speech/vision/motor/sensory/cognitive)
- pain
- falls
- incontinence (faecal/urinary)
- infections (chest/urinary tract/other)
- pressure sores
- recurrent stroke
- seizures
- venous thromboembolism
- confusion
- depression
- anxiety.

Web resources

- Scottish Intercollegiate Guidelines Network (SIGN) guidelines: www.sign.ac.uk

Electronic versions of the articles below are available at: www.thelancet.com.

- Dennis MS, Lewis SC and FOOD trial Collaboration (2005) Effect of timing and method of enteral tube feeding for dysphagic stroke patients (FOOD): a multicentre RCT. *Lancet.* **365**: 764–72.
- International Stroke Trial Collaborative Group (1997) The International Stroke Trial (IST): a randomised trial of aspirin, subcutaneous heparin, both, or neither among 19,435 patients

A woman found slumped in a chair

with acute ischaemic stroke. *Lancet.* **349**: 1569–81.

Further reading

- Fisher M and Ratan R (2003) New perspectives on developing acute stroke therapy. *Annals of Neurology.* **53**: 10.
- Hack W, Kaste M, Bogousslavsky J *et al.* (2003) European Stroke Initiative Recommendations for Stroke Management – update. *Cerebrovascular Diseases.* **16**: 311.
- NCEPOD (2004) *Scoping Our Practice – National Confidential Enquiry into Patient Outcome and Death.* NCEPOD, London. www.ncepod.org.uk
- Royal College of Physicians (2004) *National Clinical Guidelines for Stroke* (2e). Royal College of Physicians, London.
- Warburton E (2003) Stroke management. *Clinical Evidence.* **10**: 977.
- World Health Organization (2001) *International Classification of Functioning, Disability and Health.* WHO, Geneva. Available online at www3.who.int/icf/icftemplate.cfm?

3 A worrying lump

A GP receives a letter written by a patient from the practice. It explains how the patient's 35-year-old daughter has had a breast lump for several months but is unwilling to come to the GP practice, due to her fear of physical examination. The letter goes on to describe how her daughter had been sexually abused as a child. The daughter finally started a stable relationship in her late 20s, and has a son who is 6 years old. Tragically her partner died from leukaemia 2 years after the birth of their son. The letter goes on to ask if the GP would write a letter to her daughter urging her to come to the practice, since she is ignoring the problem. Her mother is especially worried as she had breast cancer herself. She was successfully treated 7 years ago and has had no recurrence.

The GP decides to write the letter, and 2 weeks later sees the patient with her mother in the practice. She still refuses to be examined. He decides to try to get the patient to describe the lump and other associated features so that he can have a clearer idea of what he's dealing with.

(a) What should he ask the patient about?

....

....

....

(b) What are some of the common problems encountered by adults who were sexually abused as children; how might they relate to this case?

....

....

....

After a lengthy discussion, her GP decides that the features that she has described warrant further investigation. He tells his patient that the breast surgeon at the local hospital is a woman, and that all examinations are carried out at a completely professional level. The patient refuses to go for further investigation. The patient and her mother then leave the surgery. However, they have been persuaded to come back in a week.

The GP is troubled by the situation and decides to call his medical defence association. Over the phone he describes the situation. The adviser asks if the GP has assessed her capacity to refuse investigation and treatment.

(c) What conditions must be met for a patient's consent to be valid?

....

....

....

(d) How should a patient's capacity to either consent to, or refuse treatment be assessed?

....

....

....

The patient and her mother return as promised the following week. The patient explains that she has had time to think about it, and she is worried about what would happen to her son if she did nothing about the lump. She agrees to see the breast surgeon at the local hospital.

(e) How will she be assessed at the local hospital?

....

....

....

(f) What other investigations may be needed?

....

....

....

The consultant in the breast clinic sees the patient and her mother the following week. She explains that the cells taken were abnormal, and that the patient is going to need further treatment.

(g) Describe the communication skills that might help in 'breaking bad news'.

....

....

....

(h) What are the principal treatment options?

....

....

....

(i) Which members of the healthcare team might be involved in her care?

....

....

....

During the consultation, the patient's mother tells the consultant that her breast cancer had been picked up on routine screening. She is concerned because her other daughter, who is 44 years old, has not had screening. She asks about the likelihood of her other daughter having breast cancer, and asks why she hasn't been screened.

(j) What are the key features of the UK NHS breast cancer screening programme?

....

....

....

(k) What are the familial risks for breast cancer, and how are they thought to arise?

....

....

....

The consultant explains that the risk of breast cancer is not entirely familial. She explains that other important factors are thought to play a role.

(l) What are the other factors that confer risk in breast cancer?

....

....

....

Staging of the lesion is reported as T2, N1.

(m) What does this mean?

....

....

....

The tumour is successfully removed during the operation and the patient makes an uneventful recovery.

(n) How regularly will she be followed up?

....

....

....

(o) What are the common psychosocial consequences that she may suffer from following
this type of surgery?

....

....

....

✓ Answers and teaching notes

Key cases
- Breast cancer
- Benign breast disease

Clinical context

In the UK over 41,000 new cases of breast cancer occur each year, of which approximately 300 are males. Encouragingly, deaths from breast cancer have fallen by 20% in the last 10 years. In general, the risk of breast cancer rises with age (progressively >30 years). Increasing parity and long periods of breast feeding lower the risks. In the UK we are still short of fulfilling 100% breast screening, especially in social classes 4 and 5. Advances in understanding the causes of breast cancer hold much promise for treatment (e.g. monoclonal antibody therapy (Herceptin)). Unfortunately, as with other cancers, the available treatment choice can be influenced by which county the patient lives in, and in some cases, which region.

This scenario explores the physical and psychological aspects of breast cancer, its treatment, screening programmes and familial risk. Breast cancer is frequently a devastating diagnosis to receive, and issues surrounding the sensitive handling of breaking bad news are also discussed.

(a) Features of breast cancer

It is important to be aware that 9 out of 10 breast lumps seen in primary care are benign. However, breast cancer is the most common cancer in women in the UK, accounting for 30% of cancers. One in nine (11%) women in the UK will develop breast cancer. Therefore, it is important to be aware of the features of a breast lump that warrant further investigation.

The features of a lump that should make you strongly suspect cancer are a discrete, hard lump with fixation, with or without associated lymph nodes. NICE guidelines advise that these patients should be urgently referred to hospital for investigation.

The key questions the GP should ask are aimed at differentiating between the features of benign and malignant breast disease:

- the size, position, edge, consistency, fixity or mobility of the lump should be asked about (these would normally be assessed on examination)
- has the lump enlarged?
- is it painful?

- does it change during her menstrual cycle?
- are there any other lumps, particularly in the armpit?
- have there been any skin changes including dimpling, or oedematous change (suggestive of peau d'orange)?
- are there any nipple changes such as inversion, or any discharge?

The GP would also want to ask about significant risk factors. These are referred to later in this question.

> 💡 Use this opportunity to revise the common causes of breast lumps. You should be aware of the tissues in which lumps may arise. How do the questions above help to differentiate between the possible causes? What are the treatment options for benign breast disorders?

(b) Issues surrounding this case

There are many difficulties surrounding this case. People who have suffered sexual abuse often suffer from:

- insecurity, and fear of members of the abuser's sex (men or women)
- anxiety, depression and low self-esteem
- sleep and eating disorders
- poor peer relationships
- suicide attempts, self-poisoning, self-mutilation
- drug or alcohol misuse
- chronic, multiple, somatic symptoms syndrome.

Issues that the GP would want to explore should include:

- the patient's thoughts and feelings regarding her fear of physical examination. Particular attention should be paid to whether consultation and examination by another woman would help her to overcome her fear
- symptoms of depression, anxiety, and hopelessness should be sought, since these may exacerbate her fears relating to physical examination
- the risks of leaving a breast lump undiagnosed should be explained fully
- the patient should be offered counselling, support and reassurance.

(c) Informed consent

Patients have both a legal and ethical right to determine what happens to them and their bodies, and valid consent is needed before any intervention (no matter how trivial it may seem).

It is important to remember that patients can give consent non-verbally (for example by presenting their arm), orally, or in writing. For the consent to be valid, the patient must:

- have the capacity to make the particular decision (*competent*)
- have received sufficient information (*informed*)
- not be acting under duress (*voluntary*).

> It is vital to have a good working knowledge of consent in medicine. How do the general ethical principles relate to consent? What forms of consent are valid? When are written forms of consent needed? What 'special' situations require additional consent?

> You should be familiar with the consent forms currently used in the NHS. Figure 3.1 shows an example.

(d) Assessment of capacity

To have the capacity to either consent to, or to refuse treatment, a patient must be able to:

- understand what the medical investigation/treatment is, and why it is being proposed
- understand the main benefits, risks and alternatives
- understand the consequences of not receiving the proposed treatment
- retain the information long enough to make an effective decision
- make a free choice and not be put under pressure.

When an adult patient lacks the mental capacity to give or withhold consent, no one else can give consent on their behalf. However, treatment may be given if it is in their 'best interests', as long as it has not been refused in an advance directive (BMA, 2003).

> Use this opportunity to revisit the concepts of capacity and competence. What are the differences? How are patients' best interests determined? What are the important points relating to minors?

(e) Triple assessment at the breast clinic

Triple assessment of a breast lesion consists of physical examination, imaging (mammography and/or ultrasonography), and sampling of the lump for cytological and/or histological assessment (fine needle aspiration cytology (FNAC) or core biopsies). This form of assessment establishes a diagnosis in 95% of patients with suspected breast cancer.

- *clinical examination* is used to provide an index of suspicion based on the findings (see (a))
- *imaging*: this consists of a mammogram and/or ultrasound. Mammography and ultrasonography are used for women over 35 years old. Those under 35 years old should be investigated using ultrasonography, as the denser breast tissue in this age group makes mammography unreliable
- *cytology*: fine needle aspiration (FNA) has many benefits. If the lump is due to a cyst, aspiration can provide relief from both pain, and the anxiety surrounding the prospect of cancer. In contrast, if the lump is solid, cells can be obtained for cytological examination. Sometimes a core biopsy may also be performed whereby small samples of tissue are obtained.

(SIGN Guideline 29, 1998)

> Some breast units are able to perform triple assessment with same-day diagnosis. Is this 'one-stop-shop' approach psychologically appropriate? What are the potential advantages and disadvantages of such an approach?

(f) Investigation of distant metastases

Minimal staging investigations for women with early breast cancer (T1–2, N0–1) and no clinical evidence of distant metastases include:

- chest X-ray
- full blood count
- serum calcium
- liver function tests and liver ultrasound scan or CT.

However, patients with symptoms that suggest site-specific metastatic spread should be investigated appropriately.

More than half of patients diagnosed with breast cancer, with no evidence of metastatic disease, will eventually die of distant disease without local recurrence.

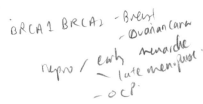
BRCA 1 BRCA 2 – Breast
– Ovarian carm
nypno / early menarche
~ late men.pause.
– ocp.

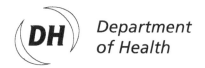

Patient agreement to investigation or treatment

(Form One)

Patient details (or pre-printed label)

Patient's surname/family name ....

Patient's first names ....

NHS number (or other identifier) ....

☐ Male   ☐ Female

Date of birth ....

Responsible health professional ....

Job title ....

Special requirements ....
(eg: other language/other communication method)

Complete and attach sticker to all Histopathology request forms

The specimen can be used for:

	YES	NO
Teaching	☐	☐
Research	☐	☐
Public Health Monitoring	☐	☐
Audit & Quality Assurance	☐	☐

WZZ 8115

To be retained in patient's notes

Figure 3.1 Consent forms used in the NHS.

Name of proposed procedure or course of treatment (include brief explanation if medical term not clear)

....

....

....

Statement of health professional (to be filled in by health professional with appropriate knowledge of proposed procedure, as specified in consent policy)

I have explained the procedure to the patient. In particular, I have explained:

The intended benefits: ....

....

....

Serious or frequently occurring risks:...

....

....

Any extra procedures which may become necessary during the procedure:

☐ blood transfusion

☐ other procedure (please specify) ....

....

I have also discussed what the procedure is likely to involve, the benefits and risks of any available alternative treatments (including no treatment) and any particular concerns of this patient.

☐ The following leaflet/tape has been provided...

This procedure will involve:

☐ general and/or regional anaesthesia ☐ local anaesthesia ☐ sedation

Signed: .... Date: ....

Name (PRINT): .... Job title: ....

Contact details (if patient wishes to discuss options later) ....

Statement of interpreter (where appropriate)
I have interpreted the information above to the patient to the best of my ability and in a way in which I believe s/he can understand

Signed: .... Date: .... Name (PRINT): ....

Top copy accepted by patient: ☐ YES ☐ NO

Please read this form carefully. If your treatment has been planned in advance, you should already have your own copy of page 2 which describes the benefits and risks of the proposed treatment. If not, you will be offered a copy now. If you have any further questions, do ask - we are here to help you. You have the right to change your mind at any time, including after you have signed this form.

I agree to the procedure or course of treatment described on this form.

I understand that you cannot give me a guarantee that a particular person will perform the procedure. The person will, however, have appropriate experience.

I understand that I will have the opportunity to discuss the details of anaesthesia with an anaesthetist before the procedure, unless the urgency of my situation prevents this. (This only applies to patients having general or regional anaesthesia).

I understand that any procedure in addition to those described on this form will only be carried out if it is necessary to save my life or to prevent serious harm to my health.

I understand that where tissue material or a specimen is obtained then it may be used for teaching, *research, public health monitoring, audit and quality assurance.
*A separate consent form may be required.

I have been told about additional procedures which may become necessary during my treatment. I have listed below any procedures **which I do not wish to be carried out** without further discussion: ....
....
....

Patient's signature: .... Date: ....
Name (PRINT): ....

A witness should sign below if the patient is unable to sign but has indicated his or her consent. Young people/children may also like a parent to sign here (see notes).

Signature: .... Date: ....
Name (PRINT): ....

Confirmation of consent (to be completed by a health professional when the patient is admitted for the procedure, if the patient has signed the form in advance).

On behalf of the team treating the patient, I have confirmed with the patient that s/he has no further questions and wishes the procedure to go ahead.

Signed: .... Date: ....
Name (PRINT): .... Job title: ....

Important notes: (tick if applicable)

☐ See also advance directive/living will (eg: Jehovah's Witness form)

☐ Patient has withdrawn consent (ask patient to sign/date here) ....

You should be familiar with the theories of breast cancer metastasis. What are the differences between Halstead's theory and embolisation theory? What are the common sites of breast cancer metastases? What are the relationships between the histological type of cancer and the likelihood of metastasis? Which genes are associated with metastasis?

(g) Breaking bad news

It is always difficult to break bad news to a patient, since it means telling them something that they don't want to hear. It can be difficult to deal with the patient's reactions, which can include anger, guilt, and blame.

Communication skills play an important part in all aspects of medicine, but a system is essential when breaking bad news. The SPIKES system (Baile *et al.*, 2000) is a useful framework to approach this unenviable but inevitable task:

- *Setting up*: breaking bad news should be done in private and in an environment with which the patient is familiar. Confirm all of the medical facts, and make sure that all of the information is at hand. Ask the patient if there is anyone they would like with them
- *Patient perceptions*: you need to know what the patient knows about the underlying illness. What does the patient think that the symptoms might mean?
- *Invitation*: you need to get permission from the patient to break the bad news. A 'warning shot' can help with this
- *Knowledge*: patients need enough information to make informed choices. Information should be given at a pace that suits the patient. Silence can be extremely useful in giving patients enough time to ask questions
- *Emotions*: you need to acknowledge a patient's emotional response to bad news. It is important to listen, and to acknowledge their reactions. Use open questions to encourage them to disclose their feelings, worries and concerns
- *Strategy and summary*: minimise anxiety by summarising and formulating a strategy and follow-up plan. It is important to discuss the future in terms of further investigations, treatment options and support. Honesty is important in these discussions rather than over-optimism.

(h) Treatment of breast cancer

Breast cancer is treated with a combination of surgery, radiotherapy, chemotherapy and endocrine therapy. Which treatment, or combination of treatments is used depends on many factors, including the tumour stage, patient age, and patient preference.

Surgery

Prognosis after breast surgery is not altered much by more extensive excisions. Consequently, surgeons are performing fewer radical operations, tending to aim towards breast conservation surgery in suitable cases. The aims of surgery are to:

- remove the local tumour and reduce local growth
- reduce the risk of metastatic spread
- provide an aesthetic result (with nipple conservation if possible).

The common surgical options include wide local excision, mastectomy, axillary sampling, axillary clearance and breast reconstruction. The exact technique or combination of techniques will depend on the features of the tumour and the patient's preferences.

A new surgical technique known as sentinel lymph node biopsy is currently being evaluated. This involves giving an injection of radioactive isotope and patent blue dye into the tissues around the primary tumour. This tracer is transported initially to the first node receiving lymph from this area – the sentinel node. This node can then be sampled and sent for histological analysis – hopefully a more reliable adjunct to staging than random axillary node sampling.

Many women are devastated by the thought of mastectomy. Discussing the possibility of breast reconstruction surgery can help. The decision to advise breast conservation surgery or mastectomy depends on many factors including the ratio of the size of the tumour to the size of the breast, the pathological features of the tumour (e.g. multiple sites), the age of the patient, the patient's general health, and the patient's preferences.

Radiotherapy

After conservative surgery, radiotherapy is frequently used, because it reduces the local recurrence rate by about two-thirds.

The key points regarding radiotherapy include:

- radiotherapy should usually be given after wide local excision
- radiotherapy should be offered after mastectomy in patients who are at high risk of recurrence
- after axillary sampling, if malignant cells are detected, options include axillary radiotherapy or axillary clearance
- radiotherapy is not normally indicated after axillary clearance, as this combination considerably increases the risk of chronic lymphoedema of the upper limb.

A worrying lump

block estrogen receptors
↳ ↓ estrogen synthesis

Chemotherapy

Chemotherapy improves survival, especially in younger patients or patients who have disease that has spread to local lymph nodes. It is also necessary with rapidly growing tumours, and when the tumour is oestrogen receptor negative.

Endocrine therapy

The aim of endocrine therapy is to reduce oestrogen activity on susceptible tumour cells (oestrogen and progesterone receptor-positive tumours). The drugs used either block oestrogen receptors (tamoxifen) or reduce oestrogen synthesis (aromatase inhibitors). Ovarian ablation can also be used. Radiotherapy or surgical removal of the ovaries has been shown to improve survival in premenopausal women, but is associated with severe side-effects (SIGN Guideline 29, Breast Cancer in Women, 1998).

> You should be familiar with the range and indications for adjuvant therapies in breast cancer. What are the side-effects of the commonly used adjuvant treatments?

(i) Multidisciplinary management

Management requires a multidisciplinary approach that may entail input from:

- surgeons
- radiologists
- pathologists
- oncologists
- breast care nurses
- counsellors
- research nurses
- patients who have been through similar experiences.

(j) Breast cancer screening programme

The NHS breast screening programme offers breast screening every three years for all women aged between 50 and 70 years. Around one-and-a-half million women are screened in the UK each year. In women over 50 years old, mammographic screening has been shown to reduce the mortality from breast cancer by at least 25%.

The main elements are:

- all women in the 50–70-year age group are screened using single oblique-view mammography
- women with mammographically detected abnormalities are investigated further in specialist breast assessment units, using triple assessment
- women under 50 years are not routinely screened. Mammography is not as reliable in pre-

menopausal women because the density of the breast tissue is higher. Additionally, the incidence of breast cancer is lower in premenopausal women.

(NHS Breast Screening Programme, www.cancerscreening.nhs.uk)

> Use this opportunity to revisit the Wilson and Jugener WHO screening principles. How does the UK breast cancer screening programme meet these criteria? Why are women over 50 the only women routinely screened? How does the screening of high-risk families conform to the general principles of screening?

(k) Genetics of breast cancer

Family history of breast cancer in a first-degree relative is one of the strongest predictive risk factors for the development of the disease. Several genes have been identified, the most common genes are:

- *BRCA1* mutation (chromosome 17), which confers a lifetime risk of 65–85% for breast cancer
- *BRCA2* mutation (chromosome 13), which confers a lifetime risk of 40–85% for breast cancer
- *TP53* mutation (chromosome 17) is associated with a high risk of breast cancer before the age of 50 years. *TP53* is also associated with other cancers.

Other genes associated with an increased risk of breast cancer include the *PTEN*, *ATM* and *CHEK2* genes.

> Use this opportunity to revise the roles of oncogenes, tumour suppressor genes and cell cycle control genes. What are their roles in the carcinogenesis of common tumours?

Other points of note concerning the familial risk of breast cancer include the following:

- the age of diagnosis in relatives, and the number of relatives who have had breast cancer are important determinants of familial risk. Other determinants of risk include the site of any tumours, whether they were multiple, and the presence of any Jewish ancestry (due to founder mutations)
- the genetic contribution to breast cancer risk has not been fully determined, since most women who have a family history do not have a mutation of *BRCA1*, *BRCA2* or *TP53* genes
- breast cancer is a multifactorial disease, probably involving complex interactions between genetic, environmental, and other unknown factors

- breast cancer is extremely common; so the likelihood of breast cancer developing in women who are related may be due to chance.

(McIntosh *et al.*, 2004)

NICE has published guidelines on the stratification of familial breast cancer risk. Their guidelines include recommendations on whether patients should be managed in primary or secondary care.

(l) Other risk factors for breast cancer

In addition to the familial risk of breast cancer, several other factors are known to be important. These include:

- *age*: the highest incidence is in postmenopausal women
- *country of residence*: incidence is high in the west, low in the east
- *race*: it is more common in Caucasians
- *social class*: highest in social class I
- *previous ovarian or endometrial cancer*
- *early menarche or late menopause*
- *nulliparity*, or being older than 30 years before having a first child
- *hormonal supplementation*: hormone replacement therapy (HRT) or the combined oral contraceptive pill (COCP)
- *obesity*: due to aromatisation in adipose tissue.

(m) Breast cancer staging

Although there are several systems for staging or classifying breast cancer (e.g. Manchester staging), patients should be staged according to the TNM classification. Clinical assessment of the tumour size generally correlates well with the final pathological assessment. Imaging provides greater accuracy.

Tumour, nodes, metastases (TNM) staging for invasive carcinoma

- T (tumour size)
  - T1: <2 cm
  - T2: 2–5 cm
  - T3: >5 cm
  - T4: fixed
- N (nodes)
  - N1: ipsilateral mobile nodes
  - N2: fixed nodes
- M (metastases)
  - M1: presence of distant metastases

Ductal carcinoma *in situ* (DCIS) is often referred to as non-invasive cancer, or sometimes stage 0. It may however transform into invasive cancer if left untreated. The likelihood of progression to invasive carcinoma is determined by the histological grade of the cancer (i.e. how abnormal the cells look under

the microscope). Treatment of DCIS depends on the size and grade of the tumour.

> You should be familiar with the major histological types of cancer. What are the differences between low-grade and high-grade tumours? How does the degree of differentiation affect the prognosis?

(n) Follow-up

The aims of follow-up are to detect recurrence in the same breast, disease in the other breast, and metastatic spread. Additionally, the close monitoring of first-degree relatives may need to be considered.

The frequency of follow-up depends on the type of surgery performed. After mastectomy the risk of recurrence declines substantially with time, so patients should be seen 6-monthly for 2 years and then yearly if there is no recurrence.

After breast conservation surgery, recurrence occurs at a fixed rate each year, and patients should be monitored every 6 months.

However, recurrence (e.g. in the scar) and metastases may become apparent between follow-up appointments. Patient education is important for the prompt identification of problems and should include:

- teaching patients how to examine themselves
- contacting the breast care nurse or GP if suspicious symptoms or signs develop.

> Follow-up is so time consuming, that the reasons for doing it must be understood by future doctors. Follow-up can be psychologically beneficial to patients. This is not true of all patients and of all cancers. Can you think of cancers where it may not be beneficial to arrange routine follow-up? How is follow-up important in terms of determining standards of care?

(o) Psychosocial consequences of breast cancer

Both the diagnosis and treatment of breast cancer can cause significant psychosocial disturbance. Issues that need to be considered include:

- *emotional issues*: following a diagnosis of breast cancer women are at risk of experiencing extreme emotional reactions. They may experience a sense of isolation, low self-esteem, anxiety, depression, hostility, and guilt

What are the components of the grief reaction? Grief can be experienced as a mental, physical, social, or emotional reaction. Can you think of examples in each category?

- *sexual issues*: issues relating to sexuality are frequently difficult for women with breast cancer. All too often these are not discussed openly, or at all. The loss of a breast, or the physical effects of chemotherapy, often exacerbated by anxiety and depression, can cause women to feel less sexually attractive. Specific difficulties include decreased libido and difficulties with sexual intercourse itself (arousal, lubrication, and orgasm). Some of these effects may be related to a reduction in circulating androgens following adjuvant therapy
- *social and family issues*: family members often describe similar emotional issues to those suffered by the patients themselves. Partners may experience loneliness, uncertainty and confusion.

Web resources

- Breast cancer guidelines: www.sign.ac.uk
- Cancer information: www.cancerbackup.org.uk
- Communication skills: www.breakingbadnews.co.uk
- Ethics website: www.ethics-network.org.uk
- Familial breast cancer guidance: www.prodigy.nhs.uk
- UK screening programmes: www.cancerscreening.nhs.uk

Further reading

- Baile W, Buckman R, Lenzi R *et al.* (2000) SPIKES – a six step protocol for delivering bad news: application to the patient with cancer. *The Oncologist.* 5: 302.
- BMA (2003) *BMA Consent Tool Kit.* BMA Publishing, London.
- Dixon JM (ed) (1999) *ABC of Breast Disease* (2e). BMJ Publishing, London.
- Hope A, Savulescu J and Hendrik J (2003) *Medical Ethics and Law.* Churchill Livingstone, London.
- Longmore M, Wilkinson I and Rajagopalan S (eds) (2004) *Oxford Handbook of Clinical Medicine* (6e). Oxford University Press, Oxford, pp. 504–5.
- McIntosh A, Shaw C, Evans G *et al.* (2004) *Clinical Guidelines and Evidence Review for the Classification and Care of Women at Risk of Familial Breast Cancer.* National Collaborating Centre for Primary Care, University of Sheffield. www.nice.org.uk
- Scottish Intercollegiate Guidelines Network (SIGN) (1998) Guideline 29. *Breast Cancer in Women.* SIGN, Edinburgh.

4 A busy haematuria clinic

A surgical SHO is on his urology rotation. His consultant is away at a meeting, and he has been asked by his registrar to help out at the busy haematuria clinic.

The first patient he sees has been referred by her GP. She is a 67-year-old woman who has suffered from recurrent urinary tract infections (UTIs). The GP has confirmed haematuria on dipstick several times, and has referred her to the clinic for possible flexible cystoscopy.

(a) What is the main cancer being sought in such a clinic?

....

....

....

(b) What is the routine work up for haematuria (excluding cystoscopy)?

....

....

....

The second patient has been referred with microscopic haematuria. She is 35 years old, had mild pre-eclampsia last year when pregnant with her third child, and has recently been put on diuretics for ankle oedema. The dipstick of her urine was strongly positive for protein and positive for blood. Her serum creatinine was 130 μmol/l but all other investigations for haematuria were normal. She still had some ankle swelling despite the diuretics.

(c) What is your working diagnosis?

....

....

....

(d) What other abnormalities on initial tests would you expect?

....

....

....

(e) How do you make a definitive diagnosis?

....

....

....

The next patient is a 64-year-old male who has atrial fibrillation and is taking warfarin. He has a 2-day history of macroscopic haematuria. On abdominal ultrasound he has a 38 mm mass jutting out of the lower pole of his left kidney. His INR is 3.1.

(f) Should this patient be cystoscoped? Give a reason for your answer.

....

....

....

(g) What pre-operative imaging would the SHO order?

....

....

....

☞ The results of the imaging suggest that the disease is localised.

(h) What specific operations could he have?

....

....

....

(i) How would you quantify this man's prognosis?

....

....

....

☞ The final patient in the clinic is a 21-year-old female student with macroscopic haematuria. No other details were supplied on the 2-week wait for cancer referral form. She was prescribed trimethoprim by her GP (which he prescribes for all his patients with haematuria). Midstream specimen and dip-stick of urine have not yet been done. In the 5 days it has taken to get her to the clinic, she has not improved. In fact, last night she says she's become all shivery, as though she has the 'flu, and has developed right loin pain.

(j) What is the most likely diagnosis?

....

....

....

(k) What should the GP have diagnosed and what symptoms should he have elicited?

....

....

....

(l) Why has her condition not improved on trimethoprim?

....

....

....

(m) How will you treat her and for how long?

....

....

....

(n) Does the loin pain need to be investigated? (If so, how?)

....

....

....

☞ She has had this problem several times before, although never so badly, and this is the first time she has had loin pain.

(o) Give one common cause for the recurrence of the condition, which may require direct questioning.

....

....

....

(p) If this does turn out to be the problem, what useful medical prophylaxis could you give her?

....

....

....

(q) What are the important non-pharmacological methods that are used to prevent UTI recurrence?

....

....

....

✓ Answers and teaching notes

A busy haematuria clinic

Key cases
- Haematuria
- Kidney tumours
- Glomerulonephritis/nephrotic syndrome
- Urinary tract infection (UTI)
- Pyelonephritis

Clinical context

Macroscopic haematuria, unless obviously due to haemorrhagic cystitis, should always be taken seriously, as should persistent microscopic haematuria. Haematuria can be due to cancer, hence it is now investigated promptly by urologists in a 'one-stop' clinic. Nearly all transitional cell carcinomas (TCCs) are diagnosed in this way. However, this scenario concentrates on some of the many other diseases that can present with haematuria. These include important medical conditions, particularly intrinsic renal disease.

(a) Bladder cancer

Histologically bladder carcinoma can be either transitional cell-, squamous cell- or adeno-carcinoma; although, in the West, the latter two are rare. TCC may occur between the renal pelvis and the urethra, i.e., they arise from the urothelium. However, the bladder is the commonest site. The typical presentation is one of painless haematuria. Other urinary symptoms the patient may experience are:

- increased urinary frequency
- urgency
- dysuria
- recurrent UTIs.

In concentrating urine, the kidneys also concentrate carcinogens which are excreted in urine. Therefore, risk factors include smoking (probably the cause in one-third of cases) some drugs (e.g. cyclophosphamide) and industrial carcinogens. The most famous was β-naphthylamine, which was used in the rubber industry, until its ability to cause bladder cancer was proved at the Michelin tyre factory in Stoke on Trent.

Diagnosis requires biopsy, normally by transurethral resection of the tumour and of the underlying detrusor (bladder) muscle. This may prove to be curative, but also allows determination of the grade of the cancer and whether it is invasive. Treatment and survival are strongly influenced by the grade and stage of the disease.

> You should be familiar with the grading and staging of bladder cancer and the implications that this has for treatment options.

(b) Work up for haematuria
- Full blood count (FBC)
- Urea and electrolytes (U&E)
- Dipstick the urine (MSU if positive for WBC and/or nitrites)
- Urine microscopy
- Urine cytology
- X-ray of the kidneys/ureters/bladder (KUB)
- Ultrasound (U/S) of the kidneys, bladder, and prostate
- PSA (men only)

FBC is particularly for the haemoglobin concentration; significant haematuria can cause iron deficiency anaemia, and patients find it difficult to say how much blood they have lost.

U&E are a useful measure of renal function.

The urine from all patients with haematuria should be tested for infection using a dipstick. Cystoscopy should be avoided in a patient with undiagnosed urinary infection as it could cause septicaemia. If the urine is infected, it is preferable to delay the cystoscopy until the infection has been cleared.

Urine microscopy is important in the investigation of both macroscopic and microscopic haematuria. The presence of dysmorphic red blood cells or casts may point to specific diagnoses.

Cytology has a particular role in detecting poorly differentiated bladder cancer cells. Such cells 'fall off' from both poorly differentiated cancers, and from carcinoma *in situ*. Well-differentiated carcinomatous transitional cells generally retain the ability to cohere to their normal counterparts until the cells die.

> You should be aware of the differences between the genetic mutations of well and poorly differentiated TCCs. Well-differentiated TCCs only become invasive when further mutations occur, whereas carcinoma *in situ* and poorly differentiated cancers start that way.

KUB can detect stones, including bladder calculi (except for radiolucent ones).

U/S of the kidneys and bladder shows up various pathologies:

- solid renal masses (and cysts, which are of no consequence and are common)
- bladder tumours over 0.5–1 cm
- hydronephrosis
- hydroureter
- stones
- chronic retention
- enlarged prostates.

It is easy to miss small renal cancers on IVU. About the only pathology that can be picked up by IVU but missed on U/S is non-obstructing TCC of the upper tracts. IVUs are therefore only required in selected cases as a secondary investigation.

PSA should be considered in all cases of haematuria in men over 50 years old, or if there is a family history of prostate cancer (*see* p. 208).

In this patient's case there is no evidence of infection. Thus cystoscopy is needed because bladder pathology, including cancers, particularly if they are necrotic, could be the reason for repeated infections (but also *see* (o) below).

(c) Glomerulonephritis/nephrotic syndrome

True pre-eclampsia is usually worst with the first pregnancy. Similar problems, such as hypertension and proteinuria, can also be due to either 'essential' hypertension or hypertension secondary to renal disease, as in this case unmasked by pregnancy. Presumably, the symptoms and signs of the underlying renal disease seemed to remit for a while after the patient's third child was born.

> Use this opportunity to revise the structure of the glomerulus. How do the normal structure and function of the capillary wall and basement membrane prevent protein leakage? What abnormalities are found in glomerular disease?

Nephrotic syndrome is due to glomerular disease causing major protein loss in the urine. It is characterised by:

- proteinuria (>3 g/24 h)
- oedema
- hypoalbuminaemia (<30 g/l).

Diabetes mellitus, amyloidosis, systemic vasculitides, Henoch–Schönlein purpura, drugs and allergies are all causes of the nephrotic syndrome. In addition, all types of glomerulonephritis can present as the nephrotic syndrome.

Further complications result from the fact that albumin is not the only protein that leaks into the urine.

> Complications of the nephrotic syndrome include hypercoagulability, hypercholesterolaemia, increased susceptibility to infection and oliguric renal failure. Can you account for these effects in terms of specific proteins lost in the urine, and the effects on plasma oncotic pressure?

(d) Results of initial tests

- Hypertension
- Proteinuria (e.g. on the dipstick test)
- Hypoalbuminaemia
- Urinary casts

Hypertension is very common in patients with glomerulonephritis and needs to be well controlled. It can speed up the decline in renal function by causing renal damage. Often, hypertension is less evident in patients with the nephrotic syndrome because of their low serum protein.

Proteinuria is almost always present in all types of glomerulonephritis, even if it is not as gross as in the nephrotic syndrome. For example, 'microalbuminuria' can be used to screen diabetics for the early stages of diabetic nephropathy.

Hypoalbuminaemia causes the manifestation of the syndrome.

Urinary casts are found by centrifuging a fresh urine specimen (the 'microscopy' of an MSU should do this). They are a sign of renal tubular damage.

(e) Definitive diagnosis

Definitive diagnosis is established through renal biopsy. This is particularly important when a specific histological diagnosis may dramatically influence management.

> Use this opportunity to reflect on the causes of glomerulonephritis. Which groups of patients should *not* have a renal biopsy and why?

(f) Renal cell carcinoma

- This patient should have a cystoscopy. Renal cancer is unlikely to be the cause of his haematuria, as it is unlikely that a 38 mm cancer of the lower pole has reached the collecting system.

It is important that a cause for the haematuria is found because serious pathology may be missed if it is simply assumed that this incidental finding is the cause of his haematuria.

The urinary tract is one of the many sites where bleeding due to over-anticoagulation can occur. However, although the reported INR is high, considering the reason for his anticoagulation, it would be very unusual for this man to develop haematuria without an underlying cause. One can almost argue that therapeutic warfarinisation can lead to earlier diagnosis of conditions which present with haematuria.

(g) Imaging studies

- CT of the abdomen
- CT of the chest

The CT of the abdomen can give the surgeon a precise idea of which operation to plan, as well as showing up intra-abdominal metastases, including:

- nodal
- suprarenal
- hepatic.

Chest CT is important because if metastases are present, the patient is effectively incurable. This is despite the fact that immunotherapy can be of some value in otherwise fit patients, particularly if the primary cancer is removed. In this particular case, the chance of finding any metastases is small but they must still be sought.

(h) Surgical treatment options

Patients with localised disease may be offered surgical treatment with a view to curing the disease. Options are:

- laparoscopic radical nephrectomy
- 'open' radical nephrectomy
- 'nephron-sparing' partial nephrectomy.

Although it takes longer to perform, and requires specific training, laparoscopic nephrectomy is now rapidly becoming the norm for the removal of technically straightforward kidney cancers, because recovery is quicker than after 'open' radical nephrectomy.

Nephron-sparing nephrectomy gives as good results in suitable cases, of which this may well be one. The cancer is simply removed with a thin covering of normal renal tissue (>2 mm to ensure tumour clearance). This operation is especially useful, in that it prevents the subsequent need for dialysis, in patients with a small cancer in a solitary functioning kidney, or who have bilateral cancers.

This man's anticoagulation should not be a contraindication for surgery. However, small renal 'incidentalomas', such as are found on an U/S scan for other reasons, can be very slow growing and very

rarely metastasise. Such growth, or lack of it, can be monitored by serial U/S scans. It is therefore sometimes appropriate to remember that part of the Hippocratic oath, which says never do harm, when such tumours are found in very unfit patients.

> Take this opportunity to revise the peri-operative management of patients requiring anticoagulation. Consider the risks of bleeding problems if anticoagulation is temporarily stopped versus developing the complication for which the anticoagulation was prescribed in the first place.

(i) Prognosis

In a patient such as this, with localised disease, the prognosis is excellent. The survival can be quoted as over 90%. Cancers up to 4 cm in diameter are now classified as T1a. T1b is 4–7 cm and T2 is >7 cm. The prognosis of the latter two is similar (>75–80%), which is why the stage T1a has been split off.

(j) UTI complicated by acute pyelonephritis

Inflamed kidneys become painful and tender. Bacteraemia occurs easily because renal tubules and capillaries are so close to one another. Such bacteraemia or, worse, septicaemia leads to pyrexia, frequently accompanied by shivering or rigors, usually followed by drenching sweats as the pyrexia subsides. Apart from the danger of septic shock, untreated, or unsuccessfully (e.g. bacterial resistance to the antibiotic prescribed) treated pyelonephritis can rapidly cause permanent renal damage, even in the absence of simultaneous obstruction. Scarring of a kidney on U/S scan is a frequent subsequent finding.

(k) (Haemorrhagic) cystitis

Patients with urinary tract infection induced cystitis usually present with some or all of:

- dysuria
- increased frequency
- strangury
- nasty-smelling urine.

Renal infection is usually secondary to lower tract infection if the kidneys are otherwise normal. It can largely be prevented by prompt treatment of the cystitis with a suitable antibiotic. Secondary pyelonephritis is usually caused by ureteric reflux, which would cause no renal damage in the absence of lower-urinary tract infection.

This diagnosis should have been obvious clinically, and easily confirmed by dipstick testing. Thus, this was an inappropriate referral to the haematuria clinic. However acute pyelonephritis after suffering the misery of haemorrhagic cystitis for 5 days will probably require a brief hospital admission.

(l) Problems with treatment

The infecting organism is probably resistant to this antibiotic. Trimethoprim is used commonly, but resistance to organisms acquired in the community is increasing. The GP should have sent off an MSU, so that if the organism did prove to be resistant, a suitable alternative could have been prescribed in the knowledge that it would be effective.

> Use this opportunity to revise the definitions of uncomplicated and complicated UTIs. What are the common infecting organisms and commonly used antibiotics? What are the complications of UTIs in adults and children, and what are the indications for further investigations?

(m) Successful treatment

If patients look well, and are able to eat and drink, changing to oral cefalexin would be acceptable. However, if they look ill, it is better to be cautious. Patients should be admitted and given 80–120 mg of gentamicin parenterally, and ofloxacin orally.

Unless about 2 weeks of antibiotics are given, the infection can recur a few days after giving too short a course of even an appropriate antibiotic. This long course of antibiotics, as opposed to the normal 3-day course for a straightforward UTI, is needed because microabscesses form in pyelonephritic kidneys. Until these have healed, they will contain living bacteria because the antibiotic cannot penetrate the abscess. Kidney infections are very prone to cause systemic symptoms, which are often severe. A simple explanation for this is the 'bursting' of microabscesses in a confined space so that toxins or even pus can gain access to the bloodstream.

A problem, which is starting to become potentially serious, is the emergence of ESBL-resistant enterobacteraceae (mainly *E. coli* and *Klebsiella*). ESBL is the abbreviation of extended-spectrum beta lactamase. In practice, this means a bacterium for which the carbapenems are the only reliable treatment. Such bacteria are still rarely present in the community.

> How can spread of ESBL bacilli be minimised, both inside and outside hospitals? MRSA is a good starting point – think about prevention of cross-infection and about whether asymptomatic carriers should be treated. Then think about how to acquire ESBL bacilli from a urology patient.

(n) Further investigation

This patient's first attack of acute pyelonephritis is clearly secondary to lower urinary tract infection. In this particular case, with prompt improvement and no relapse after stopping treatment, further investigation is not necessary. However, you could probably not be criticised for doing a renal U/S, which is safe, even if she is unknowingly pregnant.

(o) Cause of recurrent UTI

Sexual intercourse is a factor that will not be readily volunteered by many patients but may be revealed, on more direct questioning, as the cause of recurrent UTIs. Some women are simply prone to cystitis, but sex (the honeymoon cystitis of the Victorian era when more women married as virgins) is a frequent problem. During intercourse, bacteria are massaged into the bladder, and infection results despite high standards of cleanliness.

In other groups of women, risk factors for UTI include:

- pregnancy
- the contraceptive diaphragm
- postmenopausal atrophic changes
- diabetes mellitus
- abnormalities of urinary tract function such as incomplete bladder emptying, neuropathic bladder, and outflow obstruction
- immunocompromise.

UTIs in males are rare and need investigation to rule out sinister causes.

(p) Pharmacological prophylaxis

If the organisms are sensitive, a single tablet of nitrofurantoin 50 mg after intercourse frequently produces relief from the symptoms. This antibiotic is particularly appropriate because it is only useful in uncomplicated UTIs, since it only works when concentrated in urine. Its limited use has kept resistance relatively infrequent. If nitrofurantoin is unsuitable, trimethoprim 100 mg or cefalexin 250 mg are alternatives, according to bacterial sensitivities.

(q) Non-pharmacological prophylaxis

The simple measures listed below can provide relief for many patients with uncomplicated UTIs:

- cranberry juice
- wiping front to back after defecation
- voiding after sexual intercourse
- double voiding
- drinking plenty of fluids.

Web resources

- Causes of haematuria: www.gpnotebook.co.uk
- Guidance on UTI and urological malignancy: www.prodigy.nhs.uk

- Referral guidelines for suspected cancer: www.dh.gov.uk

Further reading

- Cohen RA and Brown RS (2003) Clinical practice. Microscopic hematuria. *New England Journal of Medicine.* **348**: 2330.
- Longmore M, Wilkinson I and Rajagopalan S (eds) (2004) *Oxford Handbook of Clinical Medicine* (6e). Oxford University Press, Oxford, p. 256.
- O'Callaghan C and Brenner B (2000) *The Kidney at a Glance.* Blackwell Science, Oxford.
- Rose BD (1987) *Pathophysiology of Renal Disease* (2e). McGraw-Hill, New York, p. 44.

5 A wheezy student

A 19-year-old student is admitted with a 2-day history of increasing shortness of breath. She complains of a non-productive cough, worse at night, and wheeze for the past 6 months with occasional chest tightness. Her medical history includes eczema, which is very mild, and hay fever. She has never smoked and takes no medication. On examination she has a BP of 130/70 mmHg, her pulse is 120 beats/min and regular, and her respiratory rate is 29 breaths/min. Her PEFR is documented as 45% of predicted. On auscultation of her chest, she has widespread expiratory wheeze. You notice during your assessment, she has to stop every 3–4 words to take a deep breath, and prefers to sit forward.

(a) What is the most likely diagnosis?

....

....

....

(b) How would you manage this patient? What initial investigations would you do and when?

....

....

....

Soon after arriving on the medical assessment unit, the nurse asks you to review the patient. Her pulse is 50 beats/min and regular, and her respiratory rate is 25 breaths/min. On auscultation of her chest, the expiratory wheeze you heard earlier appears to have gone. You note that she keeps pulling off her oxygen mask, and when she does, her oxygen saturations drop to 90%. Her PEFR is recorded as 30% of predicted, but she is unable to follow your instructions about how the test should be done.

(c) Do you think her condition has improved or deteriorated since she was admitted? Explain your answer.

....

....

....

(d) What is your immediate management?

....

....

....

After 15 minutes of treatment, she appears more settled and is helping the nurse readjust her oxygen mask to make it more comfortable. Her PEFR has improved to 50% predicted. She is moved off the medical assessment unit onto a respiratory ward. Two days later, she is discharged.

(e) What can be done to help prevent a relapse in her condition?

....

....

....

(f) What is meant by a multidisciplinary team? Who do you think will be in the multi-disciplinary team involved in this patient's care?

....

....

....

Key cases

- Asthma
- Acute severe asthma
- Life-threatening asthma

Clinical context

Asthma is a common condition and is increasing in prevalence (approximately 11% of UK adults between 20 and 44 years). Many preventable deaths are due to poor assessment, and failure to recognise the features of life-threatening asthma. This case provides an overview of asthma, concentrating on the clinical features, and how these reflect disease severity and management in both the acute and chronic setting.

(a) Differential diagnoses

A diagnosis of asthma is suggested by the presence of a history of episodic wheeze, shortness of breath, chest tightness, and cough. This is supported by a history of atopy.

> What are the pathophysiological mechanisms involved in asthma? Explain how the symptoms and signs of asthma arise. Which inflammatory cells are involved?

This patient has presented with signs of an acute severe exacerbation of asthma. These include:

- respiratory rate ≥25 breaths/min
- pulse rate ≥110 beats/min
- PEFR <50% predicted
- inability to complete sentences.

It is very important to assess a patient with an exacerbation of asthma properly. Patients should be regularly re-assessed to ensure continued improvement, and for early detection of any signs of life-threatening asthma. Poor assessment, or failure to identify signs of life-threatening asthma may prove fatal to the patient.

The 2001 Asthma Audit by the National Asthma Campaign reports that:

- the number of new cases of asthma each year is now three to four times higher in adults and six times higher in children than it was 25 years ago
- approximately 1500 people die from asthma in the UK each year, over one-third of whom are people under the age of 65 years

- confidential enquiries have indicated that many of these deaths could have been prevented through correct assessment of severity of the exacerbation on presentation and correct emergency management.

(b) Initial management

All patients presenting with an acute severe exacerbation of asthma should be treated as follows:

- oxygen 40–60%
- salbutamol 5 mg, or tertbutaline 10 mg via an oxygen-driven nebuliser
- ipratropium bromide 0.5 mg via an oxygen-driven nebuliser
- prednisolone 40 mg orally once a day.

If the patient's condition does not improve after 15 minutes, regular oxygen-driven nebulised salbutamol or terbutaline and prednisolone should be continued until the patient improves.

If the patient fails to improve, or develops signs of life-threatening asthma, intravenous aminophylline should be considered and the patient should be discussed with ICU for assessment and consideration of invasive positive pressure ventilation (IPPV).

The following initial investigations should be done *after* initial emergency treatment:

- an FBC will show if this patient is anaemic. If the total white cell count is raised, white cell differential will guide you on possible causes for an exacerbation, which include infection
- urea and electrolyte concentrations should be measured as the patient may be dehydrated
- blood cultures should be taken if the patient is pyrexial
- a chest X-ray may show the presence of infection, and should be done if a pneumothorax is suspected
- an ECG to exclude co-morbidities
- if the patient has a cough productive of purulent sputum, a sputum sample should be sent for microscopy and culture. This can help to detect the presence of infection and will give information on antibiotic sensitivities.

(c) Reassessment of patients presenting with exacerbation of asthma

The patient has deteriorated. Since admission, she has developed signs of life-threatening asthma. Life-threatening asthma is characterised by a PEFR <33% and *any* of the following:

- silent chest
- cyanosis
- poor respiratory effort
- oxygen saturation <90% on room air
- bradycardia
- cardiac arrhythmia
- hypotension
- confusion.

(d) Further management when the patient fails to improve

The patient should be discussed with ICU immediately so that she can be assessed for IPPV. Blood gases should be done as part of the assessment of severity. A normal or raised $PaCO_2$ indicates life-threatening asthma, and that the patient should be considered for IPPV.

> Take this opportunity to become familiar with the symptoms and signs and management of acute severe and life-threatening asthma.

(e) Discharging patients admitted with acute severe or life-threatening asthma

Clinical improvement, based on regular re-assessment is the best way to decide when a patient is 'safe' to discharge. A good indicator is when the measured PEFR is >75% of the predicted PEFR or of the best PEFR achieved before admission, and with a diurnal variation <25%.

To reduce the risk of relapse, all patients:

- should have been on their 'discharge medication' for at least 24 hours before they are discharged. For example, if a patient has required nebulised bronchodilators as an inpatient, but is to be discharged on inhaled bronchodilators, they should have these inhalers for 24 hours before they go home, without any deterioration in their clinical condition

> Why do you think it is important for a patient to have this period of observation before going home?

- should go home with a PEF meter and a written asthma plan. Before going home patients should receive education about their condition, training on the correct use of inhalers, and measuring and recording PEFR. Education should involve recognising the symptoms and signs of an exacerbation, what to do, and when to seek help

> What are the different types of inhaler device available? How are they used?
>
> You can learn about this by going to the website www.asthma.org.uk and clicking on the icon 'How to use your inhaler'.

- should complete a course of oral steroids. These should be taken for at least 5 days or until recovery
- should be seen by their GP within 2 working days and in a respiratory clinic 4 weeks following discharge from the hospital.

(f) The multidisciplinary team

A multidisciplinary team (MDT) is a team of professionals from different specialties brought together to ensure the best care is provided for the patient. An MDT approach is important in the management of asthma both in the hospital and in the community.

For asthma, the MDT may comprise:

- respiratory physician
- GP
- respiratory nurse specialist
- district nurse
- pharmacist
- respiratory technician
- smoking cessation adviser.

As you can see from the list, the MDT involves professionals based both in hospital and in the community. Some of the members, e.g. the respiratory nurse specialist, will see patients while they are in the hospital and then again in the community following discharge. An MDT approach facilitates continuation of the care commenced in the hospital, into the community.

Web resources

- 2001 Asthma audit: www.asthma.org.uk
- Management of asthma: www.brit-thoracic.org. uk

Further reading

- Holt PG, Macaubas C, Stumbles PA and Sly PD (1999) The role of allergy in the development of asthma. *Nature.* **402**: B12.
- Longmore M, Wilkinson I and Rajagopalan S (eds) (2004) *Oxford Handbook of Clinical Medicine* (6e). Oxford University Press, Oxford, pp. 184–7, pp. 794–5.
- Rees J and Kanabar D (eds) (2005) *ABC of Asthma* (5e). BMJ Publishing, London.
- Rodrigo GJ, Rodrigo C and Hall JB (2004) Acute asthma in adults: a review. *Chest.* **125**: 1081.

6 An unrousable patient in the recovery room

You are called to see Florence, an 80-year-old obese (BMI = 32) woman in the post-operative recovery room. She is unrousable after her right hemiarthroplasty. The anaesthetist tells you that she had standard anaesthetics (propofol and alfentanil), and her pulse, BP and SpO_2 were normal throughout the operation.

Looking through the notes you discover that the patient fractured her hip after a fall at home, and was unable to get up. She was found by her daughter almost 24 hours later. The patient had no recollection of what happened before the fall, although she felt she may have lost consciousness prior to falling. She regained consciousness shortly after the incident, and there was no evidence of head trauma. The patient had described feeling tired recently. There was no previous history of falls. Additionally, her daughter felt that Florence had gained weight over the previous two months, without changing her diet.

(a) What are the important components of your post-operative clinical assessment?

....

....

....

(b) What are the possible causes of delayed awakening after anaesthesia?

....

....

....

(c) What initial investigations will you request?

....

....

....

(d) Which physiological variables should be monitored for the first few hours after surgery?

....

....

....

On examination she has small pupils that are equal in size and respond slowly to light.

(e) Discuss possible causes of this finding in this patient.

....

....

....

The patient is transferred to the ICU where she regains consciousness. However her GCS is 13 (E4, V4, M5).

(f) What are the common causes of post-operative confusion?

....

....

....

(g) How could her confusion be quantified?

....

....

....

> Florence remains stable in the ICU, and returns to the orthopaedic ward later the same day.

(h) What additional post-operative investigation is needed and when should this be done?

....

....

....

(i) What underlying conditions need to be considered, given the clinical history leading up to the fall?

....

....

....

> Later that day the consultant anaesthetist questions the senior house officer's pre-operative assessment of the patient. He says that ageing affects all of the body's systems, and asks the senior house officer to give an example of effects on cardiovascular, respiratory, renal and immune system physiology which may add to the risks of anaesthesia and surgery.

(j) How would you reply to the consultant's question?

....

....

....

(k) Which significant co-morbidities should be excluded in a thorough pre-operative assessment?

....

....

....

> Florence recovered well post-operatively and was discharged 4 weeks later with a walking aid. She remained determined to stay in her own home despite being advised to consider a residential home or moving to a bungalow.

(l) Which healthcare professionals need to be involved in this patient's subsequent care?

....

....

....

Key cases
- Fractured neck of femur
- Pre-operative assessment
- Hypothyroidism
- Post-operative complications

Clinical context
The comatose patient is a common medical emergency that is challenging for the doctor. As no history is available from the patient, sources of further information need to be rapidly found. These include hospital records, relatives, or the patient's GP. As this scenario shows, the most important component of management is to ensure that the patient's ABCDE are assessed and supported by relevant resuscitative measures.

Always review any information available, and comprehensively examine the patient to provide clues to the cause of coma. This scenario has many facets including pre-operative assessment, approach to the comatose patient, and the physiology of ageing. As you work your way through the questions, try to imagine that you are the doctor involved, and ask yourself how would you approach this interesting patient's case?

(a) Assessment of the unconscious patient
Assessment should involve a review of the intra-operative history and examination of respiratory, cardiovascular, and neurological systems. As with the immediate management of *any* unconscious patient, the priority is to assess and maximise ABCDE:

- *airway*: this patient is intubated, and is therefore unlikely to require further management; however, in the initial assessment of any unconscious patient the airway should be assessed first, or in this case re-assessed, and if necessary cleared and resecured
- *breathing*: this patient is being ventilated, but monitoring chest expansion and listening for breath sounds is still necessary. SpO_2 must also be assessed
- *circulation*: check the patient's pulse (for rate, rhythm, character and volume), jugular venous pressure, capillary refill and blood pressure. Again, it is reported that the cardiovascular parameters were within normal limits during the operation, but these must be assessed again

(e.g. to assess undiagnosed bleeding or myocardial ischaemia)
- *disability*: identify immediate life-threatening conditions not already covered in the ABC assessment. The commonest causes of post-operative unrousability include drugs, cardiorespiratory, neurological, and metabolic disorders (particularly hypoglycaemia). Glasgow Coma Scale (EVM) or AVPU should be documented, even if starting at a baseline of 3 or U respectively, since the change of mental status in response to any treatment can give important information. A full neurological examination is impossible with an unconscious patient, however suspicion of a TIA or stroke may be raised by asymmetry in any of the following:
  - response to painful stimuli
  - plantar response
  - tendon reflexes
  - tone
- *environment*: check the patient's temperature and examine the skin for any evidence of a rash.

> 🔅 You should be familiar with the physiological variables that should be recorded in the care of the unconscious patient. What is the rationale for their measurement? How do they relate to stable, recovering or deteriorating patients?

(b) Failure to wake up after anaesthetic
After a successful anaesthetic, patients should wake up relatively quickly. However, the length of time it takes to regain consciousness following anaesthesia can be variable. It depends on the patient's physical condition, the anaesthetic/analgesic drugs used, and the duration of surgery. When establishing an index of clinical suspicion it is important to bear in mind:

- known pre-operative medical conditions
- peri-operative problems
- post-operative status.

Important factors include:

- *drug-related*: overdose of opioids or muscle relaxants. Remember that small or elderly patients may require lower doses of drugs. Additionally, it is important to anticipate the effects of liver and/or renal disease on drug metabolism and excretion

- *respiratory failure*: patients with underlying respiratory disease, airway obstruction, or opiate-mediated respiratory depression often retain CO_2, which can lead to deterioration of mental function and narcosis, or, as in this context, delayed awakening after anaesthesia
- *circulatory failure*: intra-operative MI or pulmonary embolism are particular risks in patients with significant risk factors. These may be undiagnosed during the surgical procedure and may present as failure to wake up after anaesthetic
- *metabolic complications*:
  - hypoglycaemia can be precipitated by the stress of surgery, particularly in diabetic patients taking insulin or oral hypoglycaemics, patients with significant liver disease, alcoholics, and septicaemic patients
  - severe hyperglycaemia may occur in diabetics i.e. hyperosmotic non-ketoacidotic diabetic coma, or diabetic ketoacidosis
  - electrolyte imbalance: hyponatraemia can produce coma. This is usually due to pre-operative or peri-operative management (e.g. overenthusiastic fluid resuscitation, or in special situations such as TURP syndrome where aqueous glycine is absorbed through the damaged prostatic vasculature)
  - myxoedema coma: this may result from the stress of surgery in an elderly patient with undiagnosed hypothyroidism
- *neurological complications*:
  - cerebral hypoxaemia will result in a reduced level of consciousness and hence failure to wake up after anaesthesia
  - haemorrhagic or embolic stroke is a particular risk of neurosurgery, cardiac surgery, or carotid surgery.

(Radhakrishnan *et al.*, 2001)

> Take this opportunity to revise the metabolic causes of coma. What features in the history and examination would help distinguish between the different possibilities?

(c) Investigations

Investigations should include those aimed at helping in the assessment of the above causes. These should include:

- arterial blood gas sampling
- ECG (12-lead and continuous monitor)
- markers of myocardial damage (troponin T, creatinine kinase, etc)
- blood glucose (and BM)
- urea and electrolytes
- thyroid function tests
- CT of the brain.

(d) Post-operative monitoring

The origin of the word monitor is from the Latin 'monere' which means 'to warn'. Post-operative monitoring is essential to provide early warning of deterioration in the patient's condition. In general, a monitoring regime should include the following:

- respiratory rate
- SpO_2
- pulse
- BP
- urine output
- Glasgow coma score
- temperature.

Nurses will usually start a suitable monitoring regime in the recovery room. When patients regain consciousness, it is essential to ensure that they are receiving appropriate analgaesia.

(e) Miosis (contracted pupil)

On examination of the patient, she had small equal pupils which had delayed response to light. The possible causes of miosis in this patient are:

- age, since nearly all elderly patients are miotic. Sluggish pupils may be found if there is co-existing cataract or glaucoma
- opioid toxicity, which classically causes 'pinpoint pupils'
- metabolic comas, which cause the pupils to be normal or mildly contracted. Pupils are never pinpoint, unless there is coexisting opioid toxicity/pontine haemorrhage. However, in this patient, the delayed response to light is a significant indicator that this could be a metabolic coma. The delayed light reflex, or hyporeflexia, is classical of hypothyroidism. This would tie in with the clinical history of weight gain and lethargy. One extreme manifestation of hypothyroidism is myxoedema coma.

Pontine lesions (e.g. pontine haemorrhage) also cause bilateral 'pinpoint pupils' through the interruption of sympathetic pathways (sympathetic stimulation dilates the pupil). However, following pontine haemorrhage the pupils are usually non-reactive to light, and there would be evidence of hyperventilation, hyperpyrexia, and flaccid tetraparesis.

> You should be familiar with the control of pupil constriction and dilation and its diagnostic importance. Use this opportunity to revise common pupil signs in neurological disease.

Myxoedema coma

This is the only emergency associated with hypo-thyroidism and is very rare. It occurs almost exclu-sively in the elderly (>65 years old). The onset can be spontaneous, although, more commonly, it is pre-cipitated by insults including cold exposure, infec-tion, surgery, MI, and stroke. The signs of myxoedema coma include:

- patient looks 'hypothyroid'
- hypoventilation
- bradycardia
- hypotension (which can rapidly lead to severe cardiac failure)
- hyporeflexia (with a slow relaxation phase)
- hypothermia
- hypoglycaemia
- hyponatraemia.

The mortality from this condition is high, and patients require full intensive care. Treatment in-volves maximising ABCDE and:

- slow intravenous T_3 (triiodothyronine), to avoid precipitating undiagnosed ischaemic heart disease
- i.v. saline, while monitoring cardiac output and central venous pressure via a central line
- nutritional support.

Any heart failure, hypothermia or infection should be treated.

> Hypothyroidism is a common endocrine disorder, often undiagnosed, particularly in the elderly. Take this opportunity to revise the clinical features and management of the disease.

(f) Post-operative confusion

Post-operative confusion occurs in a significant proportion of surgical patients, and is more common in the elderly. It has the potential to increase the length of time spent in hospital, and can interfere with effective post-operative management.

Many of the causes are similar to those that can precipitate coma. Some of the more common causes include:

- *premorbid state* (i.e. a patient with early demen-tia): this may only become apparent when dis-cussing the patient's normal state with family members or carers
- *drugs*: those used in anaesthesia and analgesia, or following the withdrawal of benzodiazepines or opiates
- hypoglycaemia
- respiratory dysfunction causing hypoxaemia or hypercapnoea

- sepsis (chest, urinary tract, wound, i.v. cannula site infection)
- urinary retention
- TIA or stroke
- MI
- undiagnosed subdural or subarachnoid bleeding
- trauma
- epilepsy
- alcohol withdrawal
- biochemical abnormalities.

> What are the symptoms of an acute confusional state and how is it managed (*see* p. 189)? You should be familiar with the roles of both treating any underlying cause and the importance of the environment in which care is provided.

(g) Assessment of confusion

A common way to assess confusion is the abbreviated mental test (AMT). It is also useful in monitoring the improvement or deterioration in a patient's mental status. Other commonly used, but more time-consuming, tests include the mini-mental state examination (MMSE) (*see* p. 190).

> What are the components of the AMT and MMSE? Why might it be more appropriate to use the AMT in patients with post-operative confusion?

(h) Check X-ray

Post-operatively the patient needs to have a check X-ray of the right hip/prosthesis before she begins to mobilise, to ensure the prosthetic hip has not dis-located. This needs to be arranged on the first or second day post-operatively (*see* p. 107 for an example). Early mobilisation has many benefits in-cluding minimizing DVT/PE risk and preventing the many other problems arising from prolonged bed-rest (*see* pp. 76 and 196).

(i) Investigation of underlying conditions

The patient has a recent history of lethargy, weight gain, and a fall. Lethargy is a very common symptom, and in isolation is a poor predictor of 'pathology'. However, in the context of this patient, the asso-ciated symptoms provide the clues to the diagnosis. The causes of weight gain in an elderly patient include:

- change in diet (increase in calorific intake)

- lack of exercise due to poor mobility
- alcohol excess
- fluid retention due to cardiac failure or renal disease
- liver failure with hypoproteinaemia
- malignant ascites
- hypothyroidism
- hypopituitarism
- Cushing's disease.

The patient should be assessed, in particular for these potential diagnoses, and investigated according to the findings.

> How would the above conditions be confirmed or refuted? History, examination, and investigation can provide the answers in all cases.

(j) Physiology of ageing and implications for surgery and anaesthesia

The process of ageing constitutes a progressive decline in physiological functioning. This change is partially mediated by replacement of active cells by inactive interstitial cells in many tissues. Additionally, the blood supply to tissues is reduced. This can be thought of as a process that results in elderly patients having little, or no physiological reserve.

Therefore, all co-morbidities in elderly patients are exacerbated by the stress produced by surgery and anaesthesia.

Specific changes in body systems include:

Cardiovascular

In the myocardium, muscle cells enlarge but are fewer in number. Collagen and fat replace a substantial volume of the muscle mass. Combined with increased calcification, the myocardium becomes less compliant, less contractile and conducts electrical impulses less efficiently. These changes reduce the cardiac output and make the ageing heart more prone to arrhythmias (see p. 178).

Progressive coronary arteriosclerosis, combined with decreased aortic compliance, and raised systolic blood pressure leads to a reduction in coronary artery blood flow. This makes the elderly more prone to myocardial ischaemia.

The same sclerosis and calcification occur within the peripheral vascular system, increasing peripheral vascular resistance and afterload, making the elderly more prone to left ventricular failure and congestive cardiac failure.

Vasomotor control decreases, making the elderly more prone to syncope. The elderly 'thrive on vagal drive', often with a limited sympathetic compensatory response.

Respiratory

Kyphosis of the thoracic spine alters the position of the ribs. Combined with weakness of the intercostal muscles, elderly patients are often unable to breathe as effectively as younger patients.

Elastic recoil, and hence compliance of the lungs is reduced, increasing the residual volume and reducing the vital capacity.

The bronchial mucosa degenerates and the cilia have difficulty clearing secretions. This makes chest infections more common in the elderly.

Renal

A decline is seen in the number of nephrons in the kidney in elderly people. A reduction in renal blood flow, combined with a decrease in glomerular filtration and concentrating ability, impairs fluid and electrolyte balance.

Immune

The elderly have a reduced T-cell response, increasing susceptibility to infections and poor wound healing.
(Horan, 2003)

> You should be aware of the effects of ageing on all body systems. What changes occur in the nervous and haematopoietic systems? What are the implications for management of pain and anaemia respectively?

(k) Pre-operative assessment

This involves a thorough history and examination. The main goals of pre-operative assessment should be to:

- evaluate and optimise patients' general health
- anticipate and avoid possible complications.

Additional investigations should be based on the clinical picture. Significant co-morbidities that need to be considered are:

- *COPD patients* require a detailed pre-operative anaesthetic consultation
- *previous MI*: depending on the procedure, elective surgery should usually be postponed until ≥ 6 months post-MI
- *angina* and *hypertension* need to be controlled before the operation
- *congestive cardiac failure* will inevitably be aggravated by surgery, therefore, pre-operative control should be optimised

- *valvular heart disease* may require long-term anticoagulation (warfarin) to be changed to heparin; and prophylactic antibiotics may be needed
- *previous DVT/PE* carries an increased risk of recurrence. Long-term oral anticoagulation may need to be stopped for a period of time before and/or after surgery. Prophylactic or therapeutic dose low-molecular weight heparin may be needed
- *atrial fibrillation*: anticoagulation needs to be stopped, usually a week prior to surgery (the exact time varies with surgical procedure)
- *insulin-dependent diabetes* is a major problem because of the starvation associated with surgery. These patients require a GKI infusion (sometimes called an Alberti regime)
- *Addison's disease/long-term steroid treatment*: these patients require extra steroid cover to help cope with the stress of surgery
- *hyperthyroidism* needs to be controlled before surgery
- *cervical spine disease*, e.g. rheumatoid arthritis, or any arthropathy, may complicate or preclude intubation
- *anaemia* needs to be corrected before surgery
- *U&E abnormalities* should be investigated and treated before surgery
- *teeth/dentures*: in anticipation of damage during airway management (particularly important from a medicolegal point of view)
- *previous anaesthesia*: any problems should be documented, including a family history of any anaesthetic problems.

(l) Healthcare professionals involved in home help

This patient has residual mobility problems following her discharge from hospital, particularly as she continues to live in her own home. Therefore, a package of care under the supervision of a multi-disciplinary team should be planned. Healthcare professionals who might be involved include:

- geriatricians (particularly orthogeriatricians)
- GPs
- occupational therapists
- physiotherapists
- district nurses
- carers
- social workers.

See p. 108 for a fuller discussion of discharge planning following fractured neck of femur.

Web resources
- Hypothyroidism: www.endocrineweb.com
- Peri-operative cardiovascular system evaluation: www.postgradmed.com
- Post-operative assessment guidelines: www.sign.ac.uk

Further reading
- Horan MA (2003) Physiology of ageing. *Anaesthesia and Intensive Care Medicine.* 4(10): 337.
- Lavelle-Jones M (ed.) (2002) *Master Medicine: surgery 1* (2e). Churchill Livingstone, London.
- Radhakrishnan J, Jesudasan S and Jacob R (2001) Delayed awakening or emergence from anaesthesia. *Update in Anaesthesia.* 13: Article 3. www.nda.ox.ac.uk
- Roberts CG and Ladenson PW (2004) Hypothyroidism. *Lancet.* 363: 793.
- Scottish Intercollegiate Guidelines Network (SIGN) (2004) Guideline 77: *Post-operative Management in Adults.* SIGN, Edinburgh, Section 2: post-operative assessment.

7 A lawyer with a drink problem

Jenny Child is a 40-year-old lawyer who attends her GP. She complains of fatigue and poor sleep. She has no significant past medical history. On questioning she admits to drinking a bottle of wine each evening. Physical examination is unremarkable. Blood tests are sent to the laboratory.

(a) Which questions would her GP ask her to establish the likelihood of problem drinking?

....

....

....

(b) What advice would the GP give to his patient?

....

....

....

(c) How many units of alcohol is she consuming per week and how does this compare to the suggested maximum alcohol intake?

....

....

....

The results of the liver function tests are normal except for a raised gamma-glutamyl transferase level. Her GP tells her the results over the phone and says that the results are likely to indicate that she is drinking too much.

(d) What are the standard tests used to assess liver disease and how do they reflect liver structure and function?

....

....

....

(e) What help could her GP offer her with cutting down her alcohol consumption?

....

....

....

She declines help, and 6 years later she attends the A&E department. She is seen by the SHO and admits to having continued to increase her alcohol intake. She says that she wants to stop, and hasn't had a drink for the last two days. She is not on any medication. She has also recently returned from South East Asia but denies both intravenous drug misuse and unprotected sex. The SHO notes that she is a little agitated and distracted. On examination she appears tremulous, icteric and pale. Her pulse is 110 beats/min and regular, BP is 140/85 mmHg, respiratory rate is 18 breaths/min, and temperature is 37.8°C. Physical examination is normal apart from a tender right upper quadrant and a tender regular liver edge 3 cm below the costal margin.

(f) What is the most likely cause of this patient's symptoms and how do the physical signs arise from the underlying condition?

....

....

....

(g) What pharmacological treatment might ease her symptoms?

....

....

....

(h) What are the possible causes of the tender enlarged liver?

....

....

....

(i) What other physical signs would the SHO look for?

....

....

....

☞ The SHO is concerned that there may be co-existing pathology causing the liver signs, and decides to send blood for a liver screen to rule out other possible causes of liver disease.

(j) What blood tests would he order to rule out the other possible causes?

....

....

....

☞ On reviewing the available results, the medical SHO decides to admit the patient to MAU, pending a referral to a gastroenterologist. He starts her on treatment and decides to order some further investigations.

(k) What management would be appropriate on MAU?

....

....

....

(l) What radiological investigations would he request?

....

....

....

☞ The consultant gastroenterologist reviews the patient the following day. On reviewing the notes, he reads that the SHO has suggested that the patient should have a liver biopsy.

(m) What are the indications for a liver biopsy in a patient with suspected alcoholic liver disease?

....

....

....

☞ In an attempt to make the patient reconsider her drinking habits, the consultant discusses the effects that alcohol has on the liver.

(n) Describe the stages of alcoholic damage to the liver. How do they arise?

....

....

....

✓ Answers and teaching notes

Key cases
- Alcohol misuse
- Alcoholic liver disease

Clinical context
Alcohol is still regarded by many as a soft, harmless drug. Despite attempts to increase the public's awareness of the problems associated with alcohol, its use is increasing, in particular binge drinking, manifested by the increasing number of alcohol-related hospital admissions.

Although one glass of red wine a day may benefit the cardiovascular system, larger volumes (>21units/ week for men, and no more than 4 units in any one day) will affect the patient and their family/friends in many ways. The health, social, and economic ramifications of alcohol use are extensive. This scenario describes the effect of alcohol on the liver. Before continuing to read the teaching notes, spend 5 minutes thinking about the health, personal, social, and economic effects surrounding a 43-year-old managing director of his own company who is married with two children. He has a £50,000 mortgage and drives after an office party. He is drunk and crashes into another car in which two passengers die. Remember alcohol use affects more than the drinker.

(a) Problem drinking
Problem drinking, alcohol-related problems, and alcohol dependence are not interchangeable terms. The definitions of these terms vary according to the individuals affected, since people are able to drink alcohol in differing amounts without necessarily suffering personal or health-related consequences. Alcoholic liver disease is a medical diagnosis and is related to the absolute amount of alcohol consumed. Not all heavy drinkers are problem drinkers, and problem drinkers may not drink as heavily as some other people. Neither group will necessarily develop alcohol dependence or alcoholic liver disease.

Problem drinkers are probably best described as those who drink alcohol in amounts which, for them, compromise their health, personality, relationships and working lives.

People may be evasive when directly asked about their alcohol use; the CAGE questionnaire provides a validated method of assessing whether someone has an alcohol-related problem.

- Have you felt the need to **Cut** down drinking?

- Have you ever felt **Annoyed** by criticism of your drinking?
- Have you had **Guilty** feelings about drinking?
- Have you ever had a drink first thing in the morning to steady your nerves or get rid of a hangover? (**Eye-opener**)

A positive response to at least two questions is seen in the majority of patients with alcoholism, and to all four questions in approximately 50%.

(b) Advice on alcohol use
The patient should be advised to reduce drinking gradually. It has been shown that advice and brief counselling from GPs can help in reducing alcohol consumption by patients.

> 💡 Use this opportunity to review the different types of counselling available to patients. What are the general stages involved in effective counselling? What is the theory behind cognitive-behavioural therapy? What are the important communication skills that are needed?

(c) Conversion of drinks to units of alcohol
It is important to be able to convert a patient's estimated alcohol usage into units, since the number of units consumed is directly proportional to the risk of developing alcoholic liver disease. Liver disease is unlikely to develop if a patient is drinking less than:

- 50 units a week for men
- 35 units a week for women.

However, the term 'sensible drinking' is more difficult to define. The risk of developing alcohol-related problems depends on the number of units of alcohol consumed per week and the relative amount drunk in one sitting. Current guidelines for sensible drinking suggest a maximum of:

- 21 units a week for men (no more than 4 units in a single day)
- 14 units a week for women (no more than 3 units in a single day).

Conversion to units
Units are measures related to the alcohol content of different drinks. A unit of alcohol is 10ml of pure ethanol. The following list is an approximation.

- 1 pint of beer = 2 units
- 1 glass of wine (125 ml) = 1 unit
- 1 measure of spirit (25 ml) = 1 unit
- 1 bottle of wine = 7 units
- 1 bottle of spirit = 32 units

- This patient is drinking 49 units of alcohol per week.
- Her intake is above both 21 and 35 units per week, therefore she is at significant risk of developing alcoholic liver disease.

It is also important to establish the duration of alcohol use, and use in the past. These are often significantly underestimated by patients.

> You should be familiar with the burden of alcohol-related problems to society. What proportion of patients in hospital have alcohol-related problems? How does alcohol consumption relate to road traffic accidents, suicides and murders? What public health policy is there relating to alcohol consumption?

(d) Liver function tests

Liver function tests are used to provide evidence of structural liver damage and impaired synthetic function. It is important to know the normal functions and relative tissue distribution of the enzymes, proteins and metabolites measured, to appreciate which tests reflect structural damage, which reflect impaired synthetic function, and how the pattern suggests a cause.

The standard components of liver function tests are ALT, AST, ALP, GGT, albumin, bilirubin, PT and glucose. These represent structural and functional integrity respectively:

Enzymes that reflect hepatobiliary structure

Hepatocellular injury of any cause results in the release of these enzymes from the intracellular compartment, or damaged membranes into the circulation.

Alanine transaminase (ALT) and aspartate transaminase (AST)

ALT and AST are enzymes that catalyse deamination of alanine or aspartate during gluconeogenesis.

ALT is a cytosolic enzyme that is relatively specific to hepatocytes. In contrast, AST is both a cytosolic and mitochondrial enzyme. It is therefore much less specific for liver damage, as the mitochondrial isoenzyme can be released from damage to many tissues (including cardiac muscle). Very high levels are found in viral hepatitis, acute cholestasis, and shock (often cardiogenic).

Gammaglutamyl transpeptidase (GGT)

GGT participates in the transfer of amino acids across cell membranes and in the metabolism of glutathione. High concentrations of this enzyme are found in the liver and bile ducts.

Raised GGT is seen in cholestasis and hepatocellular disease, but lacks specificity. It may be raised in isolation in heavy drinkers without significant liver damage.

Alkaline phosphatase (ALP)

For a discussion of causes of raised ALP *see* p. 201. Hepatic ALP is an enzyme that is present in bile duct epithelial cell membranes. The concentration rises in cholestasis, and to a lesser extent in hepatocyte damage.

ALP is therefore useful in determining diseases that structurally affect the bile ducts such as gallstones, primary biliary cirrhosis and sclerosing cholangitis. The rise in GGT and ALP confirms that the source of ALP is hepatobiliary.

Products that reflect hepatic synthetic ability
Albumin

The liver synthesises albumin. In chronic liver disease the serum albumin level is often markedly reduced, and the level correlates well with disease prognosis. However it is important to remember that albumin levels depend on a number of other factors such as nutritional status, GI/urinary losses, and systemic illness.

Prothrombin time (PT)

The synthesis of coagulation factors is another important function of the liver. The PT reflects the synthesis factors II, VII, IX, X. When interpreting a prolonged PT it is important to remember the other causes such as vitamin K deficiency and warfarin treatment.

Bilirubin

Bilirubin is formed from the breakdown of haem. Unconjugated bilirubin is transported to the liver bound to albumin. It is water insoluble and therefore is not excreted in the urine. Bilirubin conjugated in the liver to bilirubin glucuronide is water soluble. Conjugated bilirubin appears in the urine when plasma levels rise.

Normally, most of the conjugated bilirubin synthesised by hepatocytes is secreted in bile. Intestinal flora break this down into urobilinogen, which is partially reabsorbed in the terminal ileum (enterohepatic circulation). The reabsorbed urobilinogen is excreted either via the kidney, or by the liver through the biliary tree into the duodenum. The remainder is excreted in the faeces as stercobilinogen, which causes the brown appearance.

Unconjugated hyperbilirubinaemia may reflect underlying haemolysis or myoglobin breakdown from muscle injury. Equally, defects that occur in bilirubin uptake (Gilbert's syndrome), or conjugation in hepatocytes (Crigler–Najjar or Gilbert's syndrome) may cause unconjugated hyperbilirubinaemia.

> Use this opportunity to revise the more complex causes of hyperbilirubinaemia. What is the role of UDPGT? Revise the familial non-haemolytic hyperbilirubinaemias (Gilbert's syndrome, Crigler–Najjar syndrome type I and type II).

Conjugated hyperbilirubinaemia characteristically occurs in hepatocellular damage, cholestasis, and biliary obstruction.

> Use this opportunity to revise the liver's metabolic roles. You should be familiar with the role of the liver in protein, carbohydrate and lipid metabolism, protein synthesis, bile formation, conjugation and excretion of drugs, and catabolism of hormones.

(e) Help with problem drinking

Problem drinking may be provoked by adverse life events, and patients may return to normal drinking once their circumstances change. However for those who continue to drink, supportive management strategies are available:

- advice from the GP explaining the risks and advising a reduction in alcohol consumption. This must be combined with structured follow-up consultations
- Alcoholics Anonymous or other group therapies
- counselling in primary care
- referral to the community alcohol service.

The key point with all of these interventions is that the patient needs to be willing. They have to want to 'give up'.

> What are the components of an effective community alcohol service? You should be familiar with the range of services offered including information provision, support groups for patients and relatives and relapse prevention programmes.

(f) Acute alcohol withdrawal

- This patient is suffering from acute withdrawal of alcohol.
- The withdrawal state leads to increased sympathetic activity.

Persistent alcohol use causes downregulation of the benzodiazepine–$GABA_A$ receptor complex. When alcohol is withdrawn, the functional ability of GABA as an inhibitory neurotransmitter is diminished, leading to a consequent increase in sympathetic activity. This manifests clinically as tachycardia, hypertension, tremor, hyperthermia, and sweating.

The patient's condition can deteriorate and progress to delirium tremens (DT) which is diagnosed when the above symptoms are accompanied by altered mental state, e.g. confusion, hallucinations, and agitation.

Symptoms may begin within hours of alcohol abstinence, and can develop further, peaking in most cases in 48–72 hours. It is therefore important to try to proactively prevent withdrawal, and to ensure that the correct treatment is started to prevent progression to DT.

(g) Pharmacological treatment

Patients should receive treatment to counteract the increase in sympathetic activity. Benzodiazepines are the drug of choice; chlordiazepoxide (Librium) or diazepam is commonly used. The dose should be titrated so the patient is calm (many hospitals have a protocol for the safe prescription of a detoxification regimen). Care should always be exercised in patients with cirrhosis, due to the effect on the half-life of benzodiazepines.

(h) Causes of hepatomegaly

Hepatomegaly is not a very reliable sign of liver disease, because of the variability in the size and shape of the liver and the body habitus. Remember firstly to percuss the upper border of the liver, and secondly to see if this is pushed down (increased expansion of the lung).

The important causes in this case are:

- alcoholic hepatitis
- viral hepatitis
- fatty infiltration
- acute passive congestion (right ventricular failure/tricuspid regurgitation/pulmonary embolism).

> It is important to be aware of the other common causes of hepatomegaly and hepatosplenomegaly. What are the haematological, malignant, infective, cardiac, and miscellaneous causes?

(i) Physical signs in liver disease

There may be few signs in acute-onset liver disease or in advanced cirrhosis. However, the following signs should be sought:

- *jaundice*: when serum bilirubin exceeds 35 μmol/l, the skin and the sclerae may become yellow; this is especially obvious in fair-skinned people
- *spider naevi*: these are superficial, tortuous arterioles, and typically fill from the centre outwards. They are usually restricted to the arms, face, and upper torso (usually in the distribution of the superior vena cava). They can be pulsatile and difficult to detect in dark-skinned individuals
- *palmar erythema*: this is reddening of the palms, and to a lesser extent the fingertips, indicating a hyperdynamic circulation
- *gynaecomastia*: the altered catabolism of oestrogen in a damaged liver can produce breast enlargement in men. In women this may be more difficult to detect
- *peripheral oedema*: this is due to salt and water retention and lowered plasma oncotic pressure
- *ascites*: fluid accumulation in the abdomen produces abdominal distention and bulging flanks. This often indicates severe liver disease, usually cirrhosis. Fluid accumulates in the abdomen because of portal hypertension and lowered plasma oncotic pressure
- *caput medusae*: caput medusae consists of dilated collateral veins seen radiating from the umbilicus. This sign results from recanalisation of the umbilical vein due to portal hypertension
- *splenomegaly*: this is present clinically whenever the spleen can be felt protruding beneath the left rib cage. The spleen enlarges secondary to portal hypertension, since the splenic vein drains into the portal vein. If suspected, splenomegaly should be confirmed by ultrasound.

This list is not all-inclusive, patients may also present with signs including asterixis, leuconychia, parotid swelling, scratch marks, clubbing, foetor hepaticus, testicular atrophy, and, in severe cases, hepatic encephalopathy.

> Use this opportunity to revisit the anatomy of the liver and portal venous system. Where are the common portosystemic anastamoses? Why are patients with chronic liver disease frequently hypoxaemic?

(j) Investigations in liver disease

The history is important in determining the cause of abnormal LFTs, and is complemented by various blood tests including:

- *hepatitis A, B and C serology*
- *autoantibodies*: antimitochondrial antibodies (AMA) are raised in primary biliary cirrhosis. Peripheral antineutrophil cytoplasmic antibodies (p-ANCA) are raised in sclerosing cholangitis. Antismooth muscle antibodies (SMA), antinuclear antibodies (ANA) and anti-liver–kidney microsomal antibodies (LKM) are tested in chronic autoimmune hepatitis
- *serum immunoglobulins*: IgA is raised in alcoholic liver disease. IgM is usually raised in primary biliary cirrhosis
- *ferritin*: usually massively raised in haemochromatosis (genetic studies may show C282Y, H63D genotypes). The percentage transferrin saturation should also be checked
- *serum α_1-antitrypsin*: low in α_1-antitrypsin deficiency
- *serum caeruloplasmin*: low in Wilson's disease (serum copper reduced)
- *tumour markers*: α-FP for hepatocellular carcinoma.

Other abnormalities that might be seen in alcoholic liver disease include macrocytic, microcytic or mixed anaemia, and abnormalities of red cell morphology on a peripheral blood film. Remember that the liver may be involved in systemic diseases, e.g. connective tissue disorders, and is a common site for metastases.

(k) Management of alcohol withdrawal

Management of alcohol withdrawal has three main objectives: firstly, to prevent the continuous motor activity sympathetic symptoms and the potential for withdrawal seizures with benzodiazepines; secondly, to supplement vitamins, and calories in the malnourished alcoholic; thirdly to help patients to reduce their alcohol intake in the longer term.

- As previously discussed, alcohol withdrawal should be treated with benzodiazepines (chlordiazepoxide, diazepam).
- Thiamine (vitamin B_1) replacement is important since alcoholics are often deficient. Thiamine is a cofactor for many important enzymes, and deficiency results in Wernicke's encephalopathy, peripheral neuropathy and cardiomyopathy.
- Vitamin C should be replaced. This can be achieved using the intravenous compound preparation pabrinex, which contains high-dose B and C vitamins.
- Folic acid replacement should be prescribed. Dietary deficiency of folic acid is an important

feature of many alcoholics. Folic acid is an important cofactor for the enzyme required for the production of red blood cells.

- The patient is also likely to have magnesium deficiency secondary to malnutrition and malabsorbtion. Treatment with magnesium may help prevent seizures and arrhythmias due to its cell membrane-stabilising properties.
- Patients should be adequately but not over-hydrated. If oral intake is not adequate, the threshold for instituting NG feeding should be low.
- Vitamin K is usually administered to patients with a raised INR or prolonged PT, even though this is usually ineffective because coagulopathy reflects the severity of the underlying liver disease. Vitamin K should be given in chronic liver disease, not in acute hepatitis.
- Admission to HDU should be considered in the unstable patient.

(l) Imaging

The function of imaging is to define the gross anatomy of the liver and biliary tree and to confirm/identify any other abdominal pathology (e.g. splenomegaly or pancreatic pathology). Although CT and MRI scans provide detailed information, ultrasound scans can reliably detect changes in liver texture such as fatty liver, cysts and metastases, and are excellent at gallstone detection and imaging of the biliary tree. Duplex ultrasound can detect the direction of flow through the portal system.

- The imaging that would be most appropriate in this case is abdominal ultrasound scanning.

(m) Liver biopsy

Liver biopsy is indicated in patients in whom the diagnosis of alcoholic hepatitis is uncertain based upon clinical and laboratory findings.

- Patients who may have more than one type of liver disease (such as alcohol-related disease and hepatitis C) may benefit from a liver biopsy to help determine the relative contribution of the different causes.

In this patient, if the results of the liver screen are consistent with alcoholic liver disease, a biopsy is not needed at this stage because it would not benefit the patient and has associated risks. The decision to perform a biopsy should consider the strength of the clinical diagnosis, and the role that the biopsy findings would have in guiding therapeutic options.

(n) Stages of alcoholic liver disease

The key to understanding the stages of alcoholic liver disease is an appreciation of how alcohol is metabo-

lised by the liver. Alcohol is oxidised to acetaldehyde with the generation of NADH by the enzyme alcohol dehydrogenase. Prolonged and heavy alcohol use increases the amount of NADH and reduces the amount of NAD^+. This reduction in the levels of the essential coenzyme NAD^+ inhibits the ability of the hepatocytes to oxidise fatty acids, which are then esterified to triglycerides, which accumulate in the liver. There are also similar effects on protein and carbohydrate metabolism.

These effects are most profound on the most poorly oxygenated areas of liver tissue (i.e. closest to the terminal hepatic venules). As fat accumulates in this area, an attempt at repair results in the infiltration of inflammatory/immune cells, which can result in necrosis and perivenular fibrosis. These changes are indicative of alcoholic hepatitis.

Alcohol also directly stimulates stellate cells to transform into collagen-producing myofibroblast cells. These changes cause fibrosis in the subendothelial space with loss of endothelial permeability and derangement of both hepatocyte and lobular structure and function. These changes are indicative of micronodular cirrhosis. Once the architecture of the liver becomes sufficiently deranged, liver failure will follow.

The liver changes associated with alcohol are therefore:

- fatty change (reversible)
- alcoholic hepatitis (partially reversible if there is complete abstinence)
- cirrhosis (irreversible).

Web resources

- Alcohol misuse; policy and guidance: www.doh.gov.uk
- Basic liver disease information: www.britishlivertrust.org.uk
- General liver disease information: www.gpnotebook.co.uk
- LFT interpretation: http://pmj.bmjjournals.com/cgi/content/full/79/932/307

Further reading

- Ashworth M and Gerada C (1997) ABC of mental health. Addiction and dependence – II: alcohol. *British Medical Journal.* 315: 358–60.
- Beckinghan IJ and Bornman PC (2001) ABC of diseases of liver, pancreas, and biliary system [series of articles]. *British Medical Journal.* 322.
- Kitchens JM. Does this patient have an alcohol problem? (1994) *Journal of the American Medical Association.* 272: 1782.
- Kosten TR and O'Connor PG (2003) Management of drug and alcohol withdrawal. *New England Journal of Medicine.* 348: 1786.

8 A junior SHO's experience on the surgical admission unit

As a junior SHO, you see a slim, previously perfectly healthy, 18-year-old female student in the surgical admission unit (SAU) at midnight. She was sent in by her GP with a 2-day history of feeling unwell with generalised abdominal pain. Last night she went all shivery, followed by a drenching sweat. This morning, pain has developed in the right iliac fossa (RIF) and she is feeling very nauseated.

She is successfully treated but 2 years later, she returns to SAU and she recognises you. Again, she has pain in her RIF but she says it's not the same this time. She feels a bit 'blown up', which is causing constant discomfort, but the main thing is the most awful stomach cramps in the middle of her abdomen. She has vomited everything she has tried to eat or drink for the last 24 hours.

(a) Which test is essential and why?

....

....

....

(b) What is the most likely diagnosis?

....

....

(c) What other conditions would be included in your differential diagnosis?

....

....

....

(d) If this is the working diagnosis, discuss initial treatment, definitive treatment and the process leading up to that treatment.

....

....

....

(e) Which test is likely to make this common diagnosis?

....

....

....

(f) What other observations on physical examination are relevant?

....

....

....

(g) What investigations might be appropriate?

....

....

....

(h) Discuss her management (there are two main options).

....

....

....

Your next patient is a 64-year-old man, who has never missed a day's work. He arrives at A&E by ambulance, accompanied by his wife. He is clearly very ill. His wife tells you that last night he went out to the local pub, which he rarely does, to celebrate his best friend's 65th birthday. He'd not been feeling well for a couple of days but thought he should go. His indigestion had been playing up, as had his irritable bowel. This usually gave him lower abdominal pain, especially on the left side, and diarrhoea.

She had gone to bed before he got home in a taxi. He'd woken her at 7 am saying that he'd developed awful abdominal pain 'all over', had vomited (which he had also done in the pub), and felt very weak and shivery. Seeing him, his wife had dialled 999. On examination, he looks ill and dry. His pulse rate is 105 beats/min, BP is 100/50 mmHg, and his temperature is 38°C. His abdomen is distended, with generalised rebound tenderness and only the occasional bowel sound. He is breathing shallowly with a respiratory rate of 36 breaths/min.

The SHO orders an erect chest X-ray that is shown in Figure 8.1.

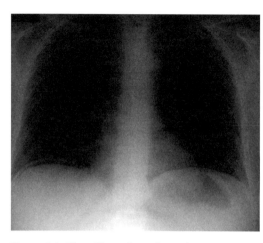

Figure 8.1 Chest X-ray from the patient.

(k) Comment on the X-ray. What does this show?

....

....

....

(i) As a surgical SHO what is your role in this man's management?

....

....

....

(l) What initial measures and investigations are required?

....

....

....

(j) What are the most likely causes of his generalised peritonitis?

....

....

....

(m) What sort of operation is needed and when? What should it achieve?

....

....

....

Key cases

- Acute abdomen
- Appendicitis
- Acute obstruction
- Perforated viscus

Clinical context

The 'acute abdomen' is a big subject. It is used to describe a spectrum of surgical, medical and gynaecological problems, ranging from the trivial to the life threatening. Medical causes of the acute abdomen have been referred to elsewhere in this book. The most common cause of abdominal pain is still idiopathic pain. Other causes include acute appendicitis, acute cholecystitis and biliary pain, peptic ulcer disease, bowel obstruction, acute pancreatitis and renal/ureteric colic.

This scenario concentrates on peritonitis (localised and generalised), and bowel obstruction. As it is so common, acute appendicitis is used as an example of localised peritonitis. Surgical causes of acute bowel obstruction are discussed, along with the diagnosis and management of generalised peritonitis within the context of a perforated peptic ulcer.

(a) Pregnancy test

A pregnancy test is an essential diagnostic step in all women of reproductive age with abdominal pain. There are two reasons for this:

- if the test is positive, measures must be taken to minimise the risk of damage to the foetus (e.g. X-rays) and of the pregnancy aborting
- a negative pregnancy test excludes bleeding from an ectopic pregnancy.

> 🔆 Use this opportunity to revisit the presentation of a ruptured ectopic pregnancy. How would this differ from a case of acute appendicitis? Which presents with signs of bleeding, and which with signs of infection?

(b) (c) Acute appendicitis

Acute appendicitis is a common condition and usually requires appendicectomy. The main question is could the acute problem be non-surgical? Several medical problems which cause acute abdominal pain have been referred to elsewhere in this book (*see* pp. 11, 42, 113, 122, 163 and 183), however these

problems do not generally cause peritonitis. Many of the conditions that mimic acute appendicitis also require surgery.

The commonest of these are:

- *ruptured ectopic pregnancy*, which has already been mentioned. It does not particularly need a gynaecologist to perform the operation
- *terminal ileitis*: this is a presentation of Crohn's disease. There is usually a history of chronic milder symptoms preceding the acute presentation (*see* p. 163)
- *carcinoma of the caecum*: often there is a mass, and this cancer is likely to have caused iron deficiency anaemia from occult blood loss (*see* p. 91)
- *ureteric colic*: this can cause rebound tenderness and vomiting. Normally, unless the stone and the urinary tract above the stone are infected, shivering/rigors and subsequent sweats are absent or are mild (*see* p. 113)
- *pyosalpinx*: this is a complication of pelvic inflammatory disease, which can mimic appendicitis
- *Meckel's diverticulitis* is rare. Normally, the diagnosis is only made at operation.

> 🔆 Use this opportunity to consider the other causes of localised peritonitis. It is worth considering what the problem could be if the localised peritonitis was in the LIF and not in the RIF.

> 🔆 Sometimes a mass is also palpable in the RIF. Consider what the mass could be and how you might investigate the cause.

(d) Treatment

Immediate treatment

The findings of the National Confidential Enquiry into Patient Outcome and Death (NCEPOD) show that operations performed in the middle of the night, often by rather junior staff, have a higher morbidity and mortality than those done the next morning. It is therefore wise to delay definitive treatment, by appendicectomy, until the next morning, as long as the patient's condition does not deteriorate. Until the operation takes place, it is necessary to keep the patient in an optimal state by management of

ABCDE (*see* p. 139). Specific actions that should be taken include:

- *i.v. fluids*: she has already vomited, is pyrexial and sweating, and is losing fluid into the inflamed area. Therefore, she is likely to become significantly dehydrated
- *i.v. antibiotics*, such as a cephalosporin and metronidazole. There is no good reason why the latter cannot be given as a suppository, but drugs taken orally are more likely to be vomited. As appendicitis is an infective condition, it would be inviting unnecessary progression, while awaiting surgery, if effective antibiotics were not started as soon as possible

> Use this opportunity to revise the use of antibiotic prophylaxis in general surgery. When should antibiotics be given? If this operation was going to be in 30 minutes' time, would you still start antibiotics and, if so, why?

- *contact the surgeon*: the surgeon will want to confirm the diagnosis, decide if further investigations are needed, and obtain written consent – especially in an emergency setting
- *order any necessary pre-operative investigations*: the minimum would be FBC, U&E, and serum glucose. Dipstick testing of the urine is also highly desirable. In an 18-year-old fit woman, the anaesthetist will not require a CXR, ECG, or any other investigations under normal circumstances

> What abnormalities might be found in the urine in acute appendicitis? If blood, protein, or even leucocytes were found would this alter the diagnosis (*see* p. 114)?

- *rectal examination*: if the appendix extends into the pelvis, there may well be tenderness high up on the right side of the rectum, which would also be the case if the problem were a pyosalpinx
- *go to theatre and book the appendicectomy on the emergency list*: it is acceptable to delay the operation until the next morning but not to delay the operation any longer than is essential
- *order hourly, or 2-hourly observations of respiratory rate, pulse, blood pressure, and temperature*: if there is a delay in an urgent operation, any unexpected deterioration in the patient's condition must be identified immediately and appropriate action taken

- *give sufficient analgesia*: it is a misconception that analgesia masks symptoms and signs. Appropriate analgesia should always be given.

Definitive treatment

This is appendicectomy.

> You should be familiar with the standard approach to removing an appendix. The anatomical position of the appendix is very variable. Take this opportunity to revise the anatomy of the appendix. How can some anatomical variations modify the presenting symptoms and signs of appendicitis, and cause technical difficulties in removing it? Histologically, what is a major component of the appendix? What is a faecolith and can it cause appendicitis?

(e) Intestinal obstruction: erect abdominal X-ray to look for intestinal obstruction

Intestinal obstruction is a common cause of an acute abdomen. It can occur at any point of the intestine and can even occur in more than one place at once, particularly if some disease process sticks several loops of bowel together (e.g. Crohn's disease). The higher the level of the obstruction, the less dilated bowel will be visible on X-ray, but vomiting will be an earlier feature. Vomiting is a relatively late feature of obstruction of the terminal ileum and colon. In contrast, the lower the level of the obstruction, the more likely that the patient will experience 'total constipation' (passing neither faeces or flatus), often accompanied by considerable distension of the abdomen by gas in the obstructed colon.

> Bowel sounds should be increased in this case. Why? Take this opportunity to review the value of listening for bowel sounds. What are 'tinkling' bowel sounds? What is paralytic ileus and what are its causes?

The erect X-ray usually shows multiple fluid levels in the dilated bowel loops.

> How can you distinguish between dilated small and large bowel? Why do you see fluid levels? Where does the fluid come from, and what implication does this have for homeostasis?

(f) Physical examination

- Full abdominal examination.

Once the diagnosis of intestinal obstruction has been made, the cause must be found. The easiest cause to diagnose clinically is when a loop of bowel enters a hernia, and the neck is too tight to allow the passage of fluid through the loop. Therefore each patient must have all potential sites of a hernia examined.

> You should be familiar with the common sites of hernias. What are the anatomical landmarks for differentiating femoral from inguinal hernias? Describe the anatomy of the inguinal canal. Which hernias obstruct more frequently, and why?

Previous abdominal surgery, including gynaecological operations, is another common cause of intestinal obstruction. This can occur in two ways:

- a hole in the mesentery ('internal' hernia)
- twisting around a band adhesion.

The other main causes are intra-abdominal disease. The bowel can become scarred by diseases, such as Crohn's disease, diverticulitis, and previous radiotherapy, and by any malignant disease of the bowel (usually the colon, but the small bowel can be secondarily involved in any other intra-abdominal malignancy). Other rarer causes include different types of intraluminal obstruction. Intussusception is commoner in children (particularly as a complication of Henoch–Schönlein purpura), but can occur in adults with an intestinal polyp. Another cause is volvulus of the sigmoid colon or caecum. This causes enormous distension of the colon, which may be visible in a thin person. It is commoner in Africans than in Europeans.

(g) Investigations

The most common investigations carried out for someone with acute abdominal pain include:

- *FBC*: this is taken for a baseline but a persistently raised WCC suggests underlying inflammation or infection
- *U&E*: useful in guiding fluid replacement
- *serum amylase*: to exclude acute pancreatitis (*see* p. 123)
- *urinalysis*
- *pregnancy test*
- *erect CXR*: to look for signs of pneumoperitoneum due to a perforated viscus
- *abdominal X-ray*: mainly to look for evidence of intestinal obstruction.

It is sometimes appropriate to perform a gastrografin enema or colonoscopy in patients with colonic obstruction.

(h) Management of intestinal obstruction

The two options are:

- conservative
- surgical.

Initial management is conservative. This consists of replacing fluid loss and decompressing the stomach and proximal small bowel with a nasogastric tube. This is often referred to as 'drip and suck'. It is appropriate to start this treatment while assessing the patient. It is also appropriate if the obstruction is only partial (e.g. if the patient is still passing flatus). The rationale for conservative management is that in some patients, such as those with adhesive obstruction, the twist in the bowel can resolve, especially if the nasogastric tube decompresses the obstructed bowel loops. However, the patient must be monitored carefully during conservative management.

There are several indications for surgery:

- failure to respond to conservative management
- reducing an 'external hernia'
- definitive management of the disease (e.g. an obstructing carcinoma) which is causing the obstruction because, clearly, such obstruction is never going to respond to 'drip and suck'
- if there is a risk, or a likelihood of bowel becoming necrotic. This is a particular risk in 'closed loop obstruction'. A typical example of this has already been mentioned – a loop in a hernia. This patient could also have a closed loop obstruction; she has right iliac fossa pain. If conservative management did not relieve this pain, it could be because the closed loop has not been decompressed. Failure to relieve such closed loop obstruction in time can mean losing a significant length of bowel or rupture of the closed loop, leading to peritonitis.

(i) Perforated viscus: your management role

Remember the 'golden hour'. As soon as you see this man, you know that:

- he is seriously ill
- he needs to be resuscitated
- he needs an operation
- the surgeon and anaesthetist should know about him as soon as possible
- any essential investigations need to be done rapidly
- you are part of a team whose members you must know.

(j) Causes of acute, generalised peritonitis

It is difficult to miss the diagnosis of generalised peritonitis, once you have seen a few cases. This man's symptoms have come on rapidly and his observations confirm what his wife could see instantly – that he is very ill. Therefore, something has happened suddenly and the likely causes are:

- *perforated peptic ulcer*: the patient's indigestion could indicate previous peptic ulcer disease
- *faecal peritonitis*: perhaps the patient's 'irritable bowel' was really diverticular disease or even (sigmoid) colon cancer
- *acute pancreatitis*: this can be alcohol induced (*see* p. 122)
- *bowel infarction*: in this patient this is an unlikely diagnosis, because there are no features to indicate either atherosclerosis or new-onset atrial fibrillation (leading to an arterial embolus). Usually extensive bowel infarction is either secondary to prolonged closed loop obstruction (discussed above), or to loss of blood supply to the infarcted segment of bowel.

The commonest cause of extensive infarction is sudden loss of flow in the superior mesenteric artery, either by an embolus (hence the mention that the patient was not in atrial fibrillation), or due to sudden occlusion, e.g. thrombosis, in the artery. A characteristic feature of significant (usually small) bowel infarction is metabolic (lactic) acidosis, which is too severe to be explained by the patient's general condition.

> What are the causes of metabolic acidosis that might need excluding? Think whether his respiratory rate is relevant. It may simply be that irritation of the diaphragm, from the inflamed peritoneum under it, is the problem. If so, what symptom should he have?

(k) Gas under the diaphragm (pneumoperitoneum)

An erect X-ray which includes the diaphragm (e.g. CXR) will show this in the majority of cases of bowel perforation. This man has gas under the right side of his diaphragm. If the patient's clinical condition precludes an erect X-ray, a horizontal X-ray is an alternative, and this should show gas under the anterior abdominal wall.

(l) Initial investigations and treatment

The important initial investigations are:

- FBC
- U&E
- blood glucose
- amylase
- group and save
- X-ray
- arterial blood gases
- ECG (routine at his age).

Initial measures

Remember your ABCDE approach (*see* p. 139). A possible sequence is as follows:

- high-flow oxygen, monitored with pulse oximetry
- insert an i.v. cannula (as large as you can). It may have to be smaller than you would like, especially in a dehydrated patient. Get a venous blood sample and send it off urgently
- start an infusion of saline as quickly as the i.v. cannula permits
- monitor blood pressure, pulse, and respiratory rate
- get an arterial blood gas sample
- start ECG monitoring and do a 12-lead ECG
- monitor his temperature and prevent hypothermia
- give an immediate dose of 2 g ceftriaxone and an infusion of 500 mg metronidazole
- get the portable X-ray done
- insert a nasogastric tube
- insert a urethral catheter to monitor urine output
- ensure that the surgeon and anaesthetist are summoned
- hand over to either the surgeon or the anaesthetist. The latter may well put up a central (venous) line and an arterial line.

(m) The operation

This patient needs an immediate laparotomy. The subsequent findings will dictate the precise nature of the operation. If the surgeon is not sure of the site of the perforation, a small midline incision is made. If the peritoneal cavity contains faeculent fluid, the incision will be extended inferiorly to deal with the source in the lower abdomen. If the problem is a perforated peptic ulcer the incision will be extended superiorly.

In the case of a perforated duodenal ulcer, the perforation can usually be closed and/or plugged with omentum (and the patient treated with *Helicobacter pylori* eradication therapy). In contrast, in faecal peritonitis, further peritoneal soiling has to be prevented. This is done by exteriorising the diseased bowel as a double-barrelled colostomy. If, however, the diseased colon is stuck to adjacent structures, a Hartman's procedure is often performed. Distal bowel is oversewn, and either an end colostomy (if the diseased bowel can be removed) or a double-barrelled colostomy, is created proximal to the diseased bowel.

Web resources

- Antibiotic prophylaxis in surgery: www.sign.ac.uk
- Management of wound infection: www.nice.org.uk
- NCEPOD website: www.ncepod.org.uk

Further reading

- de Dombal FT (1991) *Diagnosis of Acute Abdominal Pain* (2e). Churchill Livingstone, London.
- Lavelle-Jones M (ed) (2002) *Master Medicine: surgery 1*. Churchill Livingstone, London.
- Malone AJ and Shetty MR (1997) Diagnosis of appendicitis. *Lancet.* **349**: 1774.
- Russell RCG, Williams NS and Bulstrode NCG (eds) (2004) *Bailey & Love's Short Practice of Surgery* (24e). Arnold, London.

9 A diabetic patient with a leg ulcer

A 76-year-old woman is referred by her GP to the outpatient vascular clinic with a persistent ulcer on her left leg. The patient says that she knocked her leg about a month ago, and thought that it would eventually heal. However it has got worse and is now painful all of the time.

On further questioning, the woman says that she gets pain in the left calf on walking approximately 70 yards. The pain is relieved by standing still, and she finds that she can walk a little further once the pain eases. She suffers from diet-controlled type 2 diabetes, angina, and had a myocardial infarction 3 years ago. On examination the ulcer is just above the lateral malleolus.

(a) What is the most likely underlying cause of the ulcer?

....

....

....

(b) What are the other important causes of chronic leg ulceration?

....

....

....

(c) What are the main points that should be clarified in the history?

....

....

....

The consultant examines the patient.

(d) What are the key features on physical examination of the lower limbs?

....

....

....

As part of the assessment, the patient is sent down to the vascular laboratory to assess her ankle brachial pressure index (ABPI). The Doppler test shows an ABPI of 0.6 in the affected leg at rest, which falls to 0.45 following exercise.

(e) What conclusion can be drawn from this result?

....

....

....

(f) Which blood tests should be ordered?

....

....

....

(g) What are the most important *principles* of treatment in this case?

....

....

....

(h) What conservative measures would you advise?

....

....

....

👉 The patient does not improve with conservative treatment, and a bypass graft operation is done on the left leg. Three months later she presents to the A&E department complaining that she cannot feel or move her right leg. Her symptoms came on earlier in the day and have progressed rapidly.

(i) What is the working diagnosis?

....

....

....

(j) What are the important symptoms and signs that support this diagnosis?

....

....

....

(k) What is your immediate management?

....

....

....

👉 The patient is taken directly to the operating theatre for 'on-table angiography'. The angiogram is shown in Figure 9.1.

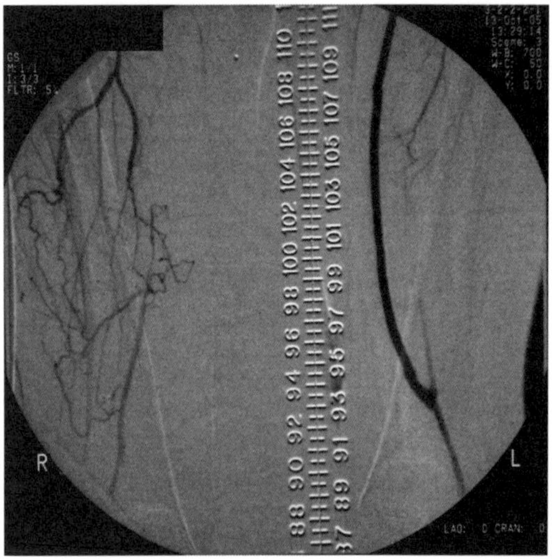

Figure 9.1 On-table angiogram.

(l) What can be seen on the angiogram?

....

....

....

(m) What are the treatment options?

....

....

....

👉 Following the procedure the patient can feel her right leg again. Clinically the leg looks perfused and the pedal pulses are palpable. Two weeks later she is discharged to the care of her GP with a follow-up appointment at the vascular clinic.

(n) How should the GP assess his patient at his review appointments?

....

....

....

Key cases

- Peripheral vascular disease (PVD)
- Chronic limb ischaemia
- Acute limb ischaemia
- Leg ulceration

Clinical context

Usually patients with PVD present *de novo* with intermittent claudication, and the majority do not have diabetes. The combination carries a much worse prognosis. Up to 70% of cases may stabilise with conservative management. Claudication is also a symptom of generalised atherosclerosis, and has wider important implications for the patient. Forty per cent of non-diabetic patients who present with intermittent claudication will be dead within 5 years from the associated complications of vascular disease (myocardial infarction, stroke etc) unless preventative treatment is started. The risks are greater in those with PVD and diabetes. It must be remembered that in the UK, there are as many undiagnosed diabetics as those who are already known to have the disease. It is therefore prudent to test the serum glucose levels of all new patients presenting with intermittent claudication. Additionally, smoking is a major risk factor for the development of claudication. If patients continue to smoke having developed this symptom, the prognosis is worse.

This scenario discusses two complications of PVD in more detail. These complications are ulceration, and local progression of occlusive vascular disease.

(a) Arterial insufficiency

Atherosclerosis is extremely common, and occlusive disease can affect most blood vessels. The most important sites, in terms of morbidity and mortality, are the coronary arteries, carotid arteries, arteries of the lower limbs, and the aorta.

Lower limb ischaemia can be acute, chronic, or, more commonly, acute-on-chronic. Chronic lower limb arterial disease due to atherosclerotic occlusive disease is considered here. In a critically ischaemic limb, the patient may have developed rest pain, gangrene or ulceration. Without intervention the limb will need amputation.

> You should be familiar with the pathogenesis of atherosclerosis. What are the key stages? What are the roles of the endothelium, intimal smooth muscle and macrophages in the development of atherosclerosis?

Arterial ulcers

These may develop after minor trauma to the legs, as skin nutrition is inadequate to achieve healing. Unlike ulcers due to other causes, arterial ulcers are usually painful. Patients will often have other symptoms and signs of significant peripheral arterial disease, such as short distance intermittent claudication and rest pain. The ulcers tend to occur anywhere below mid-calf level. It is important to assess the patient's general health, focusing particularly on any co-existing cardiovascular disease.

> It is important to be familiar with vascular examination of the leg, surface anatomy, and how to use a hand-held Doppler probe. Practise examining peripheral pulses on a normal subject, so that you can identify reduced and absent pulses in patients.

(b) Chronic leg ulceration

Skin necrosis produces an ulcer. A cell will die if deprived of oxygen, in a shorter time than the loss of its supply of nutrients, because it has a reserve of the latter. There are often multifactorial causes. These include:

- *poor quantity of blood*: a reduced blood supply occurs for the following possible reasons:
  - large- and small-vessel arterial disease
  - reduced venous drainage
  - reduced cardiac output (heart failure, shock)
  - prolonged local pressure (causing local reduction in blood perfusion leading to pressure sores)
  - pathological vasoconstriction
  - local trauma, which can disrupt adjacent blood vessels
- *failure to take avoiding action*: local pain normally results in a person taking avoiding action, such as relieving the pressure to avoid a pressure sore. Ischaemia very frequently causes pain. However,

if the patient cannot feel pain, tissue damage may occur. This can happen in peripheral neuropathy (common in diabetics), spinal cord damage (pressure sores are a big problem in paraplegics), and in the unconscious patient

- *poor quality of blood*:
  - low PaO_2 (as in COPD)
  - anaemia
- *poor-quality tissues*:
  - malnourished patients are more prone to ulceration
  - oedema – the increase of extracellular fliud forces cells to be further from their capillary blood supply
- *toxic cell damage*: this includes cell disruption by viruses, and toxins produced by bacteria and parasites. Tropical ulcers are a common example abroad. However, the damage can also be physical – for example, heat and cold
- *toxic cells and tissues*: linked to toxic cell damage is an increased risk of infection and impaired healing of tissues. This includes all forms of 'immunosuppression', including immunosuppressive drugs, malnutrition and vitamin deficiencies.

Poorly controlled diabetes is, perhaps, a special case. Many bacteria and yeasts thrive in a sugar rich environment. So patients have increased susceptibility, rather than decreased resistance, to infection.

Important causes of ulceration therefore include:

- arterial insufficiency
- venous insufficiency
- diabetic and other neuropathies
- pressure ulcers
- vasculitis
- tropical and other local infections (rare in British nationals, but common in immigrants to this country)
- haemoglobinopathies
- malignant tumours, e.g. squamous cell carcinoma
- any combination of the above.

Venous ulcers

Venous disease accounts for 80–90% of leg ulcers. Ulceration can result from either venous insufficiency due to previous thrombosis, or varicose veins causing superficial venous insufficiency. Increased hydrostatic pressure leads to fluid transudation. The skin often 'weeps' plasma, and the usually painless ulcers often fluctuate between healing and breakdown. They arise typically in the 'gaiter' area above the medial malleolus.

There may be a history of DVT, with or without other symptoms or signs of deep venous insufficiency, and/or varicose veins. Patients with varicosities and venous ulceration should be considered for varicose vein surgery to prevent recurrence once

healed; and those with deep venous insufficiency often benefit from compression stockings. The mainstay of treatment is compression bandaging, with elevation of the limb, and local treatment of infection, rather than systemic antibiotics. Any arterial component must be excluded (*see* ABPI later in this question, p. 78); otherwise compression bandaging may exacerbate the ulceration.

> Use this opportunity to revise the normal mechanisms that prevent high pressure in the superficial veins of the lower limb. What are the contributions of the muscle pump and deep vein/perforator valves? How can their function be assessed by clinical examination?

Diabetic ulcers

Diabetic ulcers tend to be painless because of sensory neuropathy (which may be the main predisposing cause). They usually occur on the foot, either as perforating ulcers on the sole beneath the metatarsal heads or at other bony prominences, such as the toes, the ball of the great toe and the malleoli. Unlike most chronic leg ulcers, which have a sloping edge, diabetic ulcers have a characteristic 'punched-out' edge with abrupt transition from normal skin to the necrotic crater. On the sole of the foot, they often have a hyper-keratinised edge in response to excess local pressure during walking. It is important to remember that ulcers in diabetic patients may have neuropathic, arterial, and venous components.

> You should be familiar with the importance of good diabetic foot care and the organisation of community services. What are the principles of good diabetic foot care? What would a community podiatrist check in an annual patient review?

Pressure ulcers

Pressure ulcers are areas of localised damage to the skin and underlying tissues. Common sites include areas overlying bony prominences (heels, sacrum, and elbows). They can be extremely painful, are at high risk of infection, and may prove very difficult to treat. It is important to assess a patient's risk of pressure sores, and hence prevent their development. Nursing staff may use a pressure sore risk score such as the Waterlow pressure sore risk assessment score.

Patients' potential to develop pressure ulcers depends on many risk factors, including immobility, reduced levels of consciousness, malnutrition, old age, peripheral neuropathy and peripheral vascular disease.

> What techniques are used to avoid pressure sores? What are the common aids used? Describe why education, positioning and seating are important.

Vasculitis

Systemic vasculitis may cause multiple leg ulcers which are usually found in conjunction with vasculitic lesions elsewhere. Vasculitic ulceration may be associated with rheumatoid disease, systemic lupus erythematosus, scleroderma, polyarteritis nodosa, and Wegener's granulomatosis.

> Use this opportunity to revisit the systemic vasculitides. Where are the other common sites of microcirculatory vasculitis? What are the common physical signs?

Tropical ulcers

Tropical ulcers and other local infections tend to follow trauma to the leg.

Malignant ulceration

Malignant tumours may cause ulceration. It is important to be aware of the features that are suspicious of squamous cell carcinoma (SCC).

A special case is 'Marjolin' ulcer, which is caused by malignant transformation occurring in a previous chronic ulcer or old scar. Any change in a chronic wound should therefore be viewed with suspicion.

(c) History in leg ulceration

A thorough history in patients with chronic leg ulceration will establish the likelihood of venous, arterial, diabetic, and other rarer causes of ulceration, and should aim to establish the severity of a patient's symptoms. It is also important to ask about other risk factors and drugs which may exacerbate arterial insufficiency and ulcer healing.

Features in the history that might suggest a venous component include:

- symptoms of venous insufficiency including leg pain, aching, swelling, pigmentation and itching (haemosiderin deposition)
- history of fracture, trauma or surgery in the affected leg
- previous DVT in the affected leg
- varicose veins.

Features that might suggest significant arterial disease include:

- intermittent claudication or rest pain
- atherosclerotic disease at other sites (e.g. ischaemic heart disease, transient ischaemic attacks, or stroke).

Previous medical history

- Diabetes
- Hypertension
- Dyslipidaemia
- Smokers with significant lung disease
- Rheumatoid disease
- Systemic vasculitides

Drug history

- Long-term steroids (reduce the skin's ability to heal)

Claudication history

- Duration of symptoms
- Is the claudication distance constant?
- Does the calf pain settle quickly (within minutes) on resting?
- Any pain in the thighs or buttocks?

Wound history

- Duration of symptoms
- Size of wound
- Thorough assessment of any pain, or lack of pain

Smoking history

- Number of 'pack years'
- Motivation to stop smoking

(d) Examination of the legs

Examination of the legs includes an assessment of the arterial supply, a systematic search for features consistent with venous insufficiency and a clinical description of the leg ulcer. Additionally, a sensory neurological examination is needed.

Assessment of the arterial supply

- Palpation of the femoral, popliteal, posterior tibial, and dorsalis pedis pulses
- Capillary refill time
- Assessment of limb temperature
- Colour of the limb

> Use this opportunity to review the structure and function of the circulation to the leg. You should be able to describe the pathophysiology and biochemistry underlying ischaemic pain. What are the contributions of anaerobic metabolism, free radicals and cellular injury?

Features of venous insufficiency

- Oedema of the lower limb, ruling out non-venous causes of unilateral and bilateral oedema (e.g. lymphoedema, hypoproteinaemia, and cardiac causes)
- Presence of varicose veins (particularly in the distribution of the long and short saphenous veins)
- Venous dermatitis
- Lipodermatosclerosis (thickened sclerotic skin)
- Discolouration
- Signs of previous DVT (*see* p. 157)

Description of the ulcer should include:

- the size of the ulcer (for future reference)
- the position of the ulcer, which gives an indication of its probable cause. Venous ulcers are usually above the medial malleolus, arterial ulcers are frequently located on the toes or lateral aspect of the calf, and neuropathic ulcers are predominantly found on weight-bearing areas such as the soles of the feet (or areas in contact with footwear)
- the ulcer edge (e.g. shallow, epithelialising)
- the base of the ulcer (e.g. granulating, sloughy, necrotic)
- a picture should be drawn in the patient's notes, or a photograph taken.

Sensory examination includes:

- light touch
- pain
- vibration
- proprioception.

⟶💡 A full cardiovascular examination is needed in anyone with peripheral arterial disease. What are the key features to exclude in the abdomen, chest and neck?

(e) Ankle brachial pressure index (ABPI)

Palpation of peripheral pulses does not exclude peripheral arterial disease. Measurement of the ABPI of both legs by hand-held Doppler is the best way to quantify arterial insufficiency, and should be used in the assessment of chronic leg ulcers and peripheral arterial disease. It also provides a measure of vessel competency. The ratio of systolic blood pressure at the ankle to that in the arm is calculated, with a value of 1 being normal.

- Patients with an ABPI <0.8 should be assumed to have arterial disease.
- Patients with an ABPI <0.5 are likely to develop

arterial ulcers, and require urgent referral with a view to possible revascularisation.

Exercise testing is useful in assessing the functional ability of the arterial supply. A limited flow of blood in the leg with an occluded arterial supply causes a fall in ankle systolic blood pressure during exercise-induced peripheral vasodilatation.

Care should be taken when assessing the ABPI in diabetic patients, since medial sclerosis causes a rigid artery, which prevents compression, producing a falsely high reading. Doppler examination allows an assessment of the waveform of the pulse, which can help to determine whether the vessel is calcified. A normal artery will have a tri- or biphasic waveform, whereas a stiff inelastic artery, or an artery with a proximal occlusion has a monophasic waveform.

(f) Blood tests

Blood tests will help to quantify the risk factors for PVD, possible clues to infection, and vasculitis.

Blood tests should include:

- *FBC*
- *CRP and ESR*: infection and/or vasculitis
- *U&E*: to check for the presence of renal disease
- *fasting blood glucose and/or HbA$_{1c}$*: to assess glycaemic control
- *fasting lipid profile.*

(g) (h) Treatment of chronic limb ischaemia

- The important principle of treatment is secondary prevention to reduce the patient's cardiovascular risk (MI/stroke). Improvement in claudication symptoms may occur as a secondary phenomenon as collateral supply develops.

The important conservative measures include:

- stopping smoking
- measures to reduce cholesterol and blood pressure: both lifestyle and pharmacological; i.e. dietary advice, weight loss and medication
- strict glycaemic control in patients with diabetes mellitus
- exercise training
- antiplatelet therapy: aspirin or clopidogrel.

Smoking is related to the development of peripheral arterial disease and to a worse prognosis.

Lipid lowering has been shown to slow the progression of peripheral arterial disease. While this may not reverse the disease, it is still an important part of conservative management.

Similarly, hypertension should be well controlled. However, caution is necessary since lowering systolic blood pressure can decrease the blood supply to already compromised muscle and skin. Blood pressure reduction has to be carefully controlled and regularly monitored.

Exercise therapy is capable of significantly improving claudication symptoms. Patients are encouraged to walk to near-maximum pain for a minimum period of 6 months. Exercise should be done at least three times a week, for a minimum of half an hour.

> You should be able to describe the effects of exercise training in chronic limb ischaemia. How do the consequences at the cellular level relate to the clinical findings?

(i) Acute limb ischaemia

The majority of acute limb ischaemia (60%) is caused by acute thrombosis in a vessel with pre-existing atherosclerosis. Emboli account for a further 30% of cases. It is important to distinguish between these causes since the management differs considerably.

> Use this opportunity to revise the management of acute limb ischaemia caused by embolisation. How might embolic ischaemia be suggested by physical examination? What are the differences in management?

(j) Clinical features of acute limb ischaemia

Inadequate blood supply causes the affected leg to be:

- pulseless
- painful
- pale
- paraesthetic
- paralysed
- perishingly cold.

It is important to recognise these features, since immediate treatment may be necessary to avoid amputation.

(k) Immediate treatment in acute limb ischaemia

The patient may need to be taken to theatre for definitive treatment. Therefore the immediate management should be aimed at maximising the patient's chances of limb survival:

- immediate resuscitation if necessary (ABCDE)
- analgaesia
- prompt call of specialist vascular surgical support

- blood tests including FBC, U&E, glucose, markers of myocardial damage, clotting, and group and save
- investigations including an urgent CXR and ECG
- i.v. low-molecular weight heparin (unless contra-indicated) to prevent propagation of the thrombus
- treat associated cardiovascular disease.

(l) Angiography

Emergency angiography is important in all cases where there is potential compromise of a limb. The image shows:

- blockage in the right superficial femoral artery
- collateral arterial supply on the right
- a patent femoro-popliteal graft on the left.

CT angiography is increasingly being performed. These scans provide detailed images and are excellent for studying peripheral arterial disease.

The CT angiograms taken from the patient in the scenario are shown in Figure 9.2.

(m) Treatment of acute limb ischaemia secondary to thrombosis

The treatment will depend on the severity of the ischaemia. This assessment can only be made by an experienced surgeon, and will dictate further treatment. The treatment options are:

- amputation if there is irreversible ischaemia with a non-salvageable limb
- intra-arterial thrombolysis
- angioplasty with stenting
- emergency arterial bypass surgery
- graft thrombectomy (in acute graft occlusions).

Intra-arterial thrombolysis requires a catheter to be placed into the thrombus, into which either streptokinase or t-PA is injected. Angioplasty with or without stent placement may then be used to ensure vessel patency.

Percutaneous transluminal angioplasty is used most successfully to treat aorto-iliac disease, and to a lesser extent short superficial femoral artery occlusions. A catheter is passed via the femoral artery into the area to be treated, and a balloon inflated to dilate narrowed/occluded arteries. Metal stents can be used. The patient should be given aspirin as an antiplatelet agent to reduce the chance of thrombus formation.

Reconstructive bypass surgery uses harvested veins from the patient or prosthetic material such as Dacron or PTFE. Surgery can be used to bypass an occluded artery. Examples include aorto-bifemoral bypass for aorto-iliac disease, and femoro-popliteal bypass for superficial femoral artery occlusions.

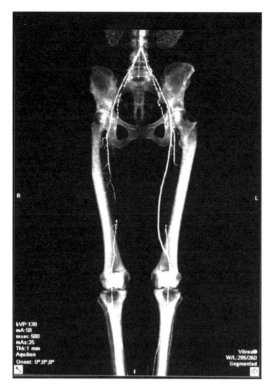

Figure 9.2 CT angiograms from the patient.

(n) Follow-up in the community

In primary care, there needs to be regular assessment and management of risk factors in patients with peripheral vascular disease. This should include all of the measures listed in section (g) (h) above.

Additionally, the extent of the impact of the arterial disease should be measured. This should include:

- assessment of walking distance
- assessment of quality of life.

Web resources

- Guidelines for the management of leg ulcers: www.prodigy.nhs.uk
- Guidelines for management of peripheral vascular disease: www.sign.ac.uk
- Guidelines for the prevention of pressure sores: www.nice.org.uk

Further reading

- Burns P, Gough S and Bradbury AW (2003) Management of peripheral arterial disease in primary care. *British Medical Journal.* **326**: 584.
- McNeely MJ, Boyko EJ, Ahroni JH *et al.* (1995) The independent contributions of diabetic neuropathy and vasculopathy in foot ulceration: how great are the risks? *Diabetes Care.* **18**: 216.
- Ouriel K (2001) Peripheral arterial disease. *Lancet.* **358**: 1257.
- Various authors (2000) ABC of arterial and venous disease [article series]. *British Medical Journal.* **320**.

10 A lorry driver with chest pain

A 56-year-old lorry driver was brought to the emergency department at his local hospital by a paramedic crew. The patient gave a 2-hour history of sudden-onset, central, crushing chest pain, with radiation to his jaw and left arm, which had woken him at 6 am. He also complained of feeling sick. On examination he is pale and clammy, his pulse rate is 84 beats/min and regular, and blood pressure is 212/134 mmHg. The cardiovascular examination is otherwise normal. The man's wife tells you that her husband is a smoker of 40/day for 30 years, and is known to have gastro-oesophageal reflux disease. She adds that her husband's father died suddenly from a heart attack when he was 55 years old.

The patient had received 300 mg of aspirin and buccal suscard during his journey to hospital. An ECG had been taken which is shown in Figure 10.1.

(a) What is your initial diagnosis?

....

....

....

(b) What changes can be seen on the ECG, and which coronary vessel is likely to be affected?

....

....

....

(c) What is your immediate management of this patient, before any investigations?

....

....

....

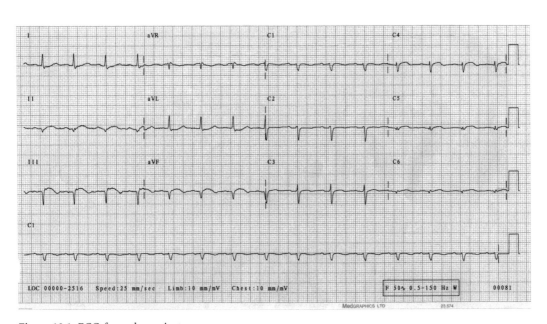

Figure 10.1 ECG from the patient.

(d) The nurse in the emergency department asks whether this man should have thrombolysis. What is your response and why?

....

....

....

> The patient continues to have chest pain. Therefore, the A&E consultant decides that this man needs urgent percutaneous coronary intervention (PCI). A glycoprotein IIb/IIIa inhibitor is given, and PCI is performed that morning by the consultant cardiologist. When the patient arrives back from the cardiac catheterisation laboratory, you are told by the nurse that the PCI was aborted because while trying to balloon the lesion the affected coronary vessel dissected. This dissection appeared to be small and the consultant decided that this man needed close monitoring rather than emergency surgery.

(e) Name the routine bedside observations you would ask the nurses to do. How often would these need to be repeated?

....

....

....

> One hour later you are called because the patient has become hypotensive (64/28 mmHg) and tachycardic (128 beats/min). On examination you confirm the tachycardia and notice that he has a markedly raised JVP at 12 cm, which had previously been normal, you also note that his blood pressure drops dramatically with inspiration.

(f) What emergency has this man developed, and how do the signs listed arise from the pathophysiology?

....

....

....

(g) What is the management of this condition?

....

....

....

> Afterwards the patient makes an uncomplicated recovery. His troponin T at 24 hours is 3.4 ng/ml and his ECG shows deep Q waves in leads II, III and aVF. After 5 days the patient is sent home.

(h) What medication can reduce both mortality and morbidity for this patient?

....

....

....

> The patient is referred for cardiac rehabilitation.

(i) Which healthcare professionals are involved in cardiac rehabilitation other than his consultant cardiologist?

....

....

....

Key cases

- Acute myocardial infarction
- Angina pectoris

Clinical context

Over one-third of patients presenting as medical emergencies have chest pain, and MI has to be excluded in all cases. This condition has significant morbidity and mortality. Early diagnosis can have a beneficial effect, reducing myocardial damage and, hence, improving patient outcome. This case shows how the diagnosis depends on the medical history, markers of myocardial injury, and changes on sequential ECGs; and how recent advances in medical therapy have significantly improved morbidity and mortality.

(a) Acute inferior myocardial infarction

This patient has presented with a textbook history of myocardial infarction. The key features are:

- sudden, severe crushing chest pain ± radiation to left arm (less commonly both arms) and/or the neck
- onset at rest, particularly in the morning hours
- constant pain, rather than episodic, and not relieved by rest (unlike angina pectoris)
- sweating (cold sweating)
- pale complexion
- nausea ± vomiting
- dyspnoea.

 How are the classical symptoms of MI produced by the underlying pathology?

The differential diagnoses to consider in a patient presenting with these symptoms are:

- *myocardial infarction*
- *angina*
- *aortic dissection*: this is an important diagnosis not to miss, since emergency surgery is the only definitive treatment. The pain is usually described as 'tearing' in nature and may start anteriorly but progresses, usually radiating to the back. Additionally, thrombolysis is absolutely contraindicated in aortic dissection
- *pulmonary embolism*: the pain usually occurs after the onset of dyspnoea and is a result of the

combination of hypoxaemia and heart strain caused by the pulmonary embolus. Pleuritic chest pain may also represent infarcted lung tissue (*see* p. 159)

- *oesophageal reflux/oesophageal spasm*
- *pericarditis*: classically the pain is worse on lying flat and relieved by sitting forwards (however, this depends on which aspect of the pericardium is affected).

 Take this opportunity to revise chest pain. What features in the history help to differentiate between all the causes listed above?

Since there is a comprehensive list of differential diagnoses to consider, the diagnosis of MI requires at least two of the following three features to be present:

- classical presentation
- typical ECG changes
- markers of myocardial injury (cardiac enzymes, particularly troponin T or I).

'Silent' MIs occur with no chest pain – although they can manifest with the other symptoms described above. These 'silent MIs' are commonly seen in diabetic and elderly patients. As with many medical conditions, young patients (i.e. the man in this question) tend to present with classical textbook symptoms and signs. In contrast, older patients often present in an indistinct and non-specific way (e.g. confusion, collapse) (*see* p. 190).

(b) Diagnosis of MI on ECG changes

- ST elevation in leads II, III and aVF, with reciprocal ST depression in I and aVL confirm the diagnosis of inferior MI in the context of the patient's history.
- This region is supplied by the right coronary artery.

The ST segment on a normal ECG is isoelectric (at the same level as the baseline). Elevation of the ST segment is seen in acute myocardial injury, and the leads in which the elevation occurs indicate the area of the myocardial damage. Therefore, specific ECG patterns occur in MI depending upon which coronary artery is occluded (*see* Figure 10.2 for a diagrammatic explanation).

> Use this opportunity to revisit the causes of ST elevation on an ECG tracing. What variations in the shape may give additional clues to the diagnosis? What are the ECG changes associated with ischaemia, injury and infarction?

Other rare causes of ST elevation are left ventricular aneurysm (persistent ST elevation post-MI), pericarditis and Prinzmetal's angina.

Specific ECG changes in MI

MI occurs when an atheromatous plaque in one of the coronary vessels ruptures and, in combination with a supra-added thrombus, critically occludes the artery. Specific ECG leads examine different areas of the heart. The site of myocardial damage can therefore be identified, and, combined with an understanding of coronary artery anatomy, the occluded vessel can be deduced (NB it is also important to realise that there is variable anatomy and dominance of the coronary arteries).

The 'standard' leads (I, II, III, aVL, aVR and aVF) look at the heart in the vertical plane, as shown in Figure 10.2:

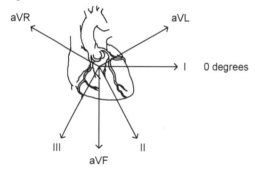

Figure 10.2 ECG lead vectors.

In this question, the ST elevation occurred in leads II, III and aVF, representing the inferior aspect of the heart. Therefore, the diagnosis is an acute inferior MI.

Furthermore, with reference to the coronary artery anatomy (*see* Figure 10.3), the inferior aspect of the heart is supplied by the right coronary artery, and this is almost certainly the vessel that has been occluded.

This information obtained from the ECG may be relevant in predicting and explaining any complications that may arise following the inferior MI, remembering that the right coronary artery usually supplies the sino-atrial node and the right ventricle.

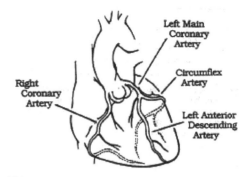

Figure 10.3 Coronary artery anatomy.

The 'chest' or V leads look at the heart in the horizontal plane from the front and left side, as shown in Figure 10.4.

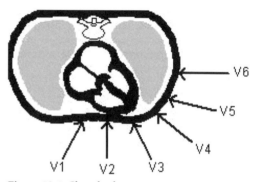

Figure 10.4 Chest leads.

Thus, leads V_1 and V_2 'look' at the right ventricle; leads V_3 and V_4, the interventricular septum; and leads V_5 and V_6 the left ventricle. As with the earlier example, the area of infarction can be deduced by the changes seen in the specific ECG leads. For example, changes in V_2–V_4 would be consistent with an anteroseptal infarction due to an occlusion of the left anterior descending coronary artery.

(c) Immediate management of MI

The immediate management of myocardial infarction is:

- analgesia with i.v. *morphine* (+ *anti-emetic*, remember the patient is often feeling nauseated even before the morphine!)
- *oxygen*: 15 l/min via tight face-mask and reservoir bag
- *nitrates*: either sublingually 2 puffs or 1 tablet
- *aspirin 300 mg*: unless clearly contraindicated. High-dose aspirin is proven to reduce mortality in acute MI.

The mnemonic *MONA* (morphine, oxygen, nitrates and aspirin) may be useful as a reminder for the immediate management of MI. In this question the patient has already had aspirin 300 mg given by the paramedic team, therefore, high-dose aspirin is not an appropriate response to (c).

(d) Thrombolysis

Thrombolysis should be considered in:

- ST elevation myocardial infarct (STEMI)
- posterior MI
- MI with new-onset left bundle branch block.

Thrombolytic therapy reduces mortality in these conditions, but, importantly, not in non-ST elevation myocardial infarctions (NSTEMI) or acute coronary syndromes (ACS). Therapy should be started within 12 hours from the onset of chest pain, but ideally at the earliest possible opportunity. The British Heart Foundation recommends <90 minutes from the onset of pain.

As the patient in this question has had an STEMI he should be considered for thrombolysis, however, there are contraindications to this intervention that must be taken into account. These include, amongst others:

- any active bleeding
- severe hypertension (>200/120 mmHg)
- suspected aortic dissection
- previous haemorrhagic stroke
- recent surgery.

This patient has a blood pressure of 212/134 mmHg, therefore he is not a candidate for thrombolysis.

> Use this opportunity to revise acute coronary syndromes (ACS) and non-ST elevation myocardial infarction (NSTEMI). What are the criteria for these conditions? How is risk stratified? What are the common ECG changes? How are these conditions treated depending on the risk scores?

Percutaneous coronary intervention/percutaneous transluminal coronary angioplasty

Percutaneous coronary intervention (PCI) or percutaneous transluminal coronary angioplasty (PTCA) is increasingly being used for recanalisation of the occluded coronary artery in acute MI. The thrombus is first visualised by angiography before balloon dilatation of the stenosis. The region may or may not be stented following balloon dilatation.

PCI complications do occur and the patient must be informed about these when obtaining consent. The major complications are:

- *contrast reaction*: as with all contrast-enhanced radiographic procedures
- *TIA/stroke/MI*: can occur but are uncommon

- *haemorrhage*: at the puncture site, particularly with the recent introduction of glycoprotein IIb/IIIa inhibition of platelet aggregation (which reduces associated MI risk post-procedure)
- *infection*
- *cardiac tamponade*: a rare but serious complication
- *dissection*.

> PCI is increasingly being used for first-line management of MI. You should be familiar with the relative merits and drawbacks of pharmacological versus invasive management strategies in MI.

(e) Routine monitoring

The coronary artery dissection during this patient's procedure should alert the doctor to the possible complication of cardiac tamponade. Monitoring should include:

- blood pressure
- pulse
- capillary refill (increasing to >2 s as cardiac output falls)
- pulse oximetry (SpO_2 decreased with falling cardiac output).

These variables should be monitored every 15 minutes.

- Continuous ECG monitoring is desirable in this patient. The ECG may show small complexes, or electrical alternans (beat-to-beat alternating height of the QRS complex) in cardiac tamponade.

(f) Cardiac tamponade

This condition is a medical emergency. Cardiac tamponade occurs when fluid (either blood or a pericardial effusion) collects between the visceral and parietal pericardium. As the outer fibrous pericardium is relatively inelastic, the heart volume is compromised by the fluid collection within the pericardial cavity. The rising intrapericardial pressure gradually reduces ventricular filling, and thus cardiac output. Eventually mechanical pump failure and death ensue.

The signs reflect the underlying pathology:

- *hypotension* occurs because, as the preload decreases, the ventricular performance falls (as per the Frank–Starling curve)
- *muffled heart sounds*: as the fluid between the heart and the parietal pericardium muffles the normal acoustics of the heart (this may be difficult to hear)

- *impalpable apex beat*: for the same reasons as above
- *raised JVP on inspiration*: since right ventricular filling is restricted
- *tachycardia* ensues in an attempt to maintain cardiac output
- *pulsus paradoxus* (systolic blood pressure falls by more than 10 mmHg on inspiration). It is important to remember that pulsus paradoxus is not paradoxical, it is an accentuation of the normal response in the pulse during respiration, in which the pulse becomes weaker during inspiration (reduced preload) and stronger during expiration.

Echocardiography is diagnostic and may enable echo-guided pericardiocentesis.

(g) Treatment of cardiac tamponade

Cardiac tamponade is a medical emergency and therefore optimisation of ABCD and E (*see* p. 139) takes initial priority. The definitive management of acute cardiac tamponade is emergency needle pericardiocentesis, which is the aspiration of pericardial fluid through a wide-bore (18G) needle. The approach is at 45° just below the xiphisternum, aiming the needle towards the tip of the left scapula. Senior help should be sought.

(Cardiologists may take a different approach in *elective* pericardiocentesis, going through the 5th or 6th intercostal space on the left, avoiding the lung and pleura by aiming for the cardiac notch of the left lung.)

(h) Secondary prevention post-MI

After MI all patients should be maintained on the following drugs (unless contraindicated) since they have secondary prevention prognostic benefits:

- angiotensin-converting enzyme inhibitors (ACE-I)
- β-blockers
- low-dose aspirin (75 mg)
- statins.

Trials have shown that cholesterol-lowering drugs substantially reduce cardiovascular mortality and morbidity, independent of cholesterol level. Currently, however, the joint UK guidelines recommend statins where total cholesterol >5 mmol/l or LDL >3.2 mmol/l.

Remember that fasting lipids need to be measured within the first 24 hours of infarct. Beyond this the serum levels are artificially raised for several weeks.

> Use this opportunity to revise the pharmacology of the common cardiac drugs. What are the mechanisms of action? What are the contraindications to their use?

(i) Cardiac rehabilitation

Cardiac rehabilitation provides a safe, controlled programme to improve cardiovascular fitness, promote secondary prevention through diet and lifestyle modification, and reduce the psychological impact of the MI. Rehabilitation programmes have been shown to reduce depression, which many patients and their family members suffer after such sudden life-threatening events.

Furthermore, early rehabilitation programmes have been shown to substantially reduce mortality in patients following MI. Therefore, all post-MI patients should be offered cardiac rehabilitation.

The healthcare workers involved in cardiac rehabilitation are:

- physiotherapists
- cardiac rehabilitation nurses
- dieticians
- smoking cessation nurses
- consultant cardiologists.

Web resources

- Acute-MI guidelines: www.eurheartj.oupjournals. org
- ECG workshop: www.fammed.wisc.edu

Further reading

- Bertrand ME, Simons ML, Fox KA *et al.* (2002) Management of acute coronary syndromes in patients presenting without persistent ST elevation: the Task Force on the Management of Acute Coronary Syndromes of the European Society of Cardiology. *European Heart Journal.* **23**: 1809.
- Hampton JR (2003) *The ECG Made Easy* (6e). Churchill Livingstone, London.
- Longmore M, Wilkinson I and Rajagopalan S (eds) (2004) *Oxford Handbook of Clinical Medicine* (6e). Oxford University Press, Oxford, pp. 120–4, 782.
- Meier MA, Al-Badr WH, Cooper JV *et al.* (2002) The new defintion of myocardial infarction: diagnostic and prognostic implications in patients with acute coronary syndromes. *Archives of Internal Medicine.* **162**: 1585.
- Resuscitation Council (UK) and ERC (2006) *Advanced Life Support Course Provider Manual* (5e). Resuscitation Council (UK) and ERC, London.
- Scottish Intercollegiate Guidelines Network (SIGN) (2002) *Guideline 57. Cardiac Rehabilitation.* Scottish Intercollegiate Guidelines Network, Edinburgh.

A teacher with intermittent rectal bleeding

11

A 67-year-old female, retired school-teacher presents to her GP with a 3-month history of intermittent rectal bleeding. She is otherwise well, although she is obese (BMI 33). Her past history comprises a previous Caesarian section, well-controlled hypertension (for which she takes bendro-fluazide), and she is a smoker. Her only other regular medication is hormone-replacement therapy.

(a) What important questions might the GP ask relating specifically to the presenting complaint?

....

....

....

(b) What specific parts of the physical examination are needed?

....

....

....

(c) What findings would the GP want to exclude on examination?

....

....

....

The examination is unremarkable, although the rectum is noted to be loaded with faeces. Given the history the GP decides to refer the patient to hospital.

(d) Does this patient require rapid access?

....

....

....

(e) What are the criteria for rapid referral?

....

....

....

(f) What is the differential diagnosis?

....

....

....

After a period of time she is seen in the surgical outpatient clinic. She has now developed diarrhoea and complains of fatigue, breathlessness and central chest pain on climbing stairs. She undergoes further investigation, and is found to have a large rectal tumour, 13 cm from the anal verge, with appearances consistent with a carcinoma.

(g) What further imaging might the consultant request?

....

....

....

On examination, the consultant notes that she has pale conjunctivae. He therefore requests some blood tests. Which abnormalities might be expected, given the patient's symptoms and history?

....

....

....

(h) Fill in the blank spaces with ↑ ↓ or ↔ for increased, decreased or normal respectively:

Haemoglobin	
Mean cell volume	
Serum iron	
Total iron-binding capacity	
Serum ferritin	

Staging investigations do not show any evidence of spread outside the rectum.

(i) Given the position of the tumour, which potentially curative surgical options would be considered?

....

....

....

The histology report on the resected specimen states that the tumour is a Duke's stage B.

(j) What does this mean about the extent of the tumour?

....

....

....

(k) What is her probable 5-year survival?

....

....

....

(l) Can you name another commonly used staging system for colorectal cancer?

....

....

....

Twelve months later, a follow-up ultrasound scan of the liver reveals that the patient has multiple metastases throughout all segments of the liver. She reports that she feels well, and is clinically asymptomatic.

(m) What treatment options may be available to her?

....

....

....

She expresses some concern that her son has increased risk of developing colorectal cancer, although there are no other family members who are known to have the disease. She asks if there is a national screening programme for colorectal cancer.

(n) Are her concerns justified?

....

....

....

(o) Is there a national screening programme for colorectal cancer in the UK?

....

....

....

Key cases
- Rectal bleeding
- Colorectal cancer
- Anaemia

Clinical context
Colorectal cancer is a common condition. It remains the third most common cancer in the UK currently with 32,000 new cases and 17,000 deaths per annum. Rectal carcinoma accounts for 37% of all large-bowel cancers; 75% of colorectal cancers are in either the rectum or distal colon; 25% are found proximal to the splenic flexure; 4–5% of patients have synchronous lesions. Sadly overall 5-year survival remains at 40%, poorer than in the countries of our European neighbours. Earlier diagnosis, prompt access to specialist investigations and treatment should improve morbidity and mortality. Screening, now to be introduced in the UK for all people aged between 60 and 70 years, should lead to diagnosis at an earlier stage. The hope is that multidisciplinary team assessment and multimodal treatment will improve outcomes.

This case illustrates the importance of early diagnosis. Five-year survival is closely related to the pathological stage, and clinicians must have a low threshold for thoroughly investigating relevant bowel symptoms.

(a) Clinical features and history of rectal bleeding
Specific questions that need to be asked of the patient presenting with rectal bleeding include:

- the colour of the blood, and whether it is on the surface or mixed with loose faeces
- whether the blood is just on the toilet tissue, or splatters the toilet bowl
- the amount, duration and frequency of any bleeding
- is defaecation painful?
- change in bowel habit
- the presence of anal symptoms such as pruritus (itching)
- pain
- tenesmus (urge)
- systemic symptoms (anorexia and weight loss)
- symptoms of anaemia
- family history of bowel cancer, ovarian cancer, breast cancer or ulcerative colitis.

Fresh blood *per rectum*, i.e. bright red as opposed to altered blood, is usually distal colonic or rectal in origin. Bleeding from the proximal colon may be darker. This must be distinguished from melaena, which is black, tarry stool, and originates from the upper GI tract. Melaena is partially digested blood, and may or may not co-exist with haematemesis. Rapid upper GI haemorrhage may cause fresh rectal bleeding rather than melaena, due to irritation of the bowel and consequent rapid transit through the intestine. These patients usually exhibit signs of haemorrhagic shock.

Occult faecal blood loss may cause iron-deficiency anaemia, without altering the appearance of the stool to the naked eye. This may explain the presentation of lethargy or decreased exercise tolerance. Other important points to elicit in the history of rectal bleeding include: amount, duration and frequency. Associated symptoms that may point towards a diagnosis include: change in bowel habit, pain, tenesmus, systemic symptoms (anorexia, weight loss) and a family history of cancer as listed above.

(b) (c) Physical examination
A bedside examination is essential and must include:

- full abdominal examination
- digital examination of the rectum.

Signs are rare in early colorectal carcinoma. However, the list of significant negatives is extensive. In this case pale conjunctivae may be present, and examination should aim to exclude tenderness, masses and distension of the abdomen.

On rectal examination, the presence of haemorrhoids and fissures should be excluded. In addition, assess anal tone, the presence of any masses, blood (fresh or otherwise) and mucus; and, when relevant, the size and character of the prostate.

> What are the components of a full abdominal examination? Which extra-abdominal features should be noted on inspection? Which lymph nodes should be palpated? What should percussion be used to assess?

(d) (e) Rapid access (2-week wait)
The Department of Health introduced the rule, in August 2000, that all patients with suspected colorectal cancers should be seen by a specialist within 2

weeks. This was thought to be a useful method for improving the early cancer detection rate.

The criteria for such a referral vary slightly from trust to trust, and include:

- a palpable right-sided abdominal mass
- a palpable rectal mass
- rectal bleeding with associated change in bowel habit, looser stools and/or increased frequency of defaecation persistent for more than 6 weeks
- iron-deficiency anaemia with positive faecal occult blood without an obvious cause (Hb < 10 g/dl)
- any change in bowel habit for longer than 6 weeks in a patient older than 45 years.

Low-risk symptoms which should not be rapidly referred include:

- rectal bleeding with anal symptoms
- change in bowel habit to decreased frequency of defaecation and harder stools
- abdominal pain without clear evidence of intestinal obstruction
- anal symptoms including soreness, discomfort, pruritus and prolapse as well as pain.

As with any disease, risk factors are important in establishing a suitable index of clinical suspicion. For colorectal cancer these include:

- *diet*: a Westernised diet containing increased amounts of animal protein and low in fibre
- *family history*: particularly if family members have developed the disease at a young age (<45 years) – families may benefit from genetic screening and counselling
- *ulcerative colitis*: risk increases over time – there is a 10–20% chance of developing cancer in patients who have had ulcerative colitis with total colonic involvement for 10 years. Distal colitis does not confer a high risk
- *adenomatous colonic polyps*: many undergo malignant change if left untreated
- *familial adenomatous polyposis coli*: multiple adenomas throughout the colon from a young age confer a very high risk, even 100% by the 4th decade
- *acromegaly*.

> What are the potential flaws of the 2-week wait ruling? What possible consequences does rapid referral have for those with or without cancer? How is it possible to ensure that the referral criteria are robust enough?

(f) Causes of PR bleeding

Common

- Haemorrhoids
- Anal fissure
- Diverticular disease
- Acute colitis of any cause
- Colonic polyps
- Colon cancer
- Colonic angiodysplasia

Uncommon

- Small bowel angiodysplasia
- Meckel's or other small bowel diverticulae
- Small bowel tumours
- Causes of upper GI haemorrhage, e.g. bleeding peptic ulcer

(g) Further investigation

When considering which investigation to choose, it is important to decide where the site of the tumour is most likely to be. The clinical presentation of colorectal cancer depends on the site of the tumour:

- *right hemicolon*: anaemia, palpable mass, tend to present later and not to cause obstruction
- *left hemicolon*: change in bowel habit, rectal bleeding, obstruction
- *rectum*: change in bowel habit, rectal bleeding, tenesmus, mucus discharge.

> How does the position of the cancer determine the symptoms and signs listed above? Why would a rectal carcinoma tend to produce tenesmus?

Imaging techniques for suspected colorectal cancer

The entire colon should always be examined to exclude a synchronous tumour, which occurs in 4–5% of cases. Furthermore, histological diagnosis should be made with a tissue biopsy of the lesion. The only instances when the whole colon should not be visualised are when a stenotic cancer prevents passage of a flexible colonoscope, or when bleeding is brisk enough that surgery should not be delayed.

This patient needs to be investigated fully, and therefore it is important to visualise the whole colon with a combination of:

- colonoscopy
- barium enema
- pelvic MRI for rectal cancer. This is clinically important to help determine the resection margins
- CT colonography. This may be used if other investigations are incomplete or inconclusive.

Most patients have CT to stage the cancer, and CT colonography for primary diagnosis is used infrequently.

These imaging investigations should also be augmented with blood investigations, e.g. FBC, LFTs and tumour markers (CEA, CA 19-9, and CA 125).

(h) Anaemia

Remember that anaemia is not a diagnosis, it is a symptom of an underlying condition. Thus, it is imperative that anaemia is fully investigated to establish its underlying cause (*see* pp. 200, 227 and 228).

Microcytic anaemia (commonly due to iron deficiency) can be due to blood loss, inadequate iron intake, or malabsorbtion. This may be the presentation of an occult GI malignancy and so should be investigated. The most common sources of blood loss include: menstruation, the GI tract and the urinary tract. Malabsorption is due to small bowel disease, mainly gluten-sensitive enteropathy (*see* p. 200). Growth, pregnancy and lactation increase the demand for iron and may expose deficiency.

Biochemical features of iron-deficiency anaemia

Haemoglobin	↓
Mean cell volume	↓
Serum iron	↓
Total iron-binding capacity	↑
Serum ferritin	↓

Treatment is usually with oral iron, e.g. ferrous sulphate, and should be continued for 3 months after the haemoglobin has returned to normal, to replenish iron stores. Occasionally patients will require either parenteral iron (e.g. venofer) and/or a blood transfusion depending on symptoms (*see* p. 229).

(i) Curative treatment

Potentially curative treatment involves resection of the bowel tumour, a margin of normal bowel, and the regional lymph nodes. In elective cases, re-anastomosis with or without a defunctioning colostomy is usually feasible. In emergencies such as obstruction or perforation of the colon, the surgeon may decide that an anastomosis has a high chance of leaking. Thus, the rectal stump may be closed and an end colostomy created (Hartman's procedure), or both ends of the bowel may be brought to the surface as an end colostomy and mucous fistula. Liver metastases are not necessarily a contraindication to surgical resection.

For rectal cancers (as in this patient) there are really only two options:

- *anterior resection*: excision of the distal sigmoid and upper rectum – if a safe margin of healthy tissue can be preserved below the tumour. This would be the preferred option in this patient
- *abdomino-perineal resection*: excision of the entire rectum and anal canal with permanent end colostomy – if the tumour is too close to the anus to perform an anterior resection.

Other operations for colonic cancers depend on the site of tumour.

> Use this opportunity to revisit the anatomy of the large intestine and abdomen. Which parts of the large intestine are supplied by the superior and inferior mesenteric arteries? Which factors influence the surgical options?

(j) (k) (l) Staging of colorectal cancer

There are two commonly used staging systems for colorectal cancer:

- TNM (tumour, node, metastases)
- Duke's stage.

Table 11.1 shows 5-year survival for the different stages.

Adjuvant chemotherapy should be considered for all patients with Duke's C disease. All patients with rectal cancers should be considered for pre-operative radiotherapy. Pre-operative chemoradiotherapy can be used to convert inoperable rectal cancers into operable ones.

Table 11.1 Five-year survival for stages of colorectal cancer

Duke's stage	Extent	5-year survival (%)
A (T1 or T2, N0, M0)	Limited to bowel wall. This is called localised cancer	85–90
B (T3, N0, M0)	Extends through muscular layer of the bowel wall, no lymph node involvement	65–70
C (any T, N1–3, M0)	Lymph nodes involved	35–50
D (any T, any N, M1)	Distant metastases	<5

(m) Liver metastases

The liver is a common site of metastatic disease. The portal vein drains the abdominal viscera and is presumably the route of spread for metastases from tumors of the colon and rectum, stomach, pancreas, biliary tree, and small intestine. Breast cancer commonly involves the liver, as does lung cancer.

Uni-lobar liver metastases may be suitable for potentially curative hepatic resection.

- The patient described has multiple metastases in all segments of the liver, and therefore is a candidate for palliation only.

> Revise the anatomy of the liver and note the relationships between the 'lobes' and the segments. How might the blood supply to a segment affect whether resection is feasible?

Palliative care

Patients with obstructing colorectal cancers who are not suitable for surgical resection may benefit from colonic stenting. All patients with metastatic colorectal cancers should be considered for palliative chemotherapy. Palliative radiotherapy can be used to treat patients with distressing pelvic symptoms. Medical measures are often employed to relieve symptoms.

Chemotherapy is not without risks, and is likely to have little effect in extensive disease. It is important to assess quality of life at the time of diagnosis of the multiple metastases. There may well be a case for supportive care, and advising the patient to enjoy her 'symptom-free period', rather than risk the hazards of aggressive chemotherapy.

(n) (o) Genetics and screening

Most cases of colorectal cancer are sporadic, occurring typically in individuals over the age of 50 years, and with no family history of the disease. A detailed discussion on colorectal cancer genetics is beyond the scope of this book, but all patients with the disease should have a detailed family history assessment, and

those considered to be at increased risk should be offered genetic screening if appropriate. Triggers, which may indicate an increased risk, include: two or more first-degree relatives with colorectal cancer or family members who developed the disease at a young age (less than 50 years). Therefore, from the information given, there is no reason to suspect that this patient's son is at increased risk of developing colorectal cancer. Family members thought to be at increased risk may be offered screening colonoscopy. There is currently no national screening programme for colorectal cancer in the UK, although there are moves to introduce such a programme in the near future.

Web resources

- British Society of Gastroenterology guidelines: www.bsg.org.uk
- CT colonography (virtual colonoscopy): www.nice.org.uk
- Guidelines for management of colorectal cancer: www.sign.ac.uk
- Improving outcomes in colorectal cancer: www.nice.org.uk
- Public Health Genetics Unit: www.phgu.org.uk
- Referral guidelines for suspected cancer patients: www.nice.org.uk
- UK colorectal cancer screening programme: www.cancerscreening.nhs.uk

Further reading

- Adam R, Delvart V, Pascal G *et al.* (2004) Rescue surgery for unresectable colorectal liver metastases downstaged by chemotherapy: a model to predict long-term survival. *Annals of Surgery.* **240**: 644.
- Toms JR (ed) (2004) *Cancer Stats Monograph 2004.* Chapter 6: Large bowel cancer. Cancer Research UK, London, p. 37.
- Lavelle-Jones M (ed) (2002) *Master Medicine: surgery 1* (2e). Churchill Livingstone, London.
- Scottish Intercollegiate Guidelines Network (2003) *SIGN Guideline 67. Management of Colorectal Cancer.* Scottish Intercollegiate Guidelines Network, Edinburgh.

12 A pensioner with 'waterworks' problems

A 75-year-old retired electrician is referred to a prostate assessment clinic by his GP. He has a medical history that includes well-controlled hypertension which is managed by his GP. He has recently been experiencing difficulty passing urine, and additionally complains of having to get up in the night to go to the toilet. On examination he has a moderately enlarged prostate. Urinalysis and his urea and electrolyte blood test are both normal.

(a) What other related symptoms might be elicited in this gentleman's history?

....

....

....

(b) How could his symptoms be assessed?

....

....

....

(c) Which special tests can be done in the clinic?

....

....

....

(d) Discuss the possible causes of nocturia.

....

....

....

The patient's symptoms are assessed as 'moderate'. However, he says that he would only have an operation as a last resort.

(e) Name two drugs that he could be given to alleviate his symptoms.

....

....

....

(f) Which of these treatments is he most likely to receive first and why?

....

....

....

He is so pleased with the results of his drug treatment that he is discharged from the clinic. Five years later he returns because he has started wetting the bed at night. Further questioning reveals he has been vomiting after food for 2 days, though he can still drink clear fluids. He has also lost 2 stone in weight and he thinks this is because he hasn't enjoyed food for some time because of a nasty taste in his mouth. He says that the treatment really only worked for 3 years, and his original complaint of difficulty passing urine has returned.

(g) What diagnosis is suggested by the patient's symptoms?

....

....

....

(h) What urological abnormalities would you look for on physical examination?

....

....

....

(i) What is the likely cause of his nocturnal incontinence?

....

....

....

(j) What are the other forms of incontinence commonly found in both men and women?

....

....

....

(k) Name the two most important blood tests that should be requested.

....

....

....

(l) What abnormalities would be expected on the blood results?

....

....

....

> While awaiting the result of the blood tests, the consultant arranges for the patient to have a urethral catheter inserted. The nurse is unable to pass the catheter, and instead a suprapubic catheter is inserted under ultrasound guidance. The catheter drains 2 l urine.

(m) How does this information help confirm the diagnosis, and help determine the prognosis?

....

....

....

(n) What imaging technique should be used to determine whether this problem is acute or chronic?

....

....

....

(o) What problems might this man develop following his initial treatment?

....

....

....

Key cases

- Benign prostatic hypertrophy (BPH)
- Chronic renal failure
- Urinary incontinence

Clinical context

Benign enlargement of the prostate is a common disease of males over the age of 65 years. It can cause unpleasant symptoms that can severely impair an individual's quality of life. Reduced urinary flow is normally associated with frequency and urgency. It is important to exclude prostate cancer before proceding with treatment of BPH.

BPH can present with a range of symptoms ranging from benign to life threatening. This scenario discusses the initial diagnosis and first-line medical treatment and explores the natural progression of the disease, going on to describe the most severe complication of bladder outflow obstruction, namely renal failure.

(a) Symptoms of BPH

Symptoms that a patient with an enlarged prostate gland may suffer include:

- hesitancy
- poor stream
- nocturia
- urgency
- increased urinary frequency
- post-micturition dribble
- pis en deux.

Patients may have a combination of symptoms of outflow obstruction (hesitancy, poor stream, pis en deux, i.e. stop start stream, after-dribble) and symptoms of bladder overactivity (nocturia, urgency, frequency). The latter are the result of the bladder (detrusor) muscle hypertrophy. As a result, in a way that is similar to idiopathic bladder overactivity, the bladder starts to 'rule' the patient, rather than the other way around.

It is important to distinguish between urge incontinence, and involuntary and unexpected incontinence (including bed wetting). The latter is secondary to chronic urinary retention. It is useful to think of this type of incontinence as a result of the bladder being full all the time and therefore unable to give the brain accurate messages of when it is going to let a little urine flow out of it.

 Use this opportunity to review the structure and function of the male lower genitourinary tract. You should know how the sphincters are controlled and the normal neuro-sensory pathway between brain, spinal cord and bladder. What are the contributions of sympathetic and parasympathetic innervation to the bladder and sphincters in the normal micturition reflex? What are the functions of alpha/beta and cholinergic receptors?

(b) The international prostate symptom score (IPSS)

The IPSS (International Prostate Symptom Score) is an internationally validated score. It is completed by patients to assess the severity of their symptoms (AUA score), and how these symptoms affect their quality of life (QoL score). Despite its limitations, it enables different units to compare patients and results. The American Urological Association (AUA) score is shown in Table 12.1.

In general, a score of:

- 0–8 indicates mild symptoms
- 8–19 indicates moderate symptoms
- 20–35 indicates severe symptoms.

In addition to the above, there is also a quality of life (QoL) or 'bother' score. A number from 0–6 is chosen to describe how bothered the patient is by his symptoms, 0 being not in any way bothered. This variable is used because some patients are remarkably unworried by symptoms that would bother other patients considerably. This can affect the decision to treat, or determine whether reassurance is all that is required.

(c) Preliminary investigations

- Urine flow rate
- Measurement of residual urine volume (RV)

The rate of urinary flow can be measured by either recording the volume of urine passed over a certain time, or more commonly by using a device known as a rotating disk mictiometer. The mictiometer uses the velocity of the stream of urine hitting a rotating disk to calculate its flow rate.
(D Small – a urodynamics homepage: www.sghurol. demon.co.uk/urod)

Table 12.1 AUA score chart

Please answer the following questions about your urinary symptoms. Write your score for each question at the end of each row.

Over the past month, how often have you . . .	Not at all	Less than 1 time in 5	Less than half the time	About half the time	More than half the time	Almost always	Your score
1 had a sensation of not emptying your bladder completely after you finished urinating?	0	1	2	3	4	5	
2 had to urinate again less than two hours after you finished urinating?	0	1	2	3	4	5	
3 stopped and started again several times when you urinated?	0	1	2	3	4	5	
4 found it difficult to postpone urination?	0	1	2	3	4	5	
5 had a weak urinary stream?	0	1	2	3	4	5	
6 had to push or strain to begin urination?	0	1	2	3	4	5	
And finally . . .	None	Once	Twice	3 times	4 times	5 times or more	
7 over the past month, how many times did you most typically get up to urinate from the time you went to bed at night until the time you got up in the morning?	0	1	2	3	4	5	
Add up your total score and write it in the box.	Total						

Format reproduced with permission from EMIS.

Measuring the rate with the result expressed in graphical form is very useful. The volume voided must also be noted, because everyone has a slower flow rate when they pass urine from a bladder that is not full. Patients should therefore wait until they really feel that their bladder is very full before measuring their flow rate.

The RV is measured with the use of an ultrasound scanner. A significantly increased RV, usually more than 500 ml, increases the patient's chance of developing acute (on chronic) urinary retention.

(d) Possible causes of nocturia

There are several mechanisms that may contribute to nocturia, and it is worth bearing these in mind before diagnosing urinary outflow obstruction:

- *polyuria*: some people simply drink so much fluid before going to bed that their kidneys make more than a bladder-full of urine while asleep. Patients with nocturia due to BPH do not always restrict the volume they drink in the evening. However, in others, there is a metabolic reason for the polyuria such as glycosuria due to diabetes, hypercalcaemia, or diabetes insipidus
- *reversal of diurnal rhythm*: patients who retain fluid during the day (right heart failure, venous insufficiency of the legs, etc) tend to get rid of the extra fluid when they lie down at night. This can be confirmed by getting them to collect two 12-hour urine specimens, e.g. from 9 am to 9 pm, and then from 9 pm to 9 am. They may well be sent to a urologist because they have nocturia, but when asked, they say they have no difficulty in passing the urine at night. An effective treatment is a short-acting diuretic, such as furosemide, taken a few hours before going to bed (*not* in the morning!)
- *chronic urinary retention*: (*see* (l) below)
- *overactive bladder*: (*see* (j) below)

- *enuresis*: enuresis is passing urine at night without waking. Thus secondary enuresis may complicate overflow incontinence. However, it is a term which is normally confined to patients whose bladders appear to be completely normal, typically in patients who have never been 'dry' at night.

(e) Medical treatment options

- α-blockers
- 5-α-reductase inhibitors

α-blocker drugs were originally developed for the treatment of hypertension. Those most commonly used for the treatment of BPH symptoms are 'selective', i.e., have minimal hypotensive side-effects, and are once-daily, sustained-release tablets, such as tamsulosin and alfusosin. It is very quickly obvious whether they are going to be therapeutic. 5-α-reductase inhibitors prevent the production of dihydrotestosterone, reducing vascularity in benignly enlarged prostates, and hence preventing haematuria. However, they take months to work if they are going to.

The side-effects and other therapeutic uses for these two medical treatments can be deduced from their modes of action.

> You should be familiar with the pharmacology of commonly used drugs. In this case, you should know the mode of action of both α-blockers and 5-α-reductase inhibitors, their side-effects and their different therapeutic uses.

(f) First-line therapy

- *α-blocker*: better side-effect profile/therapeutic effect achieved quickly.

(g) Chronic renal failure

The symptoms described are those of uraemia. These include:

- weakness
- tiredness
- ankle swelling
- vomiting
- pruritus
- anorexia
- weight loss.

Often patients do not present with these symptoms. Instead, a U&E blood test, often requested for another reason, makes the diagnosis well before the development of uraemic symptoms.

Significant uraemia is almost always caused by renal impairment. Diabetes mellitus, hypertension and urinary tract obstruction are common causes of chronic renal failure in the west. There is wide geographical variation in the causes of chronic renal failure.

Long-standing loss of renal function may be classified as mild, moderate, severe, or end-stage, depending on the glomerular filtration rate. End-stage renal failure is defined as severe enough that, without dialysis, the patient could not survive.

Unfortunately, symptoms of uraemia are relatively non-specific and frequently arise too late to prevent dialysis, either immediately or after a short postponement. It is only when significant correctable factors are present that end-stage renal failure can be prevented in an untreated patient with uraemic symptoms. These factors include:

- *pre-renal*: e.g. treating dehydration, cardiac failure, renal artery stenosis
- *renal*: treating reversible glomerular and interstitial disease
- *post-renal*: removing obstruction, or bypassing it by a catheter, nephrostomies, or ureteric stenting.

Therefore, history, examination and investigation should establish the cause of the renal impairment.

> This question has only discussed post-renal causes of impaired renal function.
>
> Use this opportunity to remind yourself of the following:
>
> (a) history, examination, investigation and treatment of immediately correctable pre-renal factors: thus uraemic symptoms are often precipitated by dehydration caused by a GI upset, diuretics, etc
> (b) diagnosis of renal causes, e.g.
> - family history of Alport's syndrome
> - two large abdominal masses (polycystic disease)
> - antiglomerular basement membrane antibodies
> - casts on urine microscopy, microscopic haematuria
> - Bence-Jones protein, other protein, or myoglobin in the urine.

(h) Examination

- A palpably enlarged bladder
- Enlarged prostate gland on rectal examination
- Palpation of the kidneys

Bed wetting is a symptom of chronic urinary retention so this patient's bladder should be palpated to see if it is enlarged. The dome of the bladder is almost always to the right of the midline, possibly 'steered' that way by the presence of the sigmoid colon on the left side. In very obese patients it may be necessary to perform a U/S scan. The other symptoms of weakness and vomiting are likely to be due to uraemia (*see* above). The kidneys may also be balloted in case they have enlarged, and the prostate gland should be assessed by rectal examination.

Other physical signs of chronic renal failure are rare. However a full physical examination may reveal:

- signs of fluid overload, e.g. peripheral oedema, pulmonary oedema, cardiomegaly
- pallor due to anaemia
- scratch marks due to uraemic pruritus (rare).

(i) Overflow incontinence

This is a symptom of chronic urinary retention. It may only be present at night. As the bladder is full all the time, you can regard it as not 'knowing' when to tell the brain that it is full. This is effectively the opposite of acute retention, when a bladder knows it is full and is screaming this fact to the brain.

(j) Other types of incontinence

- *Urge incontinence*: patients wet themselves before they have time to get to the toilet. If severe, they go on to void to completion because they cannot stop the flow of urine once it has started. The problem is aggravated by decreased mobility (Parkinson's disease, arthritis, etc). Urge incontinence is due to an overactive bladder whose contractions cannot be sufficiently inhibited voluntarily.
- *Stress incontinence*: a weak sphincter (usually in women who have had vaginal deliveries) allows urine to escape when the intra-abdominal pressure exceeds a certain limit (laughing, coughing, straining, gymnastics, etc). Stress incontinence is not due to muscular bladder activity.

(k) Blood tests

The two most pertinent blood tests that should be requested are:

- FBC
- renal profile (urea, creatinine and electrolytes).

Anaemia is almost universal in chronic renal failure due to erythropoietin deficiency and increased red cell destruction in the circulation.

Urea and creatinine are raised, and potassium may be alarmingly high at presentation. Other electrolyte disturbances include acidosis, hypocalcaemia and hyperphosphataemia.

> You should be familiar with the electrolyte problems encountered in chronic renal failure. What are the sources of urea and creatinine? Why are they commonly measured to assess renal function? What is the cause of the hyperkalaemia and hypocalcaemia seen in chronic renal failure?

(l) Interpreting the blood results

When the blood results return, you would expect to see:

- raised serum urea and creatinine
- raised serum potassium
- reduced haemoglobin (anaemia).

Usually a seemingly very high potassium level (e.g. >6 mmol/l) should respond quickly to catheterisation, so a glucose and insulin infusion, salbutamol, or calcium resonium are unlikely to be needed. In monitoring recovery, the serum creatinine normally starts to fall before the serum urea. The urea level may be disproportionally high if patients are dehydrated (remember the patient has been vomiting). Dehydration often tips the balance in uraemic patients, leading to their admission. Chronic renal failure causes a normochromic normocytic anaemia, which is usually of a severity that corresponds to the degree and duration of the chronic renal failure.

> The kidneys play a crucial physiological role in the body and you should know the actions of the kidneys and their effects on the other systems of the body. When considering treatment you should be aware of the pathophysiological mechanisms relating to anaemia, renal osteodystrophy, oedema and hypertension.

(m) Immediate measures to relieve obstruction

Passing a catheter will relieve the chronic obstruction causing this gentleman's symptoms.

- Passage of a large amount of urine on insertion of the urinary catheter helps confirm the diagnosis.
- It is also very useful for the urologist to know the volume of urine being chronically retained. This can give some idea of how quickly the bladder will regain function. A detrusor stretched by 500 ml is likely to recover well. In contrast, 5 l of urine suggests significant permanent damage to the detrusor muscle.

(n) Renal ultrasound

- Renal ultrasound scan
- Small kidneys are usually seen in chronic retention (as in this case)

Ultrasound scan provides a two-dimensional size of the kidneys. Chronic renal failure can cause the kidneys to decrease in size, the reverse is true in acute renal failure, which can cause the kidneys to enlarge. Ultrasound is also very good at showing hydronephrosis secondary to outflow obstruction.

(o) Complications

The main problems that occur after relief of a long-standing obstruction are:

- post-obstructive diuresis
- hyponatraemia due to salt-losing nephropathy
- decompression haematuria.

In practice, the first two complications can be taken together. Damage to the renal medulla means that the kidneys' ability to concentrate urine is temporarily impaired. This leads to diuresis, of which there are several components (urea-, water-, and salt-losing diureses). The important point to make about treating this diuresis is that saline and not 5% dextrose must be used to avoid severe hyponatraemia.

In mild diuresis, increased oral fluid intake should suffice; however some patients may lose large volumes of urine, becoming significantly dehydrated. This may be so severe as to cause postural hypotension or collapse. Close monitoring of urine output is necessary. If patients pass more than 200 ml of urine for a prolonged period of time (>5 hours) then i.v. replacement is necessary. Care should be taken not to 'over-replace' fluid losses since this will just lead to further diuresis. A practical fluid replacement regime is to replace half of the preceding hour's urine output with intravenous saline.

Haematuria is common as the over-stretched bladder decompresses. The blood vessels have been damaged by being stretched, but close apposition to the stretched muscle effectively tamponades the bleeding. Relieving the obstruction reduces the pressure, allowing the damaged vessels to bleed. The patient's haemoglobin level should be checked if the bleeding persists.

Web resources

- Bandolier evidence-based medicine website: www.jr2.ox.ac.uk/bandolier
- Guidance on BPH: www.prodigy.nhs.uk
- Prostate Research Campaign UK: www.prostate-research.org.uk
- Undergraduate tutorials on prostatic disease: www.bui.ac.uk
- Urodynamics website: www.sghurol.demon.co.uk/urod

Further reading

- Wasson JH, Reda DJ, Bruskewitz RC *et al.* (1995) A comparison of trans-urethral surgery with watchful waiting for moderate symptoms of benign prostatic hyperplasia. *New England Journal of Medicine.* **332**: 75.
- Webber R (2003) Benign prostatic hyperplasia. *Clinical Evidence.* **10**: 977.
- Wilt TJ (2002) Treatment options for benign prostatic hyperplasia. *British Medical Journal.* **324**: 1047.

13 A woman found on the floor by her warden

A 76-year-old retired woman is found on the floor of her flat by the accommodation warden. The warden visits every three days and before this event she reported that the lady was mobile, relatively independent and quite fit for her age. Her past medical history includes COPD with frequent exacerbations during the winter months, which have required hospitalisation and long-term steroid use, a mild degree of heart failure, and osteoporosis.

On arrival at casualty she is maintaining her airway, has a respiratory rate of 28 breaths/min and is receiving 15 l/min of oxygen via a tight-fitting facemask with reservoir bag. She is opening her eyes to painful stimulus, making incomprehensible sounds and moving her hands to push away the sternal rub.

(a) What is this patient's Glasgow Coma Score (GCS)?

Eyes:

Verbal:

Motor:

GCS =

(b) What is the minimum GCS a patient can have?

....

....

....

After initial resuscitation, it is unclear how long the patient was on the floor. It could have been up to 72 hours.

(c) What other acute medical problems could arise from this delay?

....

....

....

(d) How would you assess this patient's hydration status?

....

....

....

Physical examination shows that the patient is considerably dehydrated. The junior doctor rapidly infuses 1 litre of crystalloid and sets up another litre to run over 1 hour. Given her history of congestive cardiac failure, he is worried about giving too much fluid.

(e) What sensible precautions could he take?

....

....

....

(f) How should her response to treatment be assessed?

....

....

....

☞ She responds well to fluid resuscitation. During further examination, the left leg appears shortened and externally rotated, and passive movement produces pain. Given her history of osteoporosis and the examination findings, the SHO suspects that she has a femoral neck fracture.

(g) What are the risk factors for developing osteoporosis?

....
....
....

(h) What are the key symptoms and signs of a femoral neck fracture?

....
....
....

(i) What should you immediately check in the affected leg if you suspect a hip fracture?

....
....
....

(j) What further assessment in A&E is advisable?

....
....
....

☞ The junior doctor sends the patient for a plain radiograph of the left hip. The film is shown in Figure 13.1.

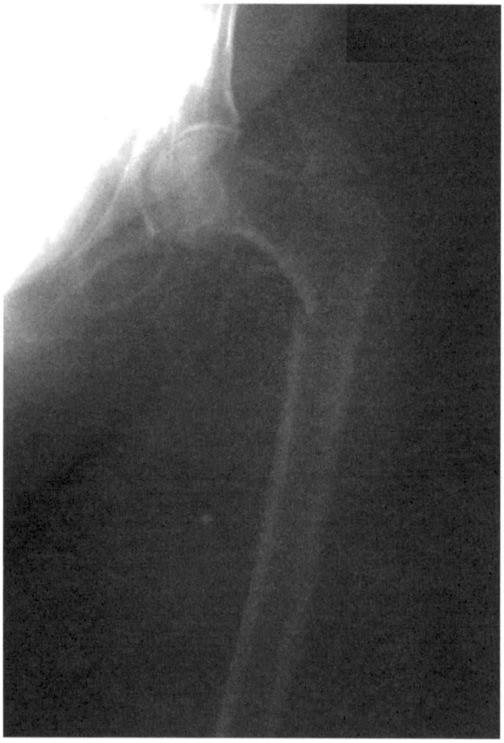

Figure 13.1 X-ray of the left hip.

(k) What are the categories for a fractured neck of femur? Which category is this fracture?

....
....
....

☞ She is taken to theatre in due course, and a dynamic hip screw is placed.

(l) What are the post-operative complications that need to be considered, and what specific measures can be taken pre-operatively to minimise the risks?

....
....
....

On the post-take ward round the consultant tells the patient that he is going to discuss her case at the multidisciplinary team meeting. He says to her that other people will be coming to talk to her to find out how she can best be cared for. He tells her that she will have an appropriate rehabilitation plan and will be back on her feet again in no time.

(m) Who should be involved in her rehabilitation?

....

....

....

(n) What are the important factors when planning this lady's discharge?

....

....

....

A woman found on the floor by her warden

Key cases

- Fractured neck of femur
- Osteoporosis
- Post-operative complications

Clinical context

Hip fracture is a common condition associated with a high morbidity and mortality. The major risk factors are female sex and osteoporosis. Consequently, population demographics forecast greater numbers of femoral neck fractures as greater numbers of females reach the 8th, 9th and 10th decades. Currently around 50,000 cases are seen each year in the UK, and there is a 10% chance of fracture in the contralateral hip. This scenario shows the importance of early diagnosis, fast pre-operative resuscitation, assessment of co-morbidity, and early and ready access to trauma lists as the preferred strategies in the management of femoral neck fractures.

The consequences range from a loss of mobility in fitter patients, to death from complications in the very frail. Despite significant improvements in the detection and prevention of osteoporosis, surgery and rehabilitation, mortality following hip fracture is still approximately 30% in the year following injury.

(a) (b) Glasgow Coma Scale/Score

Confusion and altered conscious state are common in patients presenting with hip fractures, particularly if there has been a delay (as in this case) in getting to hospital.

The Glasgow Coma Score is an easy way of communicating a patient's conscious level between members of the healthcare team. It provides an objective way of monitoring response to treatment and gives early warning of deterioration in clinical condition.

- GCS of 13–15 indicates relatively minor impairment of consciousness.
- GCS of 9–12 indicates moderate impairment of consciousness.
- GCS of < 8 indicates coma.
- GCS < 8 generally means that the patient's airway is at risk.
- Particular attention should be paid to falls in GCS, and repeated assessments are important.

The components of the Glasgow Coma Scale are eyes (E), verbal (V), and motor (M).

Eyes

- Spontaneously opening (4)
- Verbal command (3)
- To pain (2)
- No response (1)

Verbal

- Orientated (5)
- Confused sentences (4)
- Inappropriate words (3)
- Incomprehensible sounds (2)
- No response (1)

Motor

- Obeys commands (6)
- Localises to pain (5)
- Flexes to pain (4)
- Abnormal flexion (3)
- Abnormal extension (2)
- No response (1)

- Therefore this patient has a GCS of 9:
  - eyes = 2
  - verbal = 2
  - motor = 5
- Remember the lowest score a patient can have is 3/15.

(c) Complicating medical conditions

It is important to exclude co-morbidities in this patient. She has a history of chronic disease and it is not known how long she has been on the floor. A high index of suspicion is necessary.

She may be:

- hypoxaemic
- dehydrated/hypovolaemic
- hypoglycaemic
- hypothermic.

Equally she may be suffering from:

- an infection (chest, urinary tract, or sepsis from pressure sores)
- DVT or PE due to immobility
- renal failure due to CCF, hypovolaemia, or possibly rhabdomyolysis
- pressure sores
- further injuries caused by the fall
- rhabdomyolysis caused by muscle damage.

Following the assessment of ABCD and E (*see* p. 139) and appropriate resuscitation, a full examination and appropriate investigations should exclude – in particular – all of the medical conditions listed above.

(d) Hydration status

To assess fluid balance effectively it is essential to think about the important body compartments. Fluid moves between the intracellular and extracellular compartments; and in the extracellular compartment between the interstitial, venous and arterial compartments.

The body has powerful homeostatic mechanisms that regulate fluid and electrolyte balance in the vascular compartments. The result is that changes in the vascular compartments occur before those in the interstitium and intracellular compartments. Consequently the classical signs of dry mucous membranes and changes to skin turgor are late signs.

Although the vascular compartment is a closed system, changes in volume are generally first seen in the venous compartment, since two-thirds of the circulating volume is in the capacitance vessels (the peripheral and central veins). It follows that the signs of fluid depletion are first evident in the venous compartment (reduced JVP), followed by the arterial compartment (tachycardia, oliguria, hypotension) and finally the interstitial compartment (dry mucous membranes, reduced skin turgor).

The following are needed to adequately assess an individual's hydration status:

History (basics)

- Oral fluid intake/urine output (in the history setting: *roughly* how much water have you passed during the past day? Is it dark/concentrated? Does it smell? Does it hurt or sting?)
- Does the patient feel dry, especially mucous membranes?
- Concomitant medical diseases: heart failure/renal failure
- Medication: especially diuretics

Examination

- Overall inspection: is the patient unwell?
- JVP measurement
- Pulse
- Blood pressure/pulse pressure
- Capillary refill time
- Skin turgor
- Sunken eyes
- Dry mucous membrane

Investigations

- U&E
- FBC
- Urine output: initially hourly
- Central venous pressure measurement: ideal, but not essential

> Use this opportunity to revise examination of the JVP. Neck veins can be extremely difficult to see, and practice is essential. If the JVP is visible is it necessary to insert a central line? What are the risks and benefits of a central line?

(e) (f) Fluid challenge

In a patient with congestive cardiac failure it is important not to overload the failing heart. However, it is equally important to ensure that an adequate circulatory volume and hydration are achieved. One way of doing this is through appropriate monitoring of venous pressure, respiratory rate, blood pressure, urine output and capillary refill time, and how these parameters respond to small volumes (250 ml) of fluid.

Therefore, sensible measures in this patient would include:

- catheterisation
- central line insertion (either jugular or subclavian) if the JVP is difficult to see
- an intravenous fluid challenge.

The response to treatment is measured by:

- a sustained rise in venous pressure
- improvement in pulse, BP, urine output, respiratory rate etc.

If the venous pressure rises and remains elevated, but the blood pressure and urine output do not improve, then inotropes may need to be considered for circulatory support. It is vital to contact a senior colleague at this point.

> You should be familiar with the distribution of water within the various body compartments. How do you calculate fluid requirements? What are insensible losses? What are the indications for the different types of commonly used fluids?

Fractured neck of femur (NOF)

Fractured NOF is one of the most common problems encountered in orthopaedics. The main risk factors are female sex and osteoporosis.

Osteoporosis

The World Health Organization (WHO) has defined osteoporosis as a generalised skeletal disorder of low bone mass and deterioration of microarchitectural structure, leading to enhanced bone fragility and increased susceptibility to fracture. Quantitatively it is defined as a bone mineral density (BMD) 2.5 standard deviations or more below the mean value for young adults.

The prevalence of osteoporosis increases with age, being particularly common in postmenopausal women. With an increasingly elderly population, osteoporotic fractures will undoubtedly become more common.

Osteoporosis increases the risk of fractures by reducing BMD. However the risk factors for osteoporosis, falls, and fractures are all linked by one common factor – old age.

The three major sites for osteoporotic fractures are the hip, spine and forearm. However fractures of the humerus, tibia, pelvis, and ribs are also common.

(g) Risk factors for osteoporosis

- *Age*: BMD decreases, and consequently the risk of osteoporosis increases with age.
- *Sex*: women are at greater risk of osteoporosis since they have smaller bones and a lower total bone mass. Additionally, women lose bone more quickly following the menopause, and typically live longer.
- *Family history*: genetics partially determine an individual's peak bone mass.
- *Reduced oestrogen levels*: oestrogen stimulates osteoblasts and bone remodelling. Low BMD is associated with early menopause. Conversely, a late menopause or oestrogen-replacement therapy are associated with higher BMD.
- *Low weight*: smaller bones are more prone to osteoporosis.
- *Smoking*: BMD is lower in smokers.
- *Diet*: lacking in calcium or vitamin D.
- *Limited exercise and sedentary lifestyle*: exercise increases bone turnover and therefore BMD.

Additionally, medical conditions that can cause accelerated osteoporosis include:

- long-term steroid use
- coeliac disease (*see* p. 201)
- hyperparathyroidism
- osteomalacia (*see* p. 201)
- renal failure (*see* p. 98)
- inflammatory bowel disease (if the small bowel is affected, or steroids are used in disease management) (*see* p. 166)
- chronic liver disease.

(SIGN Guideline 71, 2003)

(h) Clinical features of femoral neck fracture

- Pain
- Shortened and externally rotated affected leg
- Immobility
- Inability to weight-bear

The affected leg is shortened and externally rotated because the iliopsoas pulls the femur superiorly (shortened) and the gluteus maximus laterally rotates the hip (externally rotated).

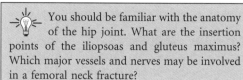

You should be familiar with the anatomy of the hip joint. What are the insertion points of the iliopsoas and gluteus maximus? Which major vessels and nerves may be involved in a femoral neck fracture?

(i) Immediate assessment

On suspicion of a fractured neck of femur, the neurovascular integrity of the leg should be checked immediately.

Examine for the femoral, popliteal, posterior tibial and dorsalis pedis pulses, and the motor, sensory and reflex components of the leg. Ensure maximum immobilisation.

(j) Further assessment in A&E

After assessment and optimisation of ABCDs – including suitable analgaesia and immobilisation – the elderly patient with a hip fracture should have a more detailed consultation aimed at preventing subsequent problems such as pressure sores and nutritional deficiencies. Additional information should be sought about continence, previous mobility, functional ability and social circumstances. All these factors have implications for both the immediate management and subsequent care of the elderly patient.

This patient has already had a detailed assessment of fluid balance and hydration status and has recovered sufficiently to give a more detailed history. SIGN guidelines suggest that early assessment, in A&E or on the ward, should include a formal recording of:

- pressure sore risk
- nutritional status
- pain
- core body temperature using a low-reading thermometer
- continence
- co-existing medical problems
- mental state
- previous mobility
- previous functional ability
- social circumstances.

(Reproduced from SIGN Guideline 56; 2002, with permission)

Further investigations include:

- *FBC, U&E*: the patient may have already had these in assessment of hydration

- *cross match*: the patient may have bled and will be going to theatre
- *12-lead ECG*: the patient has known CCF, and is at high risk of myocardial ischaemia
- *CXR*: the patient has known COPD and CCF.

An early anaesthetic review is also desirable.

(k) Categories of hip fracture

Fracture of the hip can occur at any site, however the usual classification is based around the location of the fracture in relation to the joint capsule:

- *intracapsular fractures*: described as subcapital or transcervical
- *extracapsular*: described as basicervical, trochanteric, or subtrochanteric.

Additionally, there are a bewildering number of other specialised classification systems for both intracapsular and extracapsular fractures, none of which have been unanimously adopted, e.g. Garden, Jensen, and Evans systems.

> What are the components of the articular capsule? What are the accessory ligaments? How does the anatomy affect the positions of proximal femoral fractures?

From the X-ray (*see* Figure 13.1) it can be seen that the fracture lies inferior to the trochanteric line, making this an extracapsular fracture.

The treatment of the two types is different because of the different blood supply. Intracapsular fractures often interrupt the tenuous blood supply that runs along the femoral neck from the arterial ring at the base. Consequently, the femoral head loses its main blood supply, increasing the risk of avascular necrosis (where the femoral head crumbles due to poor blood supply).

Treatment

The only definitive treatment is surgery. The method of fixation chosen depends on the location and the stability of the fracture:

Intracapsular fractures

Due to the increased risk of avascular necrosis and other complications, these fractures can be treated in two ways:

- reduction and internal fixation (using screws)
- joint prosthesis (hemi or total joint change).

Extracapsular fractures

The risk of avascular necrosis and non-union is much less than for intracapsular fractures. Therefore, this type of fracture is normally treated by use of a dynamic hip screw (DHS). The DHS consists of a metal plate with a barrel, in which another screw is placed and fixed into the femoral head. The barrel allows tiny 'micro-movements' of the fracture plates, thus promoting healing.

An X-ray of the dynamic hip screw is shown in Figure 13.2.

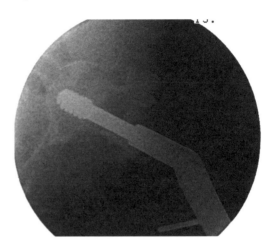

Figure 13.2 Dynamic hip screw check X-ray.

> You should be familiar with the stages of fracture healing. What are the inflammatory, reparative, and remodelling phases? How do they differ between cortical and cancellous bone? Which factors affect bone healing?

(l) Post-operative complications

General complications

- Complications of anaesthesia
- Confusion (*see* p. 189)
- Exacerbation of pre-existing conditions (COPD, CCF)
- Bleeding
- Infection (wound, pneumonia, urinary tract)
- Thrombus formation (DVT/PE)
- Hypoxaemia

Specific orthopaedic complications

- Non-union (fracture fails to heal)
- Avascular necrosis
- Dislocation
- Prosthetic wear and tear
- Infection of the DHS/prosthesis

Specific risks to this patient

- Adrenal insufficiency due to long-term steroid use for COPD
- Exacerbation of CCF/COPD

Specific measures can be initiated pre-operatively to minimise the risks of post-operative complications. These include:

- *ensuring optimal fluid and electrolyte balance*
- *optimising the treatment of any co-morbid medical conditions, e.g. CCF and COPD*: the patient may need adjustment of her diuretics and/or nebulised bronchodilators
- *antibiotic prophylaxis*: this is usually given as a single dose at the induction of anaesthesia
- *antithrombotic prophylaxis*: individual units have different policies. Low-molecular weight heparin should be given to high-risk patients (this patient)
- *supplemental oxygen*: this should be determined by regular monitoring of respiratory parameters (the patient has COPD, *see* p. 215)
- *peri-operative corticosteroid therapy* should be given. The dose should be proportional to the severity of surgical stress, and should be given for no longer than 1–3 days post-operatively.

(m) Rehabilitation

A working definition of rehabilitation is 'the reduction of functional deficits without necessarily reversing the underlying biology of the disease'.

> You should be familiar with the definitions of impairment and disability. For a comprehensive rehabilitation programme, which aspects of patient care should be considered?

Comprehensive rehabilitation needs to address a number of different levels which may be contributing to loss of function:

- the damaged system
- other body systems
- psychological attitudes
- immediate material environment (e.g. clothes)
- the near environment (e.g. housing/equipment)
- distant environment (e.g. shops)
- social support networks/family.

(From *Rehabilitation of Older People* (revised 2004) BGS Compendium Document 1.4. Reprinted with permission.)

Good rehabilitation is central to the management of hip fractures. Patients benefit from early MDT assessment by medical and nursing staff, physiotherapists and occupational therapists. The benefits have been shown to include shorter stays in hospital (which have many advantages, *see* p. 196), improved management of medical conditions, earlier functional independence, and less need for future institutional (residential or nursing home) care.

Staff who are commonly involved in rehabilitation therefore include:

- geriatricians
- surgeons
- GPs
- physiotherapists
- occupational therapists
- nurses (hospital, practice and district)
- dieticians
- social workers.

> How is quality assessed in healthcare? You should be familiar with the concepts of quality in the structure, process and outcome. Can you define effectiveness, efficiency, equity, acceptability, accessibility and appropriateness?

(n) Planning discharge

The same multidisciplinary approach should be used when planning discharge. This involves collaboration between MDT members, the patient, and the patient's family. Supported discharge schemes with liaison nurse follow-up can monitor patients' progress at home, allowing early intervention, and helping to reduce patients' fears.

General considerations when planning discharge should include (reproduced from SIGN Guideline 56; 2002, with permission):

- the patient should be central to discharge planning. Their needs and wishes, and those of their carers need to be taken into consideration
- liaison between hospital and community (including social work department) facilitates the discharge process
- occupational therapy home assessments assist in preparing patients for discharge
- the patient, carer, GP, and other community services should be given as much notice as possible of the date of discharge
- written information on medication, mobility, expected progress, pain control and sources of help and advice should be available to the patient and carer
- GPs have an important role to play in post-discharge rehabilitation and should receive early and comprehensive information on the hospital stay, services arranged and future follow-up arrangements. Complicated discharges that may have considerable impact on the primary care team should be discussed in advance with the GP
- special consideration should be given to the prevention of falls, especially potential household hazards, footwear, provision of adaptive equipment/walking aids and alarm systems (*see* p. 192).

Web resources

- Basic information: www.gpnotebook.com
- British Geriatrics Society: www.bgs.org.uk
- Comprehensive database on neck of femur fracture: www.e-radiography.net
- Full guidance on hip fracture management: www.sign.ac.uk
- Guidelines on resuscitation: www.resus.org.uk

Further reading

- Longmore M, Wilkinson I and Rajagopalan S (eds) (2004) *Oxford Handbook of Clinical Medicine* (6e). Oxford University Press, Oxford, pp. 680, 776.
- McRae R (1999) *Pocketbook of Orthopaedics and Fractures.* Churchill Livingstone, London.
- Scottish Intercollegiate Guidelines Network (SIGN) (2002) Guideline 56. *Prevention and Management of Hip Fracture in Older People.* SIGN, Edinburgh.
- Scottish Intercollegiate Guidelines Network (SIGN) (2003) Guideline 71. *Management of Osteoporosis.* SIGN, Edinburgh.
- Tallis R (1992) Rehabilitation of the elderly in the 21st Century. *Journal of the Royal College of Physicians.* **26**: 413.

14 A 32 year old with pain and urinary frequency

A 32-year-old man with no significant past history arrives in A&E with severe pain in his right iliac fossa. He states that the pain started earlier in the day and is radiating to his right loin and back. The pain is associated with an increased frequency of urination. He adds that he has also vomited and feels a bit shivery.

(a) What is the most likely diagnosis?

....

....

....

(b) Which other possible causes for this man's symptoms would it be wise to exclude?

....

....

....

(c) What information from the above history can help confirm the diagnosis; how are the symptoms related to the underlying diagnosis?

....

....

....

(d) Why does the house officer in A&E test the urine?

....

....

....

(e) Which imaging studies are appropriate?

....

....

....

(f) What specific complications may occur if infection is not excluded?

....

....

....

While waiting for the patient to be taken for imaging, the house officer prescribes dihydrocodeine for pain relief. Twenty minutes later, the patient is restless, agitated and still in considerable pain. He asks for more pain relief.

(g) Name two possible drug treatments that could be prescribed, and why is one of them particularly appropriate?

....

....

....

The drug has reduced the patient's pain.

(h) What advice would you give about oral fluid intake?

....

....

....

☞ Unfortunately, a short while later, the pain recurs and is as bad as ever.

(i) What are the indications for an invasive procedure?

....

....

....

(j) Which invasive procedures might be required?

....

....

....

☞ This patient's acute episode settles. Two months later the patient attends his follow-up outpatient visit.

(k) What blood tests should be checked?

....

....

....

(l) The tests are normal. What is the most important advice that can be given?

....

....

....

☞ Six months later, the patient reappears with his 25-year-old sister. She is experiencing the same problems as he did. She says that she is 2 months pregnant.

(m) What implications does this have for her management?

....

....

....

Key cases
- Renal/ureteric calculi
- Abdominal pain

Clinical context

Urinary tract calculi are common (8% of British males), often occurring in relatively young people. Fortunately deaths are very rare. However, if left untreated, calculi can destroy kidneys as well as causing pain, which is often unbearable. The past three decades have seen dramatic advances in minimally invasive treatment. Recurrent calculi are largely preventable, but in a minority of cases this requires treatment of important underlying diseases.

This scenario is another example of a patient presenting with abdominal pain and vomiting; however, the location and character of the pain, and presence of urinary symptoms are key features that should not be missed. Diagnostic confusion can be a common problem in cases of ureteric colic, and the causes of this are discussed, with an emphasis on understanding the pathophysiology of the condition. Complications of urinary tract calculi and contemporary management strategies are also discussed.

(a) A stone, causing renal and ureteric colic

Pain from stones obstructing the upper urinary tracts (kidney and ureter) is termed colic, but this is a misnomer. True colic is a pain which comes on in waves, lasting for a maximum of a few minutes. For practical purposes, this really only happens in the bowel. Such true colic may occur on a background of pain with colicky exacerbations, or the pain may disappear between the colicky episodes. Similar to biliary 'colic' (see p. 121), the pain from renal and ureteric stones can last for hours or days. The intensity of the pain may vary, but over hours (usually influenced mainly by pain relief starting to work and then wearing off) and, therefore, not in a colicky way.

> Use this opportunity to revise the anatomy of the urinary tract. Why are ureteric stones commonly found either at the top, middle, or lower ends of the ureters?

(b) Acute appendicitis and acute abdomen

Ureteric calculi can cause very significant GI symptoms. Nausea and vomiting are very common as is abdominal distension (with a lot of small bowel gas on X-ray). Such distension can be painful. Sometimes there is almost rebound tenderness and, if this is in the right iliac fossa, one should at least consider the possibility of GI pathology, particularly acute appendicitis. Other causes of acute abdominal pain are less likely to cause diagnostic confusion (see p. 67). It is also worth mentioning incipient rupture of an aortic aneurysm, which can present with back pain similar to renal colic. Though this is rare (usually the aneurysm has ruptured), it is an important diagnosis not to miss; however it would be very unusual in a 32-year-old man!

(c) History and examination

This man has mentioned several symptoms, some of which are likely to mean that there will be signs present on physical examination.

- *RIF pain*: patients with ureteric colic are often tender on palpating the RIF. Rebound tenderness is unusual, but is the norm in acute appendicitis. However, patients often have voluntary guarding in the RIF. The reason why ureteric pain is reasonably well localised is because the stone causes inflammation and oedema in the tissues adjacent to the ureter (which includes peritoneum). The ureter is very close to the parietal peritoneum throughout almost all its length.
- *Loin pain*: patients may well have renal pain ('colic') as well as ureteric colic. Commonly, the stone can pass along the ureter without causing symptoms. However, if the stone becomes impacted, it can block the flow of urine through the ureter causing an increase in pressure in the kidney and the renal pelvis. On examination this patient would be tender in the renal angle. Many patients think loin pain is from their kidney when, in fact, the pain is from musculoskeletal problems associated with the lumbar spine.

> ☀ Where exactly is the renal angle? How is it possible to distinguish between renal colic and musculoskeletal pain by clinical examination? What are the effects of movement?

- *Urinary frequency*: urinary frequency without dysuria is characteristic of a stone at the lower end of the ureter. What is happening is that the localised inflammation and oedema are irritating the detrusor (bladder) muscle, causing urinary frequency.
- Another symptom that can be associated with stones, usually in the lower ureter, is *testicular pain*.
- *Vomiting*: nausea and vomiting are common symptoms. They do not always represent GI pathology. This fact has been discussed in (b) above. If a patient is vomiting, parenteral or rectal drugs should be given, as absorption from the GI tract is unpredictable.
- *Feeling shivery*: rigors, *see* (f).

(d) Dipstick of the urine

- In cases of ureteric colic, the urine should be tested for blood using a bedside dipstick test.

Macroscopic haematuria is uncommon but dipstick-positive haematuria is almost always present when patients have severe symptoms. In fact, a lack of macro- or microscopic haematuria casts doubt over the diagnosis of ureteric calculi. Note, however, that asymptomatic renal/ureteric stones may well result in normal urinalysis. Although this patient has urinary frequency, his urine should be negative for nitrites and leucocytes. The urine can be abnormal (i.e. positive for leucocytes and blood) if the ureter is secondarily involved in the inflammation associated with acute appendicitis. If infection is suspected, then a midstream specimen should be sent for microscopy and culture.

> ☀ Use this opportunity to review the common urine investigations. What are the standard components of a urine dipstick test? What further investigations can be ordered?

(e) Imaging studies

- Kidney, ureter and bladder X-ray (KUB)
- Ultrasound scan: renal/abdominal/pelvic
- Intravenous urography (IVU)
- Spiral CT scan: enhanced or unenhanced

> ☀ What proportion of renal/ ureteric calculi are radio-opaque? How does the composition of the calculus affect its opacity?

A plain X-ray often confirms the diagnosis, however, difficulties that may occur are:

- phleboliths can be mistaken for stones
- stones in front of bones can be missed, especially if they are not very radio-opaque
- some stones (especially uric acid and cysteine ones) are radiolucent.

U/S scans will show hydronephrosis and are good at picking up radiolucent renal calculi. However, it requires a very good ultrasonographer to visualise a lower ureteric stone and proximal hydroureter. The advantages are that the scan is non-invasive, and contrast is not needed.

IVUs are very good at showing stones, and exactly where they are in the upper tract. There can be problems with allergy to the contrast medium, including anaphylactic shock (this is rare and usually due to iodine allergy). Care should be taken with the use of contrast in any patients with any renal dysfunction. Additionally, renal failure can occur with the use of contrast in patients with type 2 diabetes who are on metformin.

Unenhanced spiral CT scans are becoming more popular, when available at short notice. They are the investigation of choice in patients with type 2 diabetes. The patient receives more radiation with a CT scan than with a straightforward IVU. A CT scan taken from a patient with type 2 diabetes showing a left-sided vesicoureteric junction (VUJ) stone is shown in Figure 14.1.

(f) Complications of infection

The following may occur if infection is not actively sought, and treated:

- septicaemia
- rapid irreversible loss of renal function in obstructed, infected, kidneys
- perirenal/psoas abscess formation.

The kidneys are so vascular (they take a fifth to a quarter of the cardiac output at rest) that bacteria don't have to travel far to enter the blood stream. Bacteraemia is very common (positive blood cultures during periods of pyrexia). Septicaemia can then develop, and can quickly become severe.

The urine in an obstructed, infected, upper urinary tract quickly becomes purulent, and, combined with raised pressure, rapidly destroys the renal parenchyma. This process can also cause a perforation in the collecting system, with pus collecting as an

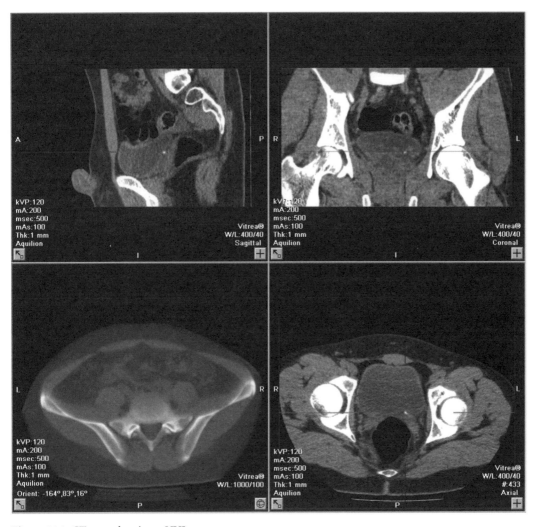

Figure 14.1 CT scan showing a VUJ stone.

abscess around the kidney. Anatomically it is then easy for the pus to enter the psoas muscle and track along the muscle sheath. When obstruction and infection are both present *without* the complications of septicaemia or perinephric abscess, it is imperative to relieve the obstruction by a percutaneous nephrostomy. The sooner the stone is removed the better, so as to avoid these complications and loss of an otherwise functioning kidney.

(g) Pharmacological treatment options

Depending on the patient and the severity of the pain, appropriate treatment would be:

- NSAID suppositories, e.g. indomethacin 100 mg, 12-hourly
- narcotic (or NSAID) injections (usually i.m.), e.g. morphine 5–10 mg, 3–6-hourly.

The main point is that GI absorption of any analgesic is totally unreliable in a patient with renal and/or ureteric colic, and who is vomiting. Although absorption is slower than by injection, the advantage of NSAID suppositories is that patients can use them at home if conservative treatment is chosen.

NSAIDs are particularly appropriate because they are anti-inflammatory analgesics and they also reduce the blood flow through obstructed kidneys. This results in decreased urine production and thus a drop in the pressure which causes the pain. Narcotic injections are usually reserved for patients in whom NSAIDS are contraindicated, or those who fail to respond to them.

Use this opportunity to revise the actions of NSAIDs. How do their actions on the arachidonic acid pathway result in a drop in GFR, and a reduction of ureteric inflammation? What are the contraindications to the use of NSAIDs?

(h) Fluid intake

- Tell him not to drink more than necessary, until he has passed the stone.

In patients who have vomited, careful fluid balance is necessary. However, drinking excessively merely causes a diuresis, which can then increase the pressure above the obstruction making the pain worse. It does *not* assist in speeding up the passage of the stone. None of us would 'treat' a blocked toilet by flushing it.

(i) Indications for surgical intervention

In general, the smaller the stone, the more likely it is to pass without surgical intervention. Stones over 5 mm in diameter are unlikely to pass.

The main indications for intervention are:

- large stones
- continuing pain despite adequate analgesia
- complete obstruction
- infection
- single kidney.

Sometimes there are non-medical reasons. For example, aeroplane pilots are forbidden from flying until the stone has been removed.

(j) Types of surgical intervention

There are three types of intervention:

- surgical removal of the stone (usually ureteroscopically)
- simple relief of obstruction (percutaneous nephrostomy)
- disintegrating the stone by extracorporeal shock wave lithotripsy (ESWL).

Ureteroscopy is the ideal way to diagnose a stone. It will also facilitate stone removal using either a dormia basket, or enabling disintegration with a lithoclast or a laser. However, if this is technically unsuccessful, it is often possible to pass a stent retrogradely, via the ureteroscope, up the ureter to relieve the obstruction.

Another way to relieve the obstruction is by percutaneous nephrostomy. This radiological procedure relieves the obstruction and preserves renal function. It is particularly important to do this urgently in the presence of infection, when a nephrostomy, rather than stent insertion, is the norm. This is done under ultrasound control, which also allows the exclusion of peri-renal and psoas abscess.

Although ESWL is frequently used to disintegrate small renal calculi as an elective procedure, it can also be used for lower ureteric stones. Most hospitals do not have a lithotripter, but can rent a mobile lithotripter, which is transported on a lorry for a planned session.

Only rarely is open surgery for stones needed, but laparoscopic ureterolithotomy is becoming increasingly available.

(k) Follow-up blood tests

The following would be required:

- renal function tests
- serum calcium (more particularly the 'corrected' serum calcium)
- serum uric acid.

A raised serum calcium or uric acid level can often cause stone formation. These can be due to either hyperparathyroidism or gout respectively, both of which can be treated. Stones are an important presentation of hyperparathyroidism, can complicate gout, and are the only presentation of cystinuria. You should be familiar with the diagnosis and treatment of all three.

> Use this opportunity to review the common causes of urinary tract stone formation. How do urinary tract infections and dehydration result in stone formation? What are the main diseases associated with hypercalcaemia, hyperuricaemia and hyperoxaluria? How might the history and physical examination reveal whether they are present?

Other more specialised tests of the urine can be requested for patients with recurrent stones (*see* below).

(l) General advice

- Drink enough fluid each day so that you make 5 pints of urine a day.

It is important to explain to patients that there are many reasons why they are more likely than others to make another stone. Examples are hyperuricosuria and hypercalciuria. In addition, there are substances in urine that retard crystal formation, even if the urine is supersaturated. This is analogous to antifreeze in a car radiator. If the antifreeze is too dilute and it is cold enough, the radiator fluid will freeze (i.e. form crystals). If the fluid intake is increased sufficiently, the chance of making another stone in the next 10 years is reduced from about 50% to 10%. Not a bad treatment! Note that this is exactly the opposite advice to that given to patients *before* they have passed their stone.

Much work has been done to try to establish why only some people form stones. However the results have relatively little impact on clinical practice. For this reason, it is only worth giving more complex treatment after a full metabolic analysis of 24-hour urine samples in patients who repeatedly form stones despite a high fluid intake. Urine may be analysed for pH, and levels of calcium, phosphate, sodium, uric acid, cysteine, oxalate, citrate, and creatinine. Some patients may then benefit from thiamine, diuretics, citrate supplements, etc.

There is no need to restrict patients' intake of calcium if they have formed a stone. The body regulates its intake of dietary calcium. Therefore, strict limitation of dietary calcium intake will serve only to increase the risk of osteoporosis.

(m) Management of urinary tract stones in pregnancy

In pregnancy, the management of ureteric stones will need to differ substantially.

- The hazards to a fetus from radiation are greatest in the first 3 months. In the third trimester, one plain X-ray is permissible.
- U/S scans are safe and can at least show hydro-nephrosis.
- NSAIDs should not be given (due to effects on the fetal ductus arteriosus).
- ESWL is contraindicated during pregnancy.
- Often it is possible to remove ureteric calculi ureteroscopically during pregnancy.

- If all else fails, a stent can be inserted until the baby has been born.

Web resources

- Diagnosis and management of renal colic: www.prodigy.nhs.uk
- Notes on renal calculi: www.surgical-tutor.org.uk
- Renal stone management: www.clinicalevidence.com

Further reading

- Coe FL, Parks JH and Asplin JR (1992) The pathogenesis and treatment of kidney stones. *New England Journal of Medicine.* **327**: 1141.
- Downey P and Tolley D (2002) Contemporary management of renal calculus disease. *Journal of the Royal College of Surgeons of Edinburgh.* **47**: 668–75. www.rcsed.ac.uk/journal/vol47_5/47500003.html
- Longmore M, Wilkinson I and Rajagopalan S (eds) (2004) *Oxford Handbook of Clinical Medicine* (6e). Oxford University Press, Oxford, pp. 264–5.
- Parmar MS (2004) Kidney stones. *British Medical Journal.* **328**: 1420.

An overweight 41-year-old multiparous smoker presents to her GP reporting a single episode of epigastric pain radiating to the right shoulder. The pain lasted for about 3 hours in the late evening, was not relieved by changes in posture, and was associated with anorexia and nausea. She says that the pain came on about 1 hour after eating her evening meal of fish and chips.

(a) Which disease processes are suggested by the history?

....

....

....

(b) What investigations would the GP consider?

....

....

....

(c) What recommendations should the GP make?

....

....

....

While waiting for her investigations, she is admitted to the A&E department with nausea, vomiting and further epigastric pain, which is severe and constant. In addition, the pain is more diffuse than before and radiates to her back. On examination she has epigastric distension, guarding and marked tenderness on palpation. She also has rapid shallow respiration.

(d) What is your differential diagnosis?

....

....

....

(e) What urgent tests would you order?

....

....

Her amylase is 1190 iu/l, and bilirubin and ALP are raised.

(f) What is the significance of these findings?

....

....

....

(g) Which tests help predict the severity of the disease?

....

....

....

(h) Briefly outline your initial management.

....

....

....

> The patient starts to deteriorate rapidly, she is now pyrexial and is showing signs of shock. The SHO institutes resuscitation measures, and calls for senior assistance.
>
> Her arterial blood gas measurements on 40% O_2 are as follows:
>
> | | |
> |---|---|
> | pH | 7.29 |
> | PaO_2 | 7.9 kPa |
> | $PaCO_2$ | 4.2 kPa |
> | HCO_3^- | 18 mmol/l |
> | Base excess | −6 |

(i) Interpret these results.

....

....

....

(j) What complication may be developing?

....

....

....

(k) How would you confirm your suspicions?

....

....

....

> She is admitted to the intensive care unit, but despite invasive ventilation her oxygen saturation is consistently recorded below 85%. After 2 weeks of progressive deterioration in ITU she is unable to breathe for herself and despite a lack of sedation her GCS is now 3.

(l) Discuss the ethical principles involved in deciding whether to continue treatment in this case.

....

....

....

Key cases

- Gallstones
- Peptic ulcer
- Acute cholecystitis
- Acute pancreatitis

Clinical context

Another case of vomiting and abdominal pain, but no apologies, it's common! Note how the site of pain can help in making your diagnosis; and this can be refined by knowing what tests to request, and how to interpret them.

Gallstones are a common reason for acute abdominal pain, and admission to hospital. There are many reasons why gallstones produce abdominal pain, some of which may be life threatening. This scenario concentrates on two conditions; acute cholecystitis and acute pancreatitis. It is important to note the numerous problems that acute pancreatitis causes, and the associated systemic manifestations. You will also realise that acute pancreatitis – like many conditions – has a high mortality and, despite comprehensive appropriate treatment, the patient in this scenario dies. This can be difficult for the relatives to accept, and members of the medical team may be similarly affected. Therefore as you read through this scenario, take a few minutes to think about how you would liaise with, and support, both the patient's relatives and your colleagues.

(a) Acute abdominal pain

In this patient the following differential diagnoses should be considered:

- biliary colic
- peptic ulcer
- pancreatitis
- muscle strain
- inferior myocardial infarction
- renal colic.

Other causes include small bowel infarction and dissecting aortic aneurysm.

In a patient presenting with abdominal pain there are several important points to consider:

- the level of pain generally relates to the origin. Foregut – upper (epigastric); midgut – middle (periumbilical); hindgut – lower (suprapubic)
- colicky pain is produced by the stretching of a hollow viscus
- constant localised pain is usually caused by peritoneal irritation

- associated back pain suggests retroperitoneal pathology
- there are important referred causes of abdominal pain (e.g. pneumonia, lumbar nerve root pathology and MI).

In any case, risk factors are essential in forming a differential diagnosis. Age, obesity and smoking are risk factors for many diseases. In the patient presenting with epigastric pain the important disease processes are gallstones producing biliary colic, peptic ulcer and pancreatitis. Multiparity is an additional risk factor for gallstones.

> You should be familiar with the common causes of acute abdominal pain. Being able to identify multiple causes for pain in each of the nine areas of the abdomen is a good start (*see* p. 67).

Biliary colic

Biliary colic is caused by the gall bladder contracting under the influence of cholecystokinin (exacerbated by fatty food), forcing a stone into the gall bladder outlet/cystic duct. This produces pain, which may be described as deep and sometimes sharp. As the gall bladder relaxes, the stone falls back from the cystic duct. This leads to cyclical waves of pain, hence the term colic.

However, the term biliary colic may be misleading. Often a stone becomes trapped in the cystic duct, or is pushed distally into the common bile duct. This pain from the passage of a stone is constant, resulting from high-pressure dilation of the biliary tree.

Biliary pain commonly occurs at night. This is probably partly due to the anatomical position of the gall bladder. When the patient is in bed the gall bladder is horizontal, allowing the stones to approach the opening of the cystic duct.

(b) Investigations

The important investigations to decide on the cause of this lady's pain would be:

- abdominal ultrasound scan (detects 90% of gallstones)
- oesophagogastroduodenoscopy (OGD) is sensitive for detecting inflammation, ulceration, and malignancy
- liver function tests

- magnetic resonance cholangiopancreatography (MRCP).

(c) Advice

At this stage the diagnosis is not known, therefore advice should be given that would be helpful for all of the possible diagnoses:

- low-fat diet
- stopping smoking
- reduced alcohol consumption.

(d) Symptoms and signs

With the previous history, the symptoms and signs listed would indicate several possibilities:

- acute cholecystitis
- inflammation/ulceration of the stomach or duodenum
- acute pancreatitis.

Acute cholecystitis

Acute cholecystitis is acute inflammation of the gall bladder, caused in 90% of cases by persistent obstruction of the cystic duct by a gallstone. It is important to recognise the symptoms and signs since it is a surgical emergency that must be distinguished from biliary colic. The complications include empyema, perforation of the gall bladder, septicaemia, and acute pancreatitis (if there are ductal calculi). Treatment is by cholecystectomy, which may be performed early, or as an elective procedure following suitable conservative management with intravenous fluids, analgaesia, and antibiotics.

Patients often have constant, severe right upper quadrant pain (which may radiate to the shoulder tip), nausea, and vomiting. On examination, the patient may be pyrexial, have shallow respiration, a tender distended abdomen and a positive Murphy's sign.

Multiple factors contribute to inflammation in an obstructed gall bladder. The bile is trapped under high pressure, causing physical and chemical irritation. Bacterial infection adds to the inflammation.

> It is important to know the cardinal symptoms and signs caused by obstruction, inflammation and infection of the structures within the biliary tree. How does the position of the stones determine the subsequent course of events?

Perforated duodenal ulcer

Most occur in patients with a history of pre-existing dyspepsia, however, a small proportion have no previous symptoms. The classic presentation is with sudden-onset epigastric pain, which generalises to the whole abdomen. Examination might reveal peritonitis with absent bowel sounds. Patients may have an associated episode of melaena or haematemesis (see p. 70).

An erect chest X-ray may show free gas under the diaphragm (see p. 66). However approximately 10% of patients do not have this finding, and if there is diagnostic doubt CT imaging may confirm the diagnosis.

Acute pancreatitis

> You should be familiar with the GET SMASHED mnemonic for the causes of acute pancreatitis. What do the letters stand for? How do these conditions cause acute pancreatitis?

Acute pancreatitis causes upper abdominal pain, nausea and vomiting. The pain is most often present in the epigastric region and right upper quadrant and may radiate to the back (remember that the pancreas is retroperitoneal). It is sometimes relieved by leaning forwards.

Pancreatitis can present with a variety of clinical features that reflect the cause of the inflammation, its severity and any systemic complications. If the inflammation is mild then epigastric tenderness may be the only sign. Conversely, patients with severe pancreatitis will have signs of generalised peritonitis (see pp. 66 and 70) and hypovolaemic shock (see p. 140).

Patients often have rapid shallow breathing. This may be due to shock, however diaphragmatic irritation can produce the same finding. Jaundice may indicate that the pancreatitis has been caused by common bile duct stones, or may reflect oedema of the head of the pancreas. Retroperitoneal bleeding can result in flank (Grey–Turner's sign) or periumbilical bruising (Cullen's sign).

Remember that the majority of cases of acute pancreatitis have a cause. This scenario has used the example of pancreatitis secondary to gallstone disease. However, patients may have signs of heavy alcohol use, chronic liver disease (see p. 63), steroid treatment, hyperlipidaemia (see p. 21) or mumps.

> How do the symptoms and signs of acute pancreatitis arise? Review the anatomy of the pancreas, its retroperitoneal position, proximity to the coeliac plexus and ganglia, and the position of the head in relation to the duodenum and common bile duct.

(e) Tests and investigations

In suspected acute pancreatitis, the following tests are indicated:

- FBC
- plasma amylase and lipase
- serum U&E
- blood glucose and urinary ketones
- C-reactive protein
- arterial blood gases
- liver function tests (liver enzymes, bilirubin, albumin) and coagulation profile (*see* p. 61)
- corrected calcium
- LDH
- lipid profile
- virology.

The initial imaging studies would be:

- *chest X-ray*: the CXR does not diagnose acute pancreatitis but it is important in ruling out perforation, which can mimic pancreatitis (*see* p. 70). Additionally, complications such as a pleural effusion or pulmonary infiltration (*see* p. 124) can be diagnosed on the CXR.
- *abdominal X-ray*: again useful in ruling out other causes of an 'acute abdomen' (*see* p. 68). Localised ileus is a common finding and generalised ileus may be seen in severe pancreatitis.

An abdominal ultrasound scan should be arranged as soon as possible.

(f) Amylase and liver function tests

- Serum amylase >1000 iu/l indicates acute pancreatitis.
- Raised alkaline phosphatase (in this instance) indicates that the pancreatitis is probably secondary to CBD obstruction by gallstones (*see* p. 201).
- Raised bilirubin is found in cases of pancreatitis secondary to biliary obstruction but also in cases where there are no obstructing gallstones (*see* p. 61).
- The most reasonable explanation for this is CBD obstruction/compression caused by the swollen head of pancreas and/or obstructing gallstone.

> You should be familiar with the elements of standard liver function tests. Which components reflect liver structure and which reflect liver function? What are the differences between cholestatic and hepatocellular abnormalities?

Serum amylase is usually greater than 1000 iu/l and increases within 6–12 hours of the onset of acute pancreatitis. It has a half-life of 10 hours and is rapidly cleared from the blood.

There are several causes of raised amylase not caused by acute pancreatitis; these include:

- perforated viscus
- renal failure
- small bowel infarction
- acidosis and diabetic ketoacidosis
- salivary gland disease
- eating disorders
- cirrhosis
- drugs.

(g) Prognostic markers in acute pancreatitis

There are several grading systems to assess the severity of acute pancreatitis. These include the Ranson criteria (for alcohol-induced pancreatitis), APACHE II and Modified Glasgow criteria for pancreatitis.

An easy way to remember the Modified Glasgow criteria is to use the mnemonic PANCREAS:

PA = PaO_2 (<8 kPa on room air)
N = neutrophils (WCC >15 × 10^9/ml)
C = calcium (Ca^{2+} <2.0 mmol/l)
R = renal (U&E, urea >16 mmol/l)
E = enzymes (LDH > 600 iu/l and AST > 200 iu/l)
A = albumin (serum albumin <32 g/l)
S = sugar (glucose >10 mmol/l).

More than three of these findings indicates a poor prognosis.

(h) Management of acute pancreatitis

The initial management of acute pancreatitis involves:

- a call for senior assistance
- nil by mouth
- high-flow O_2
- i.v. access and fluid resuscitation to correct any hypovolaemic shock (*see* p. 140)
- analgaesia with pethidine or morphine with an anti-emetic
- hourly monitoring of respiratory rate, pulse, BP and urine output
- daily monitoring of FBC, U&E, Ca^{2+}, glucose, amylase, ABG. If a scoring system is used (*see* above), daily scores are useful.

(Longmore *et al.*, 2004)

If the situation deteriorates, the patient will need to be admitted to ITU. A CT scan can demonstrate either a pseudocyst, abscess formation or pancreatic necrosis, which may require laparotomy and debridement.

Endoscopic retrograde cholangiopancreatography (ERCP) with sphincterotomy and gallstone removal may be needed if the patient shows progressive jaundice (within the first 24 hours).

(i) Arterial blood gases

The blood gases show:

- metabolic acidosis
- hypoxaemia or type 1 respiratory failure.

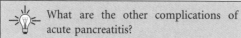 You should be able to interpret ABG results and know the common causes for respiratory, metabolic and mixed acidosis and alkalosis.

(j) Complications of acute pancreatitis

The causes of type I respiratory failure in this patient could be:

- acute respiratory distress syndrome (ARDS) (part of the systemic inflammatory response syndrome (SIRS))
- pulmonary oedema.

What are the other complications of acute pancreatitis?

(k) Acute respiratory distress syndrome (ARDS)

Physical examination, chest X-ray and repeat ABGs on 100% O_2 are needed to make the diagnosis of ARDS. The diagnostic criteria are:

- a lack of clinical congestive cardiac failure (CCF)
- chest X-ray showing bilateral infiltrates
- hypoxaemia despite high-flow O_2.

ARDS has an extremely high mortality. It can result from direct (e.g. pneumonia, aspiration, or inhalation) or indirect injuries to the lungs (e.g. acute pancreatitis or sepsis). The defining characteristic is damage to the alveoli caused by increased permeability of the pulmonary capillaries, and an acute inflammatory response. Hypoxaemia becomes progressively worse as the damage progresses. Even if the inflammation resolves there may well be residual fibrosis of the lung tissue.

Use this opportunity to revisit the components of the inflammatory response. Which immune cells are the key mediators? What is the role of cytokines?

(l) Ethics of continued treatment

Any discussion of the ethics of continuing treatment is difficult; however, some of the more relevant points could include the following:

- risks, benefits, and burdens of treatment and non-treatment must be assessed for the patient and significant others
- life has a natural end
- when death is drawing near, doctors should not strive to prolong the dying process with no regard to their patients' wishes. This is based on respect for human life and making patients' best interests the first concern
- offering life-sustaining treatment is generally in the patient's best interests, but benefits and burdens are not always limited to medical considerations
- not continuing or not initiating treatment may be indicated when it would provide no net benefit to the patient
- aim for consensus, and if this is impossible seek legal advice
- there is no legal distinction between not starting and withdrawing treatment.

Web resources

- ARDS: www.emedicine.com
- Diseases of liver, pancreas and biliary system: bmj.bmjjournals.com
- Gallstone disease: www.patient.co.uk

Further reading

- Beckinghan IJ and Bornman PC (2001) ABC of diseases of liver, pancreas, and biliary system [series of articles]. *British Medical Journal.* **322.**
- Cuscieri A (2002) Management of patients with gallstones and ductal calculi. *Lancet.* **360**: 739.
- Longmore M, Wilkinson I and Rajagopalan S (eds) (2004) *Oxford Handbook of Clinical Medicine* (6e). Oxford University Press, Oxford, pp. 478–9.
- Smotkin J and Tenner S (2002) Laboratory diagnostic tests in acute pancreatitis. *Journal of Clinical Gastroenterology.* **34**: 459.
- Swaroop VS, Chari ST and Clain JE (2004) Severe acute pancreatitis. *Journal of the American Medical Association.* **291**: 2865.

16 A history of blackouts

A 69-year-old man with a history of blackouts is found by his wife dazed, leaning forward and incontinent of urine. She telephones the GP out-of-hours service. While the GP is at the couple's house, the man has transient, uncontrolled, coarse movements of his right arm and leg. The GP calls an ambulance and the patient is admitted to the A&E department. He is now relatively stable but has not regained consciousness.

(a) What disease processes might be suggested by the above history?

....

....

....

(b) To which section of A&E should the patient be streamed?

....

....

....

Whilst being assessed in A&E the man has further convulsions, but this time they are more generalised. He is maintaining his own airway.

(c) What immediate action would the attending doctor take?

....

....

....

After initial management the patient's condition stabilises, and i.v. access is gained. The house officer sends blood to the laboratory.

(d) Which blood tests would be requested and which specific abnormalities should be excluded?

....

....

....

The patient remains stable and is transferred to the medical assessment unit. As part of his assessment, a chest X-ray is taken (see Figure 16.1). A more detailed history is taken from his wife. Apparently the patient has lost 2 stones over the past year, has had a dry cough and has suffered from shortness of breath. He has also been having headaches for some months.

(e) Comment on the chest X-ray.

....

....

....

(f) What diagnosis is most likely and what specific questions should be asked?

....

....

....

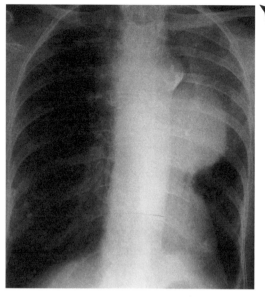

Figure 16.1 Chest X-ray.

(g) How would you explain the neurological symptoms?

....

....

....

(h) To support the working diagnosis what further symptoms and signs should be sought specifically?

....

....

....

(i) List and justify further investigations that should be done immediately.

....

....

....

The investigations confirm the suspected diagnosis and both the family and physicians agree on the futility of any curative intervention. The patient is therefore referred to palliative care services. Three months later the patient is at home in the terminal phase of his illness. He is bed-bound and cared for by his wife.

(j) Which members of the community team may be involved in his care?

....

....

....

(k) Which distressing symptoms might this man experience in the terminal phases of his illness?

....

....

....

(l) His wife reports increasing difficulty with managing the patient at home; what other options are available to them?

....

....

....

(m) What financial help are they entitled to and how should this be applied for?

....

....

....

Key cases

- Seizures/fits
- Bronchial carcinoma
- Brain tumour

Clinical context

Epilepsy affects approximately 1 in 200 people. In over 60% of cases there are no identifiable causes. However the likelihood of an identifiable cause is higher in older patients. Particular attention should be paid to the management of acute generalised seizures and the investigation of the patient with a first fit.

This scenario illustrates the management and investigation of new-onset seizures. The initial assessment and management are the same irrespective of the cause. However, appropriate investigation is aimed at early identification of treatable causes. Treatment may be straightforward, such as the correction of hypoglycaemia, however in some cases the seizure may herald a more sinister condition. There is no curative treatment for bronchial carcinoma with metastatic disease, and the scenario emphasises the importance of providing appropriate palliative care.

(a) History

This question primarily relies on knowledge of the differential diagnosis of convulsions in a 69-year-old man.

These can be considered as:

- *metabolic*: hyper- or hypo-glycaemia/natraemia/ calcaemia and hypoxaemia
- *neurological*: epilepsy (idiopathic)
- *neoplastic*: brain tumour (usually secondary)
- *vascular*: infarction or haemorrhage (stroke, TIA, haematoma or sinus thrombosis)
- *infective*: any infection, or specifically, meningitis, encephalitis or cerebral abscess
- *traumatic*: head injuries (subdural haematoma)
- *drugs*: alcoholism/withdrawal, amphetamines, cocaine.

This history provides many clues. At the age of 69, idiopathic epilepsy, drug use or infection are all unlikely. There is no report of trauma. The history favours transient ischaemic attack (TIA), stroke, undiagnosed diabetes, a space-occupying lesion, and alcohol use or withdrawal. *See* p. 20 for a fuller description of the differential diagnosis.

> Consciousness relies on the intact function of the cerebral hemispheres and reticular activating system, and adequate provision of oxygen and nutrients. Using this framework, what are the possible causes of blackouts?

(b) A&E streaming (previously triage)

This patient would be referred to either the majors or resuscitation section of A&E, since he is in need of urgent treatment and investigation, and will need to be admitted.

Streaming is a system whereby patients are allocated to different flows according to their needs. These flows are individually staffed and continue to function independently of other streams. A&E departments usually use the following classifications:

- minor case
- major case
- resuscitation.

(c) Immediate management of seizures

Seizures are caused by abnormal spontaneous electrical discharge in any part of the brain. Normal neuronal functioning is vitally dependent on the tightly regulated structural and functional environment of the neurones. Any change in this environment can provoke a seizure.

> How do the metabolic abnormalities discussed above provoke uncontrolled neuronal discharge?

Status epilepticus is defined as a seizure lasting for more than 30 minutes, or repeated seizures without any intervening consciousness. This patient has not regained consciousness and therefore has status epilepticus. The aim in management is to optimise ABCDs, maintaining airway, breathing and circulation; and to terminate the seizures as soon as possible. Once initial stabilisation has occurred, the cause can be investigated.

Treatment involves:

- maintaining the airway using adjuncts (e.g. nasopharyngeal) or intubation with the aid of an anaesthetist if necessary
- oxygen 100% and suction if necessary

- i.v. access and blood for tests (*see* below)
- correction of hypotension with fluids
- a finger prick glucose test (BM) and laboratory glucose test
- slow i.v. injection of 4 mg lorazepam to stop seizures.

If the patient is not responding it may be necessary to proceed to an infusion of an antiepileptic drug such as phenytoin, or to consider general anaesthesia and transfer to ITU with assistance from an anaesthetist.

> Use this opportunity to revise the pharmacology of drugs commonly used in the management of seizures. What are their effects on sodium channels and inhibitory and excitatory neurotransmitters? Can you predict their side-effects?

(d) Investigation of seizures

Prompt investigation is crucial to establish whether there are any treatable causes present.

Blood tests for anyone presenting with seizures should include:

- FBC for possible infection
- U&E for serum Na^+, K^+ and urea concentrations
- blood glucose
- serum Ca^{2+}/Mg^{2+}.

Additional tests include liver function tests, blood alcohol level, serum toxicology screen and arterial blood gas measurement.

Furthermore, a CT scan should be arranged as soon as possible to rule out either a primary or secondary structural cause.

(e) Chest X-ray

The chest X-ray shows a large mass in the left upper zone with nodal enlargement in the left hilum and mediastinum. There is also collapse of the left upper lobe. These changes are compatible with a bronchial carcinoma.

(f) (g) (h) Bronchial carcinoma with brain metastases

The combination of chronic respiratory symptoms, weight loss, and headaches in an elderly man – especially a smoker – suggests malignancy. Bronchial carcinoma with brain metastases would be strongly suspected.

Further specific questions will establish this patient's risk factors for bronchial carcinoma. The principal risk factors are:

- *smoking*: by far the most important risk factor for lung cancer. A full smoking history should be taken
- *asbestos exposure*: increases the risk of lung cancer by up to seven times. Additionally, people exposed are much more likely to develop mesothelioma (the chest X-ray does not suggest mesothelioma)
- *other workplace exposure*: minerals and chemicals such as uranium, arsenic, silicon, beryllium, vinyl chloride, nickel chromates, coal products, and chloromethyl ethers all increase the risk of lung cancer
- *family history*: important since there are some genetic abnormalities that increase the risk of developing lung cancer.

The four major histological types of lung cancer are listed below. Note the relative frequency of each tumour type and the different characteristics:

- *squamous cell* – 40%: central, cavitating, early-metastasising tumours that can lead to hypercalcaemia, due to bone metastases and parathyroid hormone-related peptide (PTHrP) release
- *large cell* – 10–15%: central, early-metastasising tumours carrying a poor prognosis compared with squamous cell carcinoma
- *small (oat) cell* – 20–30%: central, rapid-growing tumours. They arise from the neuroendocrine system and hence secrete ADH and ACTH
- *adenocarcinoma* – 20%: arises peripherally or in areas of lung scarring. Commonly occurs in non-smokers. Asbestos exposure is a risk factor.

> Use this opportunity to revise the effects of ectopic hormone secretion; particularly PTH, ADH and ACTH. A diagnosis of SIADH is often made prematurely on finding hyponatraemia. What urine and blood tests are needed to make the diagnosis? What are the other common causes of hyponatraemia?

Symptoms of bronchial carcinoma

Symptoms and signs can be divided up into local, distant and those caused by paraneoplastic syndromes.

Local (direct invasion)

- Breathlessness
- Haemoptysis
- Persistent non-productive cough
- Pleuritic chest pain
- Rarely Horner's syndrome (with an apical or Pancoast's tumour)
- Rarely superior vena cava obstruction with facial swelling, headache and dilated chest wall veins

Distant (metastatic effects)

- Brain metastases producing fits, headaches or hemiparesis
- Bone metastases producing pathological fractures, bone pain and symptoms of hypercalcaemia

Paraneoplastic syndromes (non-metastatic effects)

- Anorexia
- Weight loss
- Clubbing
- Peripheral neuropathy
- Muscle wasting, proximal myopathy
- Effects of ectopic hormone/peptide release
- Thromboembolism
- Functional effects, due to tumour-associated antibodies

(i) Investigation of bronchial carcinoma

Investigations for suspected bronchial malignancy will be directed by the key features in both the history and the examination:

- *neurological symptoms*: CT scan of the head (stroke or space-occupying lesion)
- *respiratory symptoms*: staging CT scan of the thorax, bronchoscopy and biopsy/washings
- *sputum cytology*
- *cytology* of pleural fluid and *histology* of associated proteinaceous clot.

(j) Palliative and community care

A palliative care service must aim to provide appropriate care to maximise the physical, psychosocial, emotional and spiritual well-being of patients with terminal illness.

The aim for all patients must be to:

- maximise the time spent at home with family and friends
- help patients to live a 'normal' life for as long as possible.

The GP and primary care team are central in providing effective palliative care. Members of the community teams that may be involved include:

- GPs
- district nurses
- health visitors
- community pharmacists
- physiotherapists
- occupational therapists
- dieticians
- social workers.

The individual's needs will vary according to the nature and stage of their illness, and inevitably there needs to be a wide range of other health services that are available. These include continence advisory services, speech and language therapists and other specialist nursing services.

What other services might be needed in the delivery of effective palliative care?

(k) Symptoms in terminal illness

Patients suffering from advanced cancer and the later stages of other chronic diseases often experience distressing physical and psychological symptoms towards the end of their lives. These include:

- pain
- weakness
- dyspnoea
- nausea and vomiting
- constipation
- confusion
- agitation and restlessness
- depression and anxiety.

All of these symptoms are potentially treatable.

How might the symptoms listed above arise in this patient's case? Use this opportunity to revise the medication commonly used in palliation of symptoms, including the WHO 'pain ladder'. How would you treat any of the symptoms listed above?

(l) Patterns of care

Although many patients will only require support at home, some may have multiple inpatient admissions alternating with time at home. Others may be unsuitable for home care because they are too ill for their family/carers to manage, or there is no one to help at home. The key to effective management is close liaison between the primary care team and hospital staff.

There are three basic patterns of care. Patients may move between these services as clinical and social circumstances change:

- *community-based*: there are a wide range of community services for patients who want to remain and die at home (*see above*)
- *community and inpatient-based*: rapid access to hospital or hospice care when necessary. The provision of day care and respite care is particularly important when certain needs cannot be met in the community

- *inpatient-based*: when patients are too ill for their carers or family to manage.

(m) Social support

There are many resources for carers to find out about financial entitlements such as attendance allowance, disability allowances, carers' allowances. GPs should be familiar with the application processes to help their patients. A social worker will advise patients on their entitlement to both financial and practical support such as home help, meals on wheels, and access to other other voluntary agencies.

This patient would be entitled to:

- *carers' allowance*, applied for from a social security office
- *attendance allowance*, applied for with the DS1500 form from a social security office.

Web resources

- BTS guidelines: www.brit-thoracic.org.uk

- Cancer NSF: www.nelh.nhs.uk
- Example X-rays: www.netmedicine.com/xray/xr.htm
- Macmillan: www.macmillan.org.uk
- Social security: www.dwp.gov.uk/lifeevent/benefits

Further reading

- Hoffman PC, Mauer AM and Vokes EE (2000) Lung cancer. *Lancet.* **355**: 479.
- Jackman DM and Johnson BE (2005) Small-cell lung cancer. *Lancet.* **366**: 1385.
- Longmore M, Wilkinson I and Rajagopalan S (eds) (2004) *Oxford Handbook of Clinical Medicine* (6e). Oxford University Press, Oxford, pp. 378–80, 812.
- Toms JR (ed) (2004) *Cancer Stats Monograph 2004.* Chapter 7: Lung cancer and smoking. Cancer Research UK, London, p. 45.

17 A problem swallowing

You are on-call and asked to clerk a 67-year-old gentleman who has been referred by his GP with a 3-month history of difficulty in swallowing.

In his past medical history he had an MI five years ago, and also suffers with moderate COPD. He has also had intermittent heartburn for several years and was diagnosed as having a hiatus hernia on gastroscopy 6 years ago.

He is a smoker of 20 cigarettes per day for 50 years and consumes approximately 30 units of alcohol per week. On examination he is obese (BMI 30), and has tar staining of his fingers. There is no lymphadenopathy. His abdomen is soft and non-tender with no palpable masses. Bowel sounds are present and normal.

(a) What mechanisms are involved in swallowing?

....

....

....

(b) Dysphagia can be broadly divided into two categories. What are they, and how do they relate to the underlying pathology?

....

....

....

(c) What further features should you enquire about in your history?

....

....

....

On further questioning the patient tells you that his symptoms have been progressively worsening, and now feels food sticking behind the middle third of his sternum. At present he can only swallow fluids. He also informs you, that on increasingly frequent occasions he has regurgitated undigested food. This happened within 30 minutes of ingestion. Once he noticed a small amount of fresh blood in the regurgitated food. He has also lost about one stone in weight since his symptoms began.

(d) What investigations would you order and why?

....

....

....

(e) What are this gentleman's risk factors for developing oesophageal malignancy, and what are the two main histological types?

....

....

....

An oesophagogastroduodenoscopy (OGD) reveals a tight, irregular stricture in the lower oesophagus. The endoscope cannot be passed through this stricture, but biopsies are taken from the affected area.

(f) What investigation would you now request?

....

....

....

☞ A few days after his OGD the oesophageal biopsies are reported as showing poorly differentiated oesophageal adenocarcinoma. Further radiological imaging has identified a mass extending from the lower oesophagus to the gastro-oesophageal junction. There are also several enlarged lymph nodes in the mediastinum, as well as multiple lesions in both lobes of the liver consistent with metastatic disease.

(g) After reconsidering this gentleman's history, what could have been the underlying premalignant condition? Are there any other premalignant conditions linked to oesophageal carcinoma?

....

....

....

(h) What treatment options are available?

....

....

....

Key cases

- Dysphagia
- Hiatus hernia
- Oesophageal cancer

Clinical context

Dysphagia is an alarm symptom that always needs immediate investigation to establish the exact cause, and start appropriate treatment. Dysphagia should never be attributed to ageing, which only causes mild abnormalities in oesophageal motility and these rarely produce symptoms.

This scenario uses the example of a patient with pre-existing upper GI disease to explore the processes involved in swallowing, and the conditions that can interrupt this tightly controlled, co-ordinated, function. Oesophageal carcinoma is possibly the most sinister cause of dysphagia; and the natural history, treatment and poor prognosis of this condition are discussed.

Dysphagia

The word dysphagia is derived from the Greek words 'dys' (with difficulty) and 'phagia' (to eat). Dysphagia is a subjective sensation that patients experience, and indicates an abnormality as liquids and/or solids pass from the mouth to the stomach. Patients' complaints range from the inability to initiate a swallow, to the sensation of liquids and/or solids 'sticking' as they pass through the oesophagus into the stomach. The term 'odynophagia' refers to pain with swallowing.

(a) Swallowing mechanisms

Swallowing is an organised, co-ordinated, sequential process that involves sensory and proprioceptive input from receptors in the mouth, oropharynx and pharynx (tongue, soft palate, fauces, tonsils, and the posterior pharyngeal wall). This input is transmitted to the swallowing centre located in the floor of the fourth ventricle through the facial (VII), glossopharyngeal (IX), and vagus (X) nerves. Information from the swallowing centre is conveyed to the muscles that are involved in swallowing through the trigeminal (V), facial (VII), glossopharyngeal (IX), vagus (X), and hypoglossal (XII) nerves.

This complex process is also co-ordinated with respiration (just imagine the consequences of breathing and swallowing simultaneously). Swallowing usually interrupts the expiration, which is completed when swallowing ends.

Swallowing comprises three phases:

- oral
- pharyngeal
- oesophageal.

Oral phase

This phase has two components. The first, or *preparatory phase*, involves the muscles of mastication that are used to form a food bolus. This process requires taste, temperature, touch, and proprioception to form a bolus of the correct size and consistency. The bolus is then held against the hard palate by the tongue. The second, or *transit phase*, is where the bolus is moved by peristaltic-like actions of the tongue towards the pharynx. This component of the swallowing process is a voluntary phase controlled by the cerebral cortex through the corticobulbar tracts. Once the bolus reaches the tonsils the pharyngeal phase is triggered.

Pharyngeal phase

As the bolus enters the pharynx, a reflex action propels the bolus towards the cricopharyngeal sphincter. Elevation of the larynx prevents food from entering the airway by closing the epiglottis, aryepiglottic folds, true vocal cords and false vocal folds. Elevation of the larynx also stretches and starts to open cricopharyngeus. Further relaxation of cricopharyngeus allows the bolus to pass into the oesophagus.

Oesophageal phase

Transit of the bolus from the pharynx to the stomach is involuntary and is controlled by the brainstem and the myenteric plexus. A peristaltic wave pushes the bolus from the upper oesophagus through the lower oesophageal sphincter into the stomach.

> Take this opportunity to revise the anatomy and physiology of the oropharynx, oesophagus and cranial nerves.

(b) Types and mechanisms of dysphagia

Dysphagia can be caused by:

- obstruction
- dysmotility.

These two categories can be used to describe pathology at any point during swallowing. Either obstruction to the passage of food through the mouth, pharynx or oesophagus; or dysfunction of the complex interaction between nerves and muscles controlling this process; or a combination of these can lead to dysphagia.

Examples include:

Obstruction

Intraluminal

- Foreign body

Intramural

- Benign/malignant tumours
- Peptic stricture
- Post-radiotherapy stricture

Extraluminal

- Bronchial carcinoma
- Mediastinal lymphadenopathy
- Atrial dilation
- Aortic aneurysm

Dysmotility

- Diffuse oesophageal spasm
- Nutcracker oesophagus
- Parkinson's disease
- Stroke
- Motor neurone disease
- Achalasia

> Use this opportunity to familiarise yourself with the above conditions and how they lead to dysphagia. You should be familiar with mediastinal anatomy, and how the structures can cause extrinsic compression of the oesophagus. What other symptoms and signs might the above disease processes cause?

(c) History in dysphagia

Key points in the history should establish an index of clinical suspicion. These include:

- solids, liquids or both
- where does it stick?
- can a swallow be initiated
- odynophagia
- regurgitation
- medication
- weight loss
- haematemesis/melaena
- symptoms of anaemia
- co-morbidities (e.g. recurrent infections).

A history of dysphagia with both solids and liquids points towards possible dysmotility. A history of rapidly progressive dysphagia from solids to liquids is more in keeping with a carcinoma (or obstruction). Further features suggestive of carcinoma include signs of upper GI bleeding (haematemesis, melaena and symptoms of anaemia) and weight loss. However, any patient who presents with dysphagia requires immediate assessment.

There are many reasons why a patient may develop recurrent chest infections. In the context of dysphagia, recurrent infection can follow regurgitation/reflux of oesophageal contents (often partially digested food), which are then aspirated.

Gastro-oesophageal reflux can cause dysphagia secondary to either oesophagitis, or peptic stricture, or dysmotility, or a combination of these. Furthermore, oesophagitis can be caused by certain drugs including bisphosphonates (alendronate), ferrous sulphate and antibiotics such as tetracycline and doxycycline.

(d) Investigations in dysphagia

Investigations are described in Table 17.1.

OGD is the preferred investigation as any mucosal lesion can be seen and biopsied for histological examination. A contrast swallow, with video fluoroscopy, is helpful in patients with unexplained aspiration. Oesophageal pH studies assess the frequency and severity of acid reflux, and help guide treatment. Oesophageal manometry provides valuable evidence when diagnosing motility disorders such as achalasia and oesophageal spasm.

Table 17.1 Investigations in dysphagia

Test	Indication
FBC	Evidence of anaemia
U&E	Dehydration or electrolyte imbalance
LFTs (including clotting and albumin)	Liver metastases
Ca^{2+}	Bone metastases
Chest X-ray	Oesophageal dilatation/aspiration pneumonia
Oesophagogastroduodenoscopy (OGD)	Visualise pathology

(e) Risk factors for oesophageal carcinoma

From the history, the patient has significant risk factors for the development of oesophageal cancer. These include:

- male
- smoking
- alcohol use
- gastro-oesophageal reflux, especially Barrett's oesophagus
- obesity.

Other risk factors include:

- occupation: asbestos workers, vulcanising industry
- genetic factors including coeliac disease.

The types of oesophageal carcinoma are:

- adenocarcinoma
- squamous cell carcinoma.

Most oesophageal cancers are either adenocarcinoma (AC) or squamous cell (SCC). The incidence of SCC is decreasing in the UK. In contrast, the incidence of AC is rising dramatically. The prognosis for both types of cancer is poor. Five-year survival is less than 10%, although patients diagnosed with early-stage disease may be cured by either surgery and/or combination therapy.

> ☀ Are the risk factors for development of AC or SCC the same? How do they differ in their anatomical distribution and microscopic appearance? Does the natural history differ?

(f) Further investigation

- Staging CT of the thorax and abdomen

After diagnosis, the extent of the disease has to be assessed or 'staged'. A CT scan of the thorax and abdomen will determine the size and site of the primary tumour (important in this case as the scope could not pass through the stricture to determine its distal end), and also the presence or absence of lymphadenopathy and distant metastases.

In comparison with CT, endoscopic ultrasound gives more in-depth information about the local extent of the tumour. A high-frequency ultrasound transducer provides detailed images of the oesophageal lesion, the surrounding oesophageal wall and local lymph node involvement.

(g) Premalignant conditions related to oesophageal cancer

From the history outlined in the scenario, this patient is at high risk of having suffered from:

- Barrett's oesophagus.

Other pre-malignant conditions include:

- oesophageal web/ring (Plummer–Vinson syndrome)
- coeliac disease (see p. 202).

Barrett's oesophagus is a premalignant condition caused by chronic reflux of gastric contents into the oesophagus. It causes glandular metaplasia of the epithelium within the oesophagus (transforming from squamous cells to small intestinal columnar cells). These cells can become dysplastic or even neoplastic with time.

> ☀ Use this opportunity to revise the differences between metaplasia, dysplasia, and neoplasia. What are other common sites of metaplasia in the body? What can cause these cells to transform?

In patients with Barrett's oesophagus, various studies have shown a 30–60-fold increased risk of developing adenocarcinoma. The majority of adenocarcinomas arise from segments of Barrett's mucosa.

However, adenocarcinoma of the oesophagus remains a rare disease. The incidence of adenocarcinoma in Barrett's oesophagus is estimated to be between 0.5% and 1% per year.

> ☀ Bearing this in mind, what are your thoughts regarding screening programmes for patients with Barrett's oesophagus? What do the NICE guidelines recommend?

(h) Treatment options in advanced oesophageal cancer

- Palliative radiotherapy
- Palliative chemotherapy
- Stenting
- Referral to palliative care team/cancer nurse specialists

The initial assessment for surgical resection is usually CT of the chest and abdomen, and endoscopic ultrasound (EUS). The presence of either lung or liver metastases precludes curative resection. Patients who have symptoms indicative of either bone or brain metastases warrant a bone scan or brain CT respectively; otherwise, these tests are not routinely recommended. Radiographic criteria of resectability for patients without overt metastases vary, depending upon the location of the primary tumour. Each patient has a detailed treatment plan produced by the multidisciplinary team.

What symptoms might patients present with that indicate the presence of bone or brain metastases? *See* p. 206 and p. 127.

Unfortunately this gentleman had widespread metastases at the time of presentation and therefore is not a suitable candidate for surgical resection. His underlying ischaemic heart disease and COPD also make him an anaesthetic risk.

Radiotherapy or combined chemoradiotherapy has a role in the management of inoperable oesophageal cancer, both for the palliation of dysphagia, and to attempt to control local disease. However, sustained remission and improved survival are rarely achieved with either and they are not without risks. Severe systemic side effects may occur with chemotherapy and there is an increased risk of tracheo-oesophageal fistulae with external beam radiation.

Stenting of the stricture, either endoscopically or radiologically, may also be possible. This procedure can be performed purely for palliation of symptoms or in conjunction with chemo- or radiotherapy.

Support for both the patient and relatives is also an important area, and referral to the palliative care team and Macmillan nurses will be beneficial.

Web resources

- Improving outcomes in upper GI cancers: www.nice.org.uk
- Referral guidelines for suspected cancer: www.doh.gov.uk

Further reading

- British Society of Gastroenterology and British Association of Surgical Oncology (2002) *Guidelines for the Management of Oesophageal and Gastric Cancer*. British Society of Gastroenterology and British Association of Surgical Oncology, London.
- De Vita VT, Hellman S and Rosenberg SA (2001) *Principles and Practice of Oncology* (6e). Lippincott, Williams and Wilkins, Philadelphia.
- Gray MR, Donnelly RJ and Kingsnorth AN (1993) The role of smoking and alcohol in metaplasia and cancer risk in Barrett's columnar line oesophagus. *Gut.* **34**: 727.
- Souhami R and Tobias J (2003) *Cancer and its Management* (4e). Blackwell Science, Oxford.

18 A motorcycle accident

A 17-year-old boy is brought to the A&E department by ambulance 30 minutes after a road traffic accident. He was riding a motorcycle that was involved in a collision with a car. He sustained significant impact on his right side, with injuries to his arm and leg, chest wall, clavicle, and the side of his head. The patient is strapped to a long spine board, with in-line immobilisation of his cervical spine, and is receiving 15 litres of oxygen via a tight-fitting face-mask and reservoir bag.

(a) What are your priorities in the immediate assessment of this patient?

....

....

....

The patient has a respiratory rate of 30 breaths/min, a pulse of 120 beats/min, and a blood pressure of 92/54 mmHg.

(b) What is this likely to indicate?

....

....

....

(c) Which clinical measurements can assess the severity of this patient's condition?

....

....

....

(d) What is the immediate management in this case?

....

....

....

As part of the continuing assessment, the patient was found to have a GCS of 7/15 (E1, V2, M4), a BM reading of 5.6 mmol/l and his pupils were equal and reactive to light. The patient was given rapid sequence induction, intubated and ventilated.

As part of a secondary survey, the SHO notices that the patient has CSF and blood leaking from his nose.

(e) What is the diagnosis? What other signs might support this diagnosis?

....

....

....

(f) What are the indications to request a CT scan of the head?

....

....

....

(g) Should this patient have a CT scan of the head?

....

....

....

Twenty minutes later while waiting for the CT scan, the SHO notices that it is becoming harder to ventilate the patient. It is difficult to squeeze the bag and the pulse oximetry reading is showing 87% saturation despite 100% oxygen. On respiratory examination, the patient has reduced breath sounds in the right upper region, and his trachea is deviated to the left.

(h) What is the likely diagnosis, and how are the physical signs produced by the underlying pathology?

....

....

....

(i) Should you order further imaging to confirm the suspected diagnosis before treating the patient?

....

....

....

(j) What is the immediate treatment of this condition?

....

....

....

A police officer telephones the A&E department and asks the SHO if he has a patient who has been involved in a head-on collision. He says the motorcycle had been stolen and that the driver of the car involved in the RTA has significant injuries. He asks the SHO if he has anyone in the department who he suspects was involved in the accident.

(k) What actions should you take when asked by a police officer to disclose details over the phone?

....

....

....

(l) Are you obliged to release the patient's name and address to the police?

....

....

....

(m) Should you release clinical details?

....

....

....

(n) Who could you discuss your decisions with?

....

....

....

Key cases

- Haemorrhagic shock
- Head injury
- Pneumothorax

Clinical context

The patient with major trauma has the potential for many immediately life-threatening injuries. Their identification and management have been revolutionised by the development of a 'structured approach' to the trauma patient. This ABCDE concept is designed to 'identify and treat' the conditions that are most likely to kill the patient, in the order that they occur. A (airway) has to be assessed and an obstruction relieved. This takes priority over B (breathing), e.g. detect and treat tension pneumothorax before C (circulation), identify and manage haemorrhagic shock etc.

This concept is the basis of this scenario. However this is only the initial assessment of the trauma patient, and the beginning of what is often a long, difficult, and complicated management strategy.

(a) Initial assessment of any emergency/trauma

All emergency assessment of acutely ill patients relies on the fundamentals of the ABCDE approach. There are many courses for healthcare professionals operating at different levels, including basic life support (BLS), advanced life support (ALS), advanced trauma life support (ATLS) and MedicALS; however the basics remain the same and have been referred to elsewhere in this book.

The implementation of ATLS principles differs slightly from ALS. The leaning is more towards trauma; however the framework is useful in any situation where patients are acutely ill or deteriorating rapidly:

- primary survey and resuscitation (assess, resuscitate and monitor)
  - A: airway *and* cervical spine in-line immobilisation
  - B: breathing *and* oxygen delivery
  - C: circulation *and* haemorrhage control
  - D: disability (AVPU or GCS)
  - E: exposure
- secondary survey and immediate management
- definitive treatment
- transfer.

It is important to keep re-assessing ABCDE in the trauma patient, since further complications are likely to occur, depending on the severity of the trauma.

(b) Haemorrhagic/hypovolaemic shock

Inadequate delivery of oxygen and nutrients to tissues is now recognised as the definition of shock. Therefore, it is important to realise that shock can result from problems with airway and breathing as well as circulation. Examples include airway obstruction and tension pneumothorax.

The first step in the assessment of circulation in a trauma patient is to recognise shock. The consequences of shock for all organ systems can rapidly become disastrous and irreversible.

In trauma, the victim could have several types of shock (e.g. cardiogenic or neurogenic). However, almost all will have a hypovolaemic component; consequently this should be treated first, in particular by stopping and preventing further blood loss (e.g. external compression, fracture reduction).

Every trauma patient has a high probability of bleeding, leading to haemorrhagic/hypovolaemic shock. These may be obvious bleeds into the external environment, or occult internal bleeds. There is a system to classify blood loss according to the clinical signs (*see* below).

(c) Clinical signs of shock

The clinical signs that should be used to assess shock and monitor the response to resuscitation include:

- respiratory rate
- pulse rate
- pulse pressure/blood pressure
- urine output
- mental state and CNS examination.

Table 18.1 shows the American College of Surgeons' classification for signs of shock.

One way to remember these 'percentages of volume loss' is to think of the scores in tennis. At 15% there is a tachycardia, at 15% to 30% there is increased diastolic blood pressure (narrow pulse pressure), at 30% to 40% there is lowered systolic blood pressure, and if interventions do not prevent further tissue hypoxaemia, it's game over.

There are certain key things that need to be remembered. These include:

- tachypnoea – does not always mean a B problem
- tachycardia – is often the first sign in shock, but nearly all patients in A&E have tachycardia

Table 18.1 The American College of Surgeons' classification system for shock signs according to blood volume loss

	Class I	*Class II*	*Class III*	*Class IV*
% Blood volume loss	Up to 15%	15–30%	30–40%	>40%
Blood loss (ml) (70 kg adult)	Up to 750 ml	750–1500 ml	1500–2000 ml	>2000 ml
Clinical signs				
heart rate (beats/min)	<100	>100	>120	>140
systolic blood pressure	Normal	Normal	Decreased	Decreased
pulse pressure	Normal	Decreased	Decreased	Decreased
respiratory rate (breaths/min)	14–20	20–30	30–40	>35
urine output (ml/h)	>30	20–30	5–15	Negligible
mental status	Slightly anxious	Mildly anxious	Anxious and confused	Confused and coma

- approximately one-third of the circulating volume must be lost before a fall in BP is observed
- all classification systems represent a stylised version of reality. Patients do not fit neatly into these categories
- look at the clinical signs of shock; there is not just one
- in assessing shock it is vital to be wary of the physiological effects of age, training, drugs and temperature.

(d) Initial management

The initial management of 'C' consists of:

- haemorrhage control
- fluid resuscitation.

Haemorrhage control is the first step in managing 'C'. This may be achieved with, e.g. pressure, splinting, pelvic sling. Remember that the site of blood loss may not be initially apparent. Examples include blood loss in the chest, abdomen, retroperitoneal compartment and thigh. This may be detected clinically, on the chest X-ray, or on abdominal ultrasound.

Aggressive fluid resuscitation to correct tissue hypoperfusion within 24 hours of injury is associated with improved clinical outcomes. Initial volume expanders of choice are crystalloids, but there is no evidence to suggest that colloid expanders are any better or worse in this function. Blood and blood products may also be used in patients with severe blood loss.

When using crystalloids an initial infusion of 1–2 litres is recommended, followed by an infusion of volume at a 3:1 ratio of crystalloid: blood volume lost. Some papers state that a ratio as high as 10:1 is appropriate in continued blood loss, due to capillary leakage and reduced plasma oncotic pressure.

The debate will continue to rage over the use of colloid solutions. Colloid solutions have the theoretical advantage of raising the plasma oncotic pressure, causing fluid shift from the interstitial space into the intravascular space. This theoretically minimises the total fluid volume of resuscitation, and thereby reduces the likelihood of tissue oedema. There have been studies showing colloid or crystalloid to be superior to one another, but after systematic review, no benefit was shown in reducing mortality or pulmonary oedema. This, accompanied by the higher cost of colloids, leads to the recommendation that crystalloids should be used for initial fluid resuscitation.

In short, if a patient is severely shocked, the protein in colloid solutions will be of no benefit.

> Use this opportunity to revisit the fluid distribution within the body compartments (*see* p. 105). How do different classes of fluid affect this balance?

> Use this opportunity to think about the other management issues in shock. What are the appropriate investigations involved? When is anticoagulation indicated?

> It is vitally important to be wary with the terminology used in shock. What are the definitions of haemodynamically normal, stable and unstable? How do these definitions relate to treatment options?

(e) Base of skull fracture

Clinically, the base of the skull lies on a line joining the corner of the eye to the mastoid process. The signs of a fracture occur along this line, which is a useful aide mémoire.

Signs that indicate a base of skull fracture include:

- *fluid from the ears/nose*: this can be colourless with or without blood (CSF otorrhoea/rhinorrhoea with or without blood)
- *racoon eyes*: black eyes with no associated damage around the eye
- *scleral/retinal haemorrhage*
- *loss of hearing in one or both ears*
- *Battle's sign*: bruising over the mastoid behind one/both ears
- *penetrating injury signs*, or visible trauma to the skull.

Battle's sign, racoon eyes and CSF otorrhoea/rhinorrhoea are indicative of basal skull fracture, and are particularly important when considering airway adjuncts or instrumentation of the nasopharynx. Basal skull fracture is a contraindication to inserting either a nasopharyngeal airway or nasogastric tube.

(f) (g) Indications for a CT head scan

With the advent of spiral CT scanning, it is tempting to consider scanning every patient to rule out serious injury. However, CT scans are not without risk, and unnecessary exposure of patients to large radiation doses should be avoided.

Additionally, care in the transfer of trauma patients is vital. Monitoring must be kept *in situ*, and particular attention must be paid to observing the patient while they are in the scanner, which can be difficult.

The National Institute for Clinical Excellence (NICE) published guidelines in 2003 for referral for a CT head scan. Patients considered suitable for a CT scan include those who have sustained a head injury and any of the following signs:

- GCS <13 at any point since the injury
- GCS of 13 or 14 at 2 h after the injury
- suspected open or depressed skull fracture
- any sign of basal skull fracture (mentioned earlier)
- post-traumatic seizure
- focal neurological deficit
- more than one episode of vomiting
- amnesia for greater than 30 minutes of events before impact
- age >65 years
- coagulopathy: bleeding diathesis or warfarin treatment.

If the patient has experienced some loss of consciousness or amnesia, and the mechanism of injury is regarded as dangerous (e.g. pedestrian struck by vehicle, fall greater than 1 metre, occupant ejected from vehicle in RTA) then a CT scan should be requested.

This patient has two of the criteria for referral. He currently has a GCS <13/15, and he has a suspected skull fracture; it is not known if the suspected fracture is depressed or open.

> Use this opportunity to revisit the possible consequences of a head injury. You should be familiar with the structures involved and common signs of subdural haemorrhage, subarachnoid haemorrhage and raised intracranial pressure. How are cerebral perfusion pressure (CPP) and cerebral blood flow regulated? What are the difficulties in maintaining CPP while not increasing bleeding elsewhere?

(h) (i) Tension pneumothorax

A 'B' problem has developed. This demonstrates the need to continually re-assess ABCDE.

- The signs given would indicate a right-sided tension pneumothorax.

This is the classical presentation of a tension pneumothorax, which may develop some time after the initial injury. Injury to the visceral pleura is thought to act as a one-way valve, allowing air into the pleural space (and not out into the atmosphere) on expiration. The result is an expanding air mass, causing pressure on the ipsilateral lung and eventually the mediastinum. Correspondingly, breath sounds are reduced, chest expansion is reduced on the affected side (which may be fixed and hyperinflated), and the affected side is hyper-resonant to percussion.

The eventual result is mediastinal shift, the trachea is deviated away from the side of the pneumothorax; compression of the vena cava and right heart structures causes decreased diastolic filling and cardiac output. This can lead to pulseless electrical activity (PEA) and eventually asystole. There is also shunting of blood to underventilated areas of lung, causing a ventilation–perfusion mismatch. The result is hypoxaemia, acidosis, and further impairment of tissue oxygenation.

> Use this opportunity to revisit the anatomy and physiology of the lungs and mediastinal structures. You should be able to relate the physiological effects outlined above to the underlying structures. Why is blood shunted to underventilated areas of the lung?

Approximately 5% of multiple trauma patients have pneumothoraces. Furthermore, a common cause for tension pneumothorax is positive pressure ventilation on a background of chest injury. In this scenario, right-sided chest injury with a fractured clavicle is likely to indicate underlying lung injury.

A tension pneumothorax causes rapid deterioration in a patient's clinical condition; arranging a chest X-ray would delay treatment with possible fatal repercussions. Thus the immediate management is based on the clinical diagnosis.

(j) Treatment of tension pneumothorax

This is treated by:

- needle decompression (needle thoracostomy)
- followed by insertion of a chest drain (tube thoracostomy).

Needle decompression with a large-bore cannula, or other commercially manufactured device is needed immediately. Historically the site has been the mid-clavicular line in the second intercostal space, on the upper edge of the third rib; however recent reports have highlighted the inability to penetrate the parietal pleura in patients with thick muscle, or excessive subcutaneous tissue.

The American College of Surgeons has recommended use of the anterior axillary line in the fourth or fifth intercostal space (the position for insertion of a chest drain). ATLS guidelines suggest the best position is just anterior to the mid-axillary line. Currently, either position will be acceptable until further guidelines are published.

Points to remember are that needle decompression converts a tension pneumothorax into a simple pneumothorax. Thus patients still need a chest drain. Additionally, before inserting a chest drain, it is important to have i.v. access, since major trauma patients will invariably have coexistent haemothoraces.

(k) Disclosure and confidentiality

Confidentiality is an integral part of all medical interactions. It is underpinned by almost all general ethical principles, and is vital to maintain the trust between doctors and patients. Breaches of confidentiality are taken very seriously by the statutory governing bodies (e.g. GMC). All doctors need to be aware of the situations when they are legally obliged to breach confidentiality.

> ☀ How do the general ethical principles of beneficence, non-maleficence, autonomy and justice apply to the absolute precedence of confidentiality? Equally, how can they be used to justify disclosure in the situations outlined below?

These include:

- where a person constitutes a real risk to themselves or others
- where asked to by a court of law
- when statutorily obliged (*see* below).

It is advisable to be wary in these situations; not everybody is concerned with the patient's best interests and they may be trying to gain information unlawfully. Furthermore a person making a call may not be who they say they are. Therefore sensible precautions include:

- write down the caller's name, rank and police station
- ask the caller for information regarding the request; why are they asking for information? What is the crime under investigation?
- request a crime scene number
- say you will phone back and hang up the receiver
- find out if there is a patient fitting the description in your department
- discuss the matter with a senior doctor
- check the phone number given to you from an independent source, and then phone the police back.

(Hope *et al.*, 2003)

(l) Statutory disclosure

The Road Traffic Act of 1988 requires disclosure of information in cases where this disclosure could assist in identifying a driver alleged to have committed a traffic offence.

(m) Disclosure of clinical details

Any disclosure of information regarding a patient should be considered carefully, and should be kept to the minimum to fulfil requirements. In this scenario, clinical details are not necessary to identify the driver; therefore this information should not be released.

(n) Help with medico-legal problems

It is always advisable to seek counsel from somebody more experienced in these situations, and your defence union can be an invaluable source of medico-legal help. People who may be able to help include:

- senior doctors
- peers
- Medical Defence Union
- Medical Protection Society.

Web resources

- Best Evidence in Emergency Medicine: www.best bets.org
- Ethics link: www.ovid.bma.org.uk
- Resuscitation Council: www.resus.org.uk

Further reading

- Advanced Life Support Group (2000) *Acute Medical Emergencies: the practical approach*. BMJ Books, London.
- American College of Surgeons (1997) *Advanced Trauma Life Support (ATLS) Manual* (7e). The American College of Surgeons, Chicago.
- Driscoll P, Skinner D and Earlham R (eds) (2000) *ABC of Major Trauma* (3e). BMJ Publications, London.
- Gwinnutt CL and Driscoll PA (2003) *Trauma Resuscitation: the team approach*. Bios Scientific Publishers, Oxford.
- Hope T, Savulescu J and Hendrick J (2003) *Medical Ethics and Law: The Core Curriculum*. Churchill Livingston, London, p. 92.

19 An Asian woman with blurred vision

Mrs Singh is a 61-year-old Asian woman who presents to her GP complaining of 'blurry' vision. She has noticed a gradual loss of clarity particularly in brightly lit environments, and complains that she has problems in seeing objects that are far away. She is overweight, with a BMI of 30, and has a sedentary lifestyle. She has had impaired glucose regulation for 5 years, for which she has received lifestyle and dietary advice from her GP.

(a) What key symptoms are important to ascertain in an ophthalmic history?

....

....

....

(b) What are the major components of the eye examination?

....

....

....

After the GP has examined her eyes, he looks at her computer records and notices that she did not attend her last review. He asks her to return to the practice the following week to have some blood tests. At the same time he arranges for her to see the community optometrist.

(c) What is the classification for diagnosing impaired glucose regulation?

....

....

....

(d) What are the complications associated with impaired glucose regulation?

....

....

....

On reviewing the results, her GP notes that her HbA_{1c} is 8.2%, random serum cholesterol is 6.3 mmol/l and blood pressure is 162/95 mmHg. The result of her 2-hour oral glucose tolerance test was 12 mmol/l. He tells Mrs Singh that her control over her sugar levels has worsened and that he would like to send her to a review clinic at the local hospital.

(e) What are the results likely to indicate?

....

....

....

(f) What symptoms might indicate worsening glycaemic control?

....

....

....

(g) What medication might he consider prescribing?

....
....
....

(h) How is she likely to be reviewed in secondary care?

....
....
....

On visiting the optometrist, Mrs Singh is found to have early stage bilateral cataracts and hence ophthalmoscopy was difficult. However, there was the suspicion of pre-proliferative diabetic retinopathy. The optometrist decides that routine referral to the hospital ophthalmology department is appropriate.

(i) Describe the components of diabetic retinopathy and their pathophysiology.

....
....
....

(j) How are cataracts classified?

....
....
....

(k) What are the risk factors for cataracts?

....
....
....

After a considerable delay she is seen in the hospital by the consultant ophthalmologist, who schedules her for surgery. However, there is a long waiting list.

(l) What are the indications for cataract surgery?

....
....
....

(m) While she is waiting, what help is available to her?

....
....
....

(n) How are patients registered partially sighted or blind?

....
....
....

Key cases

- Type 2 diabetes
- Cataracts
- Diabetic retinopathy
- Visual impairment

Clinical context

There are over 800,000 people with diagnosed type 2 diabetes in England and Wales, with an estimated 1,000,000 undiagnosed cases. This is often because the levels of hyperglycaemia may not be high enough to cause symptoms. Type 2 diabetes often follows a period of impaired glucose regulation, which may be associated with dyslipidaemia, hypertension and obesity, now recognised as the metabolic syndrome. Type 2 diabetes predisposes to significant micro-vascular and macrovascular disease. Lifestyle change, optimal glycaemic control, and risk factor modification remain the most effective preventative and treatment measures.

Impaired vision and failing eyesight are important issues to the health and well-being of many people. In the UK, cataracts remain the most common cause of visual impairment in the elderly. Cataract extraction continues to be one of the most common and successful surgical procedures, largely due to the development of small-incision surgery and faster rehabilitation. Diabetes predisposes to the early development of both cataracts and retinopathy, and visual impairment is frequently a feature of the disease. This scenario uses the backdrop of type 2 diabetes to explore visual impairment, specifically cataracts and diabetic retinopathy.

(a) History in visual problems

The huge diversity of eye diseases commonly manifest with a combination of a relatively small number of symptoms. One of the most common symptoms is visual loss, which may be acute or chronic. History and examination are directed at determining the level of visual impairment and finding the cause.

There are several pertinent points to elucidate and include in the history, which are specific to the eye. Additionally, it is important to remember that systemic diseases such as hypertension, diabetes mellitus, and AIDS can present with ocular symptoms and/or signs; hence they may be diagnosed by a relevant history and examination of the eyes.

The symptoms that should be asked about in any ophthalmological history include:

- visual loss
- diplopia
- red eye
- floaters and flashing lights.

Points to consider in a history of visual loss include:

- *pre-existing refractive error*: diabetic patients can have wild refractive changes due to abnormal blood glucose levels
- *one or both eyes*: both eyes implies systemic pathology, whereas one eye is more suggestive of ocular pathology
- *gradual loss of vision versus acute loss*: gradual loss implies chronic pathologies such as cataract or retinopathy; acute visual loss is always an emergency, and is usually traumatic or vascular in origin
- *painful versus painless eye*: e.g. painful acute glaucoma
- *nature of the visual loss*: central loss suggests macular pathology; however this may be more readily revealed on examination
- *red eye*: allergic or infective conjunctivitis, acute glaucoma or iritis
- *haloes*: glaucoma
- *flashes and floaters*: vitreous detachment. Vitreous detachment does not normally affect visual acuity unless a floater is in front of the macula
- *trauma*.

Previous medical conditions that should be asked about include:

- diabetes mellitus
- vascular pathology: peripheral vascular disease, ischaemic heart disease, stroke
- hypertension
- previous ophthalmic surgery
- multiple sclerosis.

(b) Eye examination

It is important to become proficient at eye examination. This relies on practice. There are essential components that can be completed by most doctors, and other more specialised tests that are usually performed by ophthalmologists or optometrists.

The key points on examination are:

- *inspection of the external appearance*: this should be done with adequate lighting. Work from outside the eye inwards, examining for any obvious deviation, strabismus, ptosis, swellings, bruising, haemorrhage, inflammation, discharge, gross loss of corneal clarity or difference in pupil size

> Use this opportunity to revise the external structures of the eye. You should be familiar with the blood supply and lymphatic drainage. Which lymph nodes should be examined if viral conjunctival infection is suspected?

- *visual acuity*: a Snellen chart should be used at 6 m. If the patient cannot read the first line of the Snellen chart, use picture or shape charts. If the patient cannot see these, can they count fingers, discern movement, or discriminate between light and dark?

The interpretation of a Snellen chart is very important. Most people know that 6/6 vision is good vision. If x/y equates to the interpretation value, x is the distance from the chart (i.e. 6 m), y is the distance from which a 'normal' person can see that letter.

- *visual fields*: visual field examination is important since the pattern of visual loss (e.g. homonymous or bitemporal hemianopia or quadrantanopia) can suggest particular pathologies. Each eye should be systematically tested with a white pin. If an abnormality is found in one quadrant then the search should be refined further

> You should be familiar with the route of the visual pathways and causes of visual field loss. What type of visual field loss is commonly produced by pituitary gland enlargement? How is it possible to distinguish between neglect and visual field defects?

- *cranial nerve function*: cranial nerves II, III, IV, VI should be tested. Testing of the optic nerve (II) includes visual acuity, visual fields, direct and consensual pupil responses to light and accommodation, and inspecting the fundus (particularly the optic disc). Cranial nerves III, IV and VI are tested together by examining all of the eye movements

> Use this opportunity to revise the ocular muscles. Which nerves supply the superior oblique, and lateral rectus muscles? Which nerves carry the afferent and efferent pathways for pupil and lens control?

- *fundoscopy including examination of the red-reflex*: fundoscopy is used to detect abnormalities, progressing from the front of the eye to the retina. The red-reflex is present if light is reflected by the retina. The commonest cause of an absent red-reflex is a cataract. However, occasionally a concentric ring of red-reflex can be present around the cataract. Fundoscopy is dreaded by many. This is usually due to poor teaching, lack of practice, and difficulty in visualising the fundus through an inadequately dilated pupil

> Refresh your technique of fundoscopy. Take this opportunity to revise the structures of the retina that are visible on fundoscopy. What are the positions and significance of the macula and optic disc?

- *slit lamp examination if possible*: most doctors will never use a slit lamp. However, slit lamps enable binocular examination of the entire retina when suitably trained in the use of a Volk lens. Additionally, direct intra-ocular pressure can be measured using a Perkins device. Modern slit lamps allow digital photography, which is very useful in the sequential assessment of progressive conditions such as diabetic retinopathy.

(c) Classification of impaired glucose regulation

Impaired glucose regulation is a metabolic state between normal glucose regulation and overt diabetes. There are two distinct forms of impaired glucose regulation, which can co-exist:

- *impaired glucose tolerance* (IGT) is present in patients where blood glucose levels do not meet the criteria for diabetes, but are too high to be called normal (fasting plasma glucose < 7.0 mmol/l and oral glucose tolerance test (OGTT) > 7.8 mmol/l but < 11.1 mmol/l)
- *impaired fasting glycaemia* (IFG) is present in patients whose fasting glucose level is below the diagnostic level for diabetes but too high to be considered normal (> 6.1 mmol/l; < 7.0 mmol/l).

IGT and IFG are different abnormalities of glucose regulation. IGT represents peripheral insulin resistance after eating, whereas IFG is caused by increased hepatic glucose output in the fasting state and defective insulin secretion.

IGT is more common than IFG, with IGT more common in women, and IFG more common in men. IGT becomes more common with increasing old age, whereas the prevalence of IFG levels out in middle age.

(d) Complications of impaired glucose regulation

The complications of impaired glucose regulation include:

- progression to diabetes
- development of microvascular and macrovascular disease.

IGT and IFG are associated with a significantly increased risk of developing diabetes, microvascular, and macrovascular disease, especially where both are present. A significant proportion of people with type 2 diabetes will have had IGT or IFG before the onset of their disease.

(e) Progression to diabetes

The blood results indicate progression to type 2 diabetes, and probably the development of the metabolic syndrome, as shown by the additional presence of dyslipidaemia, obesity and hypertension.

The diagnosis of diabetes is a straightforward one, and follows the WHO guidelines, which are:

- random plasma glucose >11.1 mmol/l accompanied by typical symptoms (polyuria, polydipsia etc)
- fasting plasma glucose >7.0 mmol/l
- post-2-hour OGTT value of >11.1 mmol/l.

> Use this opportunity to review the metabolic syndrome. What are the components? What are the risk factors? How can the metabolic syndrome be prevented? What are the cardiovascular risks?

(f) Symptoms of diabetes

Poorly educated patients may not be aware of the symptoms of poor glycaemic control. It is important to ask about:

- polyuria
- polydipsia, particularly drinking water at night
- nocturia
- infections, particularly candidal infection and urinary tract infections in women
- blurred vision
- weakness, abdominal pain, generalised aches
- anorexia and nausea
- tiredness.

(g) Drugs commonly used in type 2 diabetes

The priorities in management are to improve glycaemic control and treat patients' risk factors for developing microvascular and macrovascular complications. The keystone of management remains lifestyle modification. In this scenario, the medications that the GP would want to consider include:

- oral hypoglycaemics
- a statin (or fibrates if triglycerides are disproportionately raised)
- antihypertensives: probably an ACE inhibitor, calcium channel blocker or thiazide diuretic
- antiplatelet therapy (aspirin or clopidogrel) since these patients are at high risk of atherosclerosis, ischaemic heart disease, and stroke.

In new-onset type 2 diabetes, the most suitable drugs to lower plasma glucose would be oral hypoglycaemics. These work in one of three ways; firstly by increasing insulin secretion, secondly by targeting insulin resistance, and thirdly by reducing glucose absorption from the intestine.

Sulphonylureas (e.g. gliclazide) and the newer meglitinides (e.g. nateglinide) are insulin secretagogues that increase insulin secretion by pancreatic β-cells. They are useful in patients who have some remaining pancreatic function. They have the disadvantage of causing weight gain.

The biguanide metformin increases insulin-stimulated transport from the circulation into cells. It also reduces hepatic gluconeogenesis. These actions of metformin help to reduce blood glucose levels and reduce stress on pancreatic β-cells. Metformin does not increase insulin secretion and has been shown to promote weight loss. This would probably be a good choice of drug for the patient in the scenario.

Rosiglitazone and pioglitazone also target insulin resistance but through a different mechanism. These drugs are peroxisome proliferator-activated receptor-gamma (PPAR) agonists. PPAR receptors are found in tissues important for insulin action such as adipose tissue, skeletal muscle, and liver.

Acarbose is an α-glucosidase inhibitor that prevents digestion of carbohydrates. Acarbose is only effective if it is taken at the same time as food.

(h) Diabetic review clinic

Review can be in primary and/or secondary care. Most GP-led diabetes clinics and hospital diabetes clinics will have an agreed protocol for care, and a proforma for initial and annual assessment.

> How are the standards for diabetes care determined? How is the National Service Framework (NSF) for diabetes implemented in both primary and secondary care?

Initial and annual assessment should include:

- *diagnosis and co-morbidity*
- *diabetic and other medication review*
- *review of self-monitoring results*
- *weight and BMI* (+/– waist-to-hip ratio)
- *urinalysis*: blood, glucose, ketones and especially protein for the presence of microalbuminuria
- *assessment of glycaemic control*: HbA_{1c}, BM diary, hypoglycaemic episodes per week
- *eye checks*: visual acuity and retinal screening
- *blood pressure and renal profile*: U&E, albumin creatinine ratio (ACR) and cardiovascular risk
- *lipids/LFTs*: cholesterol, triglycerides (TGs), HDL, LDL
- *foot check*: pulses, monofilament neuropathy check, ulcers
- *injection site checks* for lipodermatosclerosis
- *alcohol and smoking.*

> Use this opportunity to revise the main complications of diabetes, relating them to the components of the diabetic review.

(i) Diabetic retinopathy

Retinopathy is a common microvascular complication amongst diabetics, and hence regular screening is needed. This occurs both in the community and in hospital.

The pathogenesis of retinopathy involves damage to the microvasculature of the retinal vessels. Abnormal retinal blood flow leads to vascular occlusion and leakage. Occlusion, or retinal hypoxaemia leads to neovascularisation (new-vessel formation). These vessels are tortuous and friable, and are therefore more likely to rupture causing vitreous haemorrhage. New vessels can grow into the vitreous, which can subsequently cause retinal detachment.

Occlusion of the blood vessels causes ischaemia, and hence death of nerve endings. This is clinically evident as cotton wool spots. Neovascularisation as well as the abnormal blood flow within the retinal vessels causes leakage. High pressure and vessel wall weakness are responsible for microaneurysm formation (dots). These aneurysms can rupture causing flame shaped or superficial retinal haemorrhages, or blot (deep in the retina) haemorrhages. As the blood leaks out from the ruptured vessels, so does lipoprotein, resulting in exudates.

Classification of diabetic retinopathy

- *Background retinopathy*: dots, blots, exudates and microaneurysms
- *Pre-proliferative*: cotton wool spots, venous beading and looping
- *Proliferative*: neovascularisation of the disc and elsewhere

- *Maculopathy*: oedema at the macula
- *Advanced disease*: vitreous haemorrhage and retinal detatchment

See Figure 19.1.

> You should be familiar with the treatment options for diabetic retinopathy. What are the current guidelines on screening? What are the indications for prophylactic laser treatment in pre-proliferative retinopathy?

It is important to remember that the primary treatment for all diabetic complications remains good glycaemic control.

(j) Classification of cataracts

Cataracts remain the most common cause of blindness worldwide and the most common cause of visual loss in the elderly. The problem lies within the lens; the anatomy is shown in Figure 19.2. The lens is an isolated structure constructed of specialised epithelial cells encased in an elastic capsule. The majority of the lens consists of lens fibres (elongated lens epithelial cells that have lost their nuclei and many of their organelles). Between the capsule and the outermost layer of lens fibres is a single layer of epithelial cells. These metabolically active lens cells divide, to create new lens fibres. The oldest lens fibres remain in the centre of the lens forming the 'nucleus' of the lens. New lens fibres are laid down around this 'nucleus'. The lens capsule is an elastic basement membrane secreted by the lens epithelial cells that surround the cells of the lens.

Classification of cataracts depends on the position of the opacity within the lens. There are three categories of cataract:

- *nuclear*: within the nucleus of the lens – common in the elderly
- *cortical*: localised and lying within the visual axis
- *subcapsular*: just deep to the lens capsule – common in diabetics, those on steroids, and following trauma.

It is worth remembering that these types of cataract can co-exist in one lens.

> Use this opportunity to revise common surgical techniques for cataracts. What are the associated complications?

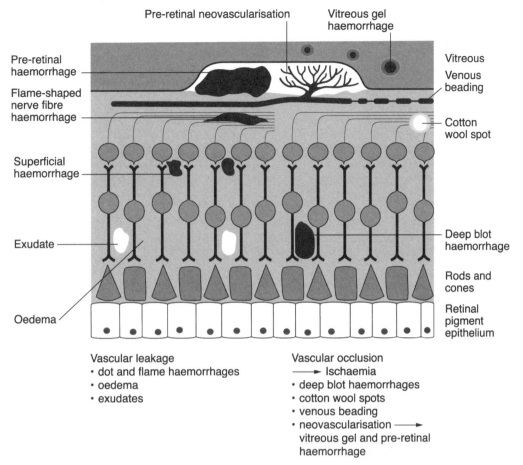

Figure 19.1 Diabetic retinopathy. (Reprinted from Batterbury M and Bowling B (2002) *Ophthalmology: an illustrated colour text*, Figure 1, p. 50, with permission from Elsevier.)

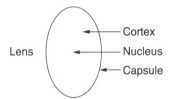

Figure 19.2 Cataracts.

(k) Risk factors for cataracts

The causes of cataracts are multifactorial. Age remains the most important; however, there are a number of other risk factors including:

- female sex
- diabetes mellitus
- UV light
- corticosteroid treatment
- nutrition and socio-economic status
- lifestyle: smoking and alcohol.

(Royal College of Ophthalmologists, 2004)

Although the risk factors for cataracts are established, there is no proven medical treatment. Surgical removal of the lens is still the only way to improve vision.

(l) Indications for cataract surgery

The suitability of a patient for cataract surgery should involve the assessment of:

- visual disability (this is more important than absolute visual impairment)
- the extent of the lens opacification
- the presence of co-morbid eye pathology (e.g. retinopathy), and deciding on the visual potential of the eye
- whether cataract surgery is likely to benefit the patient.

The Royal College of Ophthalmologists states that cataract surgery should be done whenever:

'There is sufficient cataract to limit the patient's quality of life, ability to work or drive, irrespective of the Snellen acuity, and the patient wishes to consider surgery (having received advice about the likely benefit).'
(Royal College of Ophthalmologists, 2004)

Apart from the above, there may be other indications for cataract surgery, for example to aid the treatment and monitoring of retinal disease (e.g. laser treatment for proliferative diabetic retinopathy).

> What are the issues surrounding waiting lists? How should patients' needs be assessed? What are the prioritisation scoring systems used? What governmental initiatives have been aimed at reducing waiting times?

(m) Help for partially sighted patients

The treatment of choice for cataracts is surgical. However it is important to realise that partially sighted or blind patients may benefit from a number of other interventions such as guide dogs, talking books, and home help. Elderly patients may have multiple sensory defects (e.g. sight, hearing, proprioception), and to restore one of these has a dramatic, beneficial effect on the patient.

- *Conservative*: in some very elderly patients with many co-morbidities this may be the appropriate choice.
- *Surgical*: the treatment of choice (phacoemulsification versus extracapsular cataract extraction).
- *Psychological*: the adjustment in coming to terms with visual impairment. Help may be achieved through counselling. It is important to look for concurrent psychological disorders, which may be amenable to treatment (i.e. depression due to an inability to leave the house).
- *Social*: extremely important with regards to the visually impaired. There are many ways to improve the functionality of day-to-day objects

and actions through occupational therapists. Disability living allowance and other benefits can be provided through a social worker (*see* p. 130).

(n) Registration of partial sight or blindness

Partially sighted or blind patients are registered by the local authority. This requires assessment by a consultant ophthalmologist ($<6/12$ – impaired vision, $<6/60$ – 'legal' blindness). The assessment also considers visual field loss.

Registration provides certain concessions and access to resources e.g. talking books. The Royal National Institute for the Blind (RNIB) – a registered charity – will advise on guide dogs in relevant cases.

Web resources

- Blood glucose management in type 2 diabetes: www.prodigy.nhs.uk
- Guidelines on diabetes management: www.sign.ac.uk
- Royal College of Ophthalmologists (2004) Cataract Surgery Guidelines: www.rcophth.ac.uk

Further reading

- Alberti KG and Zimmet PZ (1998) Definition, diagnosis and classification of diabetes mellitus and its complications. Part 1: diagnosis and classification of diabetes mellitus provisional report of a WHO consultation. *Diabetic Medicine*. 15: 539.
- Asbell PA, Dualan I, Mindel J *et al.* (2005) Age-related cataract. *Lancet*. 365: 599.
- Batterbury M and Bowling B (2002) *Ophthalmology: an illustrated colour text*. Churchill Livingstone, London.
- Eckel RH, Grundy SM and Zimmet PZ (2005) The metabolic syndrome. *Lancet*. 365: 1415.
- Elkington A and Khaw P (2002) *ABC of Eyes*. BMJ Publications, London.

20 A patient with calf pain

Amanda is a 32-year-old fitness trainer who goes to her GP on Monday morning after a weekend away with friends. She complains of pain and swelling in her left calf that developed over the weekend. She has not visited the surgery for over 2 years. Her only medication is the combined oral contraceptive pill, which she receives on repeat prescription. The only other point her GP notes from her practice record is the fact that she is a smoker.

(a) What further questions would he ask?

....

....

....

On physical examination her left calf is swollen and is mildly tender to palpation. Her GP wants to rule out a deep venous thrombosis (DVT), and decides to send her to the new nurse-led walk-in DVT centre at the local hospital for appropriate investigation.

(b) What advantages might a specific DVT walk-in service offer to both patients and doctors?

....

....

....

(c) How will she be assessed at the hospital?

....

....

....

The tests prove positive and she is started on suitable treatment.

(d) What are the management principles?

....

....

....

(e) How should her response to treatment be monitored?

....

....

....

Amanda makes a good recovery. Two years later she is on her honeymoon in Port Elizabeth, South Africa and notices that she's becoming increasingly breathless on exertion. Her husband insists that she attend the local hospital to get herself checked out. The consultant orders a CXR, an ECG and ABG sample (shown below).

The CXR is reported as normal.
The ABG sample is as follows:

pH	7.5
PaO_2	6.8 kPa
$PaCO_2$	3.6 kPa
HCO_3^-	27 mmol/l
Base excess	2

The ECG is shown in Figure 20.1.

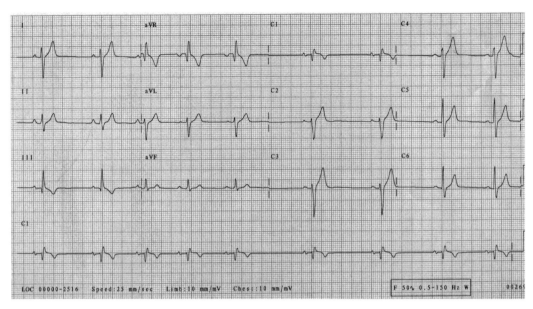

Figure 20.1 ECG recorded from the patient.

(f) Comment on the results of her investigations. Do they fit with the clinical presentation?

....

....

....

(g) Are there any other investigations that might help confirm your diagnosis?

....

....

....

(h) What other clinical features might help confirm or refute your diagnosis?

....

....

....

> The diagnosis is confirmed by subsequent investigations and the consultant discusses the treatment options. Amanda is given the choice between alternatives. The consultant suggests that she be given an infusion of alteplase.

(i) What therapeutic alternatives would be offered to Amanda and how might they relate to her case?

....

....

....

> On returning to the UK Amanda and her husband are worried. The ordeal on their honeymoon has shaken them up. They go to visit Amanda's GP with articles printed from the internet. They are worried about 'clotting defects', and the risks of thrombosis and its treatment during pregnancy.

(j) What are the key points her GP would want to discuss regarding thrombosis in pregnancy?

....

....

....

(k) Which investigations form the basis of a 'thrombophilia screen'?

....

....

....

(l) What needs to be considered before testing?

....

....

....

Key cases

- Deep venous thrombosis (DVT)
- Pulmonary embolism (PE)
- Thrombophilia

Clinical context

The incidence of DVT is 1.6/1000 of the population and is increasing. The number of patients that will develop a subsequent pulmonary embolus remains unknown. Thus DVT is a common medical condition that can produce a potentially life-threatening sequel.

The diagnosis of both of these conditions can be difficult and relies on a high index of suspicion and relevant investigations. This scenario describes the causes, assessment, investigation, and management of both DVT and PE. Furthermore, the important issues of DVT prevention, and DVT/ PE in pregnancy are discussed.

Deep venous thrombosis (DVT)

It is important not to attribute all painful swollen legs to venous thromboses. A thorough history should either establish the likelihood of DVT, including risk factors, or aim to provide an alternative diagnosis.

The differential diagnoses include:

- cellulitis
- superficial thrombophlebitis
- ruptured Baker's cyst
- muscle haematoma
- dependent oedema
- post-thrombotic syndrome
- lymphatic obstruction
- fracture
- compression of major vein.

DVT results from a complex series of events involving coagulation factors, platelets, red blood cells and the vessel wall. The components of Virchow's triad can be used to predict the risk factors for developing thrombosis and its pathogenesis:

- venous stasis
- hypercoagulability
- vessel wall disease.

Venous stasis

- Immobility (travel/bedridden/paralysis/paresis or plaster immobilisation)
- Recent surgery or trauma (which can also cause hypercoagulability)

- Abdominal or pelvic malignancy, or pregnant uterus compressing proximal vessels
- Varicose veins
- Cardiac failure

Hypercoagulability

There are many causes of hypercoagulability, including:

- Pregnancy: stasis and increased clotting factors
- Oral contraceptive pill (OCP) or hormone replacement therapy (HRT): increased clotting factors
- Ongoing infection and inflammation: thrombocytosis
- Nephrotic syndrome: reduced antithrombin III levels
- Malignancy
- Dehydration: including DKA.

A positive family history or previous history of DVT or PE may suggest an inherited or acquired thrombophilic state:

- factor V Leiden (3–5% of western population)
- antithrombin III deficiency
- protein C deficiency
- protein S deficiency
- antiphospholipid syndrome.

Vessel wall disease

- Congenital defects
- Trauma

> 🔆 Use this opportunity to revisit the mechanisms of haemostasis. How are the normal coagulation mechanisms physiologically regulated to prevent unchecked thrombus formation in vessels? How do these regulatory mechanisms relate to the thrombophilic states listed above?

(a) Specific points in the history

Provide clues to an alternative diagnosis:

- activities on holiday. Any history of trauma? Was the onset acute as in a torn muscle?
- any cuts, possible focus of infection, or fever?
- is there any history of arthritis or preceding swelling of the knee that might suggest a Baker's cyst?

Identify risk factors for thrombosis:

- *mode of transport and duration of journey*: to assess the likelihood of any significant immobility
- *possibility of pregnancy*: she takes the OCP, but has she been taking it? When was her last menstrual period?
- *previous or family history of DVT/PE* that might suggest a thrombophilic state
- *possibility of malignancy*: weight loss, muscle wasting, muscle weakness, systemic symptoms such as fever, night sweats, bruising, bleeding
- *any symptoms of infection*: respiratory, genito-urinary or GI symptoms.

In older patients a history of stroke, cardiac failure, dehydration, drug history and recent surgery should be sought.

> Think of a patient you have seen with knee swelling. How would the history be altered if the clinical suspicion favoured the alternative diagnoses listed above?

(b) DVT walk-in service

The complications of DVT can be life threatening; therefore a range of investigations are needed to confirm or refute the diagnosis. In the past a lengthy hospital visit was followed by admission for intravenous heparin and venography. Now a trained team provides rapid assessment for patients with suspected DVT. Most patients are successfully managed in the community. Only those with proximal DVTs and risk of embolism are admitted to hospital.

Advantages of a dedicated DVT walk-in centre include:

- highly trained specialist nurses provide evidence-based care. Doctors can see other cases
- reduction in hospital admissions
- they alleviate patients' anxiety, since they are managed in a calmer (non-MAU) environment
- the service can be patient focused and, where possible, appointments can be tailored to patients' daily commitments
- GPs can make a same-day referral
- diagnosis can be streamlined and a patient can be assessed and appropriately treated within a few hours, according to protocol
- the majority of patients with confirmed DVT can be treated and monitored as outpatients.

> What is the concept of enhanced-level services within primary care? What more specialised services need to be in place for effective anticoagulation monitoring in primary care? What other examples are there of enhanced-level services? Who funds these services?

(c) Assessment of DVT

Whether assessment is at a dedicated walk-in centre or an MAU, the format is generally the same and relies on a combination of:

- pretest clinical probability scoring system for DVT
- D-dimer assay
- compression or duplex ultrasonography.

Physical examination and risk assessment scoring system

It is important to remember that clinical examination is not a reliable way to diagnose DVT. The differential diagnoses are extensive, and difficulties arise because DVT can complicate many of these conditions. Further investigation is needed; however key features in the physical examination that suggest DVT include:

- calf warmth and erythema
- localised tenderness over the deep veins (anterior and posterior tibial, popliteal or femoral)
- calf swelling (usually measured 10 cm below the tibial tuberosity; >3 cm difference is significant)
- pitting oedema confined to the affected leg
- superficial, dilated, collateral veins; but not varicose veins.

Most hospitals will have a specific DVT pathway, with a proforma that combines significant risk factors and physical findings into a probability scoring system. A commonly used system is that developed by PS Wells *et al.* (*see* Further reading, p. 160).

D-dimer assay

D-dimers are variable-sized segments of cross-linked fibrin that are found in the circulation when fibrin is degraded by plasmin. They are non-specific, but levels are elevated following thrombus formation.

The debate still rages regarding the use of D-dimers, and views vary. D-dimers are sensitive but not specific for thrombosis or thromboembolism. A negative result is therefore reassuring, but a positive result is not confirmatory. Many argue that a positive D-dimer test does not provide any additional information. The D-dimer test is intended for use in people without multiple risk factors presenting with symptoms suspicious of DVT.

Key points regarding the D-dimer test

- D-dimer levels are raised in the presence of a recent thrombus, pregnancy, infection or malignancy.
- A negative D-dimer practically excludes an acute DVT.
- The test is a useful way to decide on whether ultrasound scanning of the deep veins should be done.

Ultrasound

Compression ultrasound examination or duplex Doppler ultrasound can reliably detect proximal vein thrombosis (sensitivity = 94%; specificity = 100%), but is less reliable in the more distal deep veins (sensitivity = 73%; specificity = 86%). The technique assesses the compressibility of the veins, the venous flow (by Doppler), and allows direct visualisation of any thrombus.

> Use this opportunity to revisit the concepts of sensitivity and specificity. Using the data above, calculate the numbers of false positives and false negatives if 100 patients with DVT and 100 patients with an alternative diagnosis are tested using duplex Doppler ultrasound.

(d) (e) Management of DVT

Different hospitals have different protocols for DVT management. The hospital anticoagulant service should be consulted if you are unsure about indications, drug doses, or interactions, and also to arrange outpatient monitoring. However, in general, the principles are:

- pain and swelling should be relieved with appropriate analgesia, leg elevation, and compression stockings
- propagation of the thrombus and/or embolisation to the lungs should be prevented with appropriate anticoagulation (initially low-molecular weight heparin (LMWH) e.g. tinzaparin 175 iu/kg), continued with warfarin until the INR is in the target range (2–3)
- specialist investigations may be needed for DVT with no obvious risk factors, since it may herald malignancy, or may be due to an inherited thrombophilic state, or other conditions that will affect the long-term management
- duration of treatment is influenced by the presence of continuing risk factors (e.g. certain coagulation defects, malignancy, chronic infection, inflammatory bowel disease, nephrotic syndrome). If risk factors persist, long-term anticoagulation and specialist referral may be necessary.

> Who should be investigated further for DVT? How do the number of episodes of thrombosis and the age of the patient guide further investigations?

Monitoring

Different haematology services have different protocols. However, the INR should be monitored before the first loading dose of warfarin, daily during loading, and then at intervals determined by the stability of the results.

> Use this opportunity to revisit pharmacological anticoagulation. What are the advantages of LMWH versus unfractionated heparin? What are the contraindications to warfarin therapy? How do these drugs work in relation to the normal coagulation pathways? How can their effects be reversed in an emergency?

Pulmonary embolism

The presentation of pulmonary embolism can be highly variable depending on the extent to which the pulmonary circulation is compromised, and how quickly this occurs. Breathlessness and/or tachypnoea are the classical findings, with or without pleuritic chest pain. However, the spectrum includes small emboli, which may be clinically insignificant; multiple emboli, which, if chronic may cause pulmonary hypertension, and right heart failure; or massive emboli, which may cause infarction of the lung and/or cardiac arrest with pulseless electrical activity (PEA).

(f) Initial investigations

When PE is suspected clinically, general immediate investigations should include an ECG, chest X-ray and arterial blood gas sampling. These investigations are not specific, but either provide support to the diagnosis of PE or help exclude conditions that may mimic acute PE.

- The ABG sample shows hypoxaemia with a normal $PaCO_2$ (type I respiratory failure).
- The ECG shows right bundle branch block, and the rarer S wave in lead I, Q wave in lead III, and T wave inversion in lead III. These ECG findings are consistent with acute cor pulmonale (right heart strain). The signs arise from acute volume overload of the right ventricle.

> Use this opportunity to revisit ECG interpretation. Use the diagrams in the MI question (see p. 84) to work out the ECG signs of right-sided heart strain. Which leads 'look at' the right ventricle? How might volume overload cause repolarisation abnormalities? What are the other causes of right heart strain?

(g) Further investigations

Rapid evaluation and diagnosis are needed for PE. The key investigations are:

- ventilation/perfusion scanning
- CT pulmonary angiography (CTPA)
- echocardiography
- duplex Doppler ultrasound scan of the deep veins of the legs (*see above*).

Even with the advent of CTPA, ventilation/perfusion ($\dot{V}/\dot{Q}$), or just perfusion ($\dot{Q}$) scanning is still an important option for diagnosing PE, not least because many hospitals have a nuclear medicine department. Perfusion is decreased without affecting ventilation, causing a 'mismatch'. However, in a massive PE, a significant proportion of patients will not have a high-probability $\dot{V}/\dot{Q}$ scan.

CTPA images the pulmonary arteries and the lung tissue at the same time. It is advocated by the British Thoracic Society (BTS) as the investigation of choice in PE. This is particularly true if the patient has known co-existent lung disease (e.g. COPD, pneumonia), or an abnormal chest X-ray. CTPA is highly effective in detecting proximal PEs, but is less capable of detecting smaller ones.

Echocardiography can evaluate right-sided pressures and function (as well as left ventricular and valvular function).

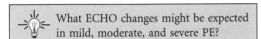

What ECHO changes might be expected in mild, moderate, and severe PE?

(h) Symptoms and signs

The signs and symptoms of PE can be non-specific, and may mimic those found in other diseases. In this scenario the patient is a young smoker, on the OCP with a history of DVT and recent immobility. However in a more elderly patient with chronic disease it may be difficult to differentiate between the symptoms of a PE and MI, COPD, pneumonia or CCF. The dilemma is usually solved with careful questioning and appropriate tests.

In PE, dysponea, tachypnoea and tachycardia are common. The patient may also complain of pleuritic chest pain (if there is infarcted lung tissue). Other symptoms include cough, haemoptysis and those of an associated DVT.

Examination may reveal signs of right heart failure such as raised JVP, and peripheral oedema. There may be a parasternal heave, pleural rub, and signs of DVT.

Relate these symptoms and signs to the underlying structure and function of the heart and lungs. How do the symptoms and signs vary in (a) acute PE, and (b) chronic pulmonary hypertension secondary to recurrent emboli?

The Prospective Investigation of Pulmonary Embolism Diagnosis (PIOPED) study showed the type and frequency of symptoms in proven PE was approximately:

- breathlessness   73%
- pleuritic pain   66%
- cough   25%
- haemoptysis   13%.

Interestingly, many of the patients who did not have PE in the study reported a similar frequency of these symptoms.

(i) Treatment options

Oxygen, analgesia and anticoagulation are the mainstays of treatment. Once a diagnosis of PE is considered, LMWH should be given, and oral warfarin should be started once the diagnosis is proven (as long as there are no contraindications to anticoagulation).

However, in massive PE thrombolytic therapy should be considered for patients who are haemodynamically compromised, those with right ventricular dysfunction, and young patients despite a normal right ventricle on echocardiography.

Other treatment options include placing an inferior vena caval filter if the thrombus has originated from the deep veins of the legs, and unstable thrombus remains.

The issues that are important in this patient include:

- could she be pregnant?
- contraindications to anticoagulation?
- contraindications to thrombolysis?
- is the PE confirmed as originating from a DVT?
- is she haemodynamically compromised?
- ECG shows right ventricular dysfunction (cor pulmonale).

(j) PE in pregnancy

The key points relating to PE in pregnancy include:

- pregnancy should be prevented while on warfarin, and contraceptive advice should be given
- PE is a major cause of pregnancy-related maternal death in the developed world
- pregnancy increases the chances of developing a DVT or PE (*see above*)
- women with thrombophilia have an increased

risk of pregnancy-associated thromboembolism, pre-eclampsia, and foetal loss

- warfarin should not be used in the first trimester and last 6 weeks of pregnancy
- anticoagulation with LMWH (sometimes with additional aspirin) can be used for the treatment of PE in pregnancy when closely supervised by haematologists and obstetricians
- anticoagulation should usually be continued for approximately 3 months after delivery to cover the additional risk of hypercoagulability during the puerperium.

(k) Thrombophilia

Thrombophilia is a propensity to form thromboses. There are many known, and presumably unknown, causes of hypercoagulability. Some of the more common genetic and acquired causes were listed in the opening section of this question. The need for thrombophilia testing should be discussed with haematologists, and should be considered when there is spontaneous thrombosis in a younger person (<45 years), recurrent thrombosis, familial tendency to thromboembolism, or recurrent miscarriage.

Therefore, this patient should be offered appropriate laboratory testing which could include:

- FBC (for platelets)
- PT/APTT
- factor V Leiden gene
- protein C levels
- protein S levels
- antithrombin III levels
- plasminogen level
- prothrombin gene mutation
- anticardiolipin/antiphospholipid antibodies and lupus anticoagulant testing.

(l) Pre-test counselling

Before a patient is investigated for thrombophilia, the following should be considered:

- is the patient able to give valid informed consent (see p. 29)?
- the patient needs to be aware of the nature of the tests (i.e. what is being tested?)
- she should be made aware of limitations of the investigations, particularly that a 'normal' throm-

bophilia screen does not mean no increased risk of thrombosis, since there are likely to be genetic defects yet to be discovered. Other important limitations include the effect of other medical conditions and medication on the results (e.g. liver disease, pregnancy, the oral contraceptive pill and anticoagulation)

- the implications of a positive test should be discussed, including potential long-term anticoagulation, and dangers associated with pregnancy. There may also be implications for first-degree relatives.

(British Heart Foundation, 2002)

Web resources

- Management of DVT: www.prodigy.nhs.uk
- Prevention of DVT and antithrombotic guidelines: www.sign.ac.uk
- Thrombophilia guidelines: www.bcshguidelines.com

Further reading

- British Heart Foundation (2002) *Thrombophilia Factfile 02/2002*. Available online at: www.bhf.org.uk/professionals/uploaded/feb02.pdf
- British Thoracic Society Standards of Care Committee Pulmonary Embolism Guideline Development Group (2003) British Thoracic Society guidelines for the management of suspected acute pulmonary embolism. *Thorax*. **58**: 470.
- Gorman WP, Davis KR and Donnelly R (2000) ABC of arterial and venous disease. Swollen lower limb-1: general assessment and deep vein thrombosis. *British Medical Journal*. **320**: 1453.
- Longmore M, Wilkinson I and Rajagopalan S (eds) (2004) *Oxford Handbook of Clinical Medicine* (6e). Oxford University Press, Oxford, pp. 446, 194, 802.
- Walker ID, Greaves M and Preston FE (2001) Investigation and management of heritable thrombophilia. *British Journal of Haematology*. **114**: 512.
- Wells PS, Anderson DR, Bormanis J *et al.* (1997) Value of assessment of pretest probability of deep-vein thrombosis in clinical management. *Lancet*. **350**: 1795.

A 19-year-old female is referred by her GP with a 3-week history of diarrhoea, lower abdominal pain and weight loss. On further questioning she tells you that she has been passing watery to 'porridge' consistency motions occasionally mixed with some fresh blood (up to ten times a day). She has also had several episodes of nocturnal defaecation.

She is a university student and has no significant past medical history. She is not taking any medication currently, but smokes approximately 15 cigarettes a day. She has recently returned from a holiday in Thailand.

On examination she is afebrile and dehydrated. Her pulse is 96 beats/min and blood pressure 110/60 mmHg. Her abdomen is soft with tenderness in the right iliac fossa and suprapubic regions. There are no masses palpable and bowel sounds are normal – as is the rectal examination.

(a) What would be your differential diagnosis for this patient?

....

....

....

(b) What initial investigations would you request?

....

....

....

(c) What markers can help predict the severity of the disease?

....

....

....

After admission, the initial blood test results are: Hb 10.5 g/dl (MCV 80 fl), WCC 7.9×10^9/l, CRP 86 µg/l. Three stool cultures are negative. After flexible sigmoidoscopy, the endoscopist writes in the notes 'appearances consistent with Crohn's disease of the sigmoid colon'. The biopsy report confirms this clinical diagnosis. She also has a barium meal and follow-through that shows findings compatible with Crohn's disease of the terminal ileum.

(d) What features would help you differentiate Crohn's disease from ulcerative colitis: endoscopically, histologically and radiologically?

....

....

....

(e) What treatment would you start?

....

....

....

The patient makes good progress with this treatment and is discharged. She returns to clinic 8 months later with a rash affecting both legs. On examination you find several firm raised red nodules on the anterior aspect of both shins. On further questioning she tells you that she has had increasingly frequent diarrhoea for the last 2 weeks.

(f) What is the rash, and how is it treated?

....

....

....

(g) What are the other extra-intestinal features associated with Crohn's disease?

....

....

....

She is seen in clinic at 3-monthly intervals over the next year. At her most recent visit she tells you that her symptoms have recurred and her GP has prescribed a course of steroids a few days before her clinic visit. This is her third course of steroids in the last year. She has also noticed a peri-anal discharge over the last few weeks.

(h) What other medication would you consider? What advice would you give the patient, and what blood tests should you check? What are the major side-effects of this drug, and how would you monitor its effects?

....

....

....

(i) What complication of Crohn's would explain the peri-anal discharge?

....

....

....

(j) List other intestinal complications.

....

....

....

The disease continues to cause significant distressing episodes and the patient eventually enquires about the possibility of surgery.

(k) What are the indications for surgery in Crohn's disease?

....

....

....

(l) What is the prognosis after surgical treatment?

....

....

....

Key cases

- Crohn's disease
- Ulcerative colitis
- Infective colitis

Clinical context

Bloody diarrhoea and weight loss are two symptoms that indicate significant intestinal pathology. Irrespective of the patient's age, malignancy must feature in the differential diagnosis along with infective and inflammatory conditions.

Other causes of these symptoms have been referred to elsewhere in this book (*see* pp. 87 and 199). When reading this scenario think of the main diagnoses in patients aged 20 years, 50 years, and 80 years presenting with these symptoms. Consider the questions in the history that provide clues to the correct diagnosis in each of these patients. It is important not to forget about risk factors, and to reflect on the relationship between infection, inflammation and malignancy in the intestine.

Inflammatory bowel disease

There are two main forms of inflammatory bowel disease (IBD); Crohn's disease and ulcerative colitis (UC). Crohn's disease can affect any part of the GI tract from the mouth to the anus, whereas UC is limited to the colon where it almost always affects the rectum.

Both conditions share many common clinical, endoscopic, histological, and radiological features. In approximately 10% of patients who have colitis, a definite diagnosis cannot be made. These patients are often described as having 'indeterminate colitis'. The prevalence of Crohn's disease is 50–60 per 100,000 compared with 80–120 per 100,000 for UC. Both have a peak age of onset anywhere between 20 and 40 years, although a second peak has been reported in Crohn's mainly affecting women over 60 years. Both sexes are equally affected in Crohn's, while in UC there is a slight female predominance.

The exact cause of these conditions is not fully understood, but both genetic and environmental factors are involved. This scenario explores the gastrointestinal and extra-intestinal features of Crohn's disease, and discusses the management issues and complications of Crohn's disease that can be refractory to medical/drug treatment.

(a) Differential diagnosis

- Inflammatory bowel disease
- Infective/traveller's diarrhoea
- Coeliac disease

The clinical manifestations of Crohn's disease are much more variable than those of UC, due to transmural involvement, and both the site and extent of the disease. Diarrhoea, abdominal pain and weight loss, with or without rectal bleeding, are typical features of Crohn's disease. However, as many as 10% of patients do not have diarrhoea. Failure to thrive due to malabsorption is common in children and may be seen before other features of the disease become evident. A patient may present with a fistula or an abscess; the clinical features will depend on the location, extent and severity.

As this patient has recently returned from holiday in the Far East, infective causes for her symptoms should be sought. Hence, stool should be sent for microscopy, culture, cysts, ova and parasites, in particular to exclude *Salmonella*, *Shigella*, *E. coli* and amoebiasis.

> You should be familiar with the common organisms causing infectious diarrhoea, both in the community and in hospital. What is the difference between endotoxins and exotoxins? Why is *Clostridium difficile* a particular threat to inpatients with IBD?

(b) Initial investigations

These will be baseline measurements, and will also monitor the response to treatment. They should include:

- FBC and blood film
- U&E
- LFT including albumin
- CRP/ESR
- amylase
- abdominal X-ray
- stool culture and microscopy ($\times 3$)
- endoscopy.

Anaemia is common in patients with IBD. This can be microcytic due to iron deficiency secondary to blood loss, or iron malabsorbtion in proximal small bowel Crohn's disease. This can also cause folate malabsorption producing a macrocytic anaemia;

however, macrocytic anaemia can be due to vitamin B_{12} deficiency in terminal ileal Crohn's disease. A mixed picture can occur due to a combination of malasorbtion of iron/folate/B_{12} and blood loss. Electrolytes should be checked, as profuse diarrhoea can lead to both dehydration and potassium loss. Albumin can be low, as proteins are often lost in diarrhoea. Inflammatory markers (CRP/ESR) are useful in determining if the disease is responding to treatment. An abdominal X-ray is important if you suspect either obstruction or toxic dilatation of the large bowel. An erect CXR would be useful to exclude perforation of a viscus.

Stool should always be sent for microscopy and culture – and in this case cysts, ova and parasites – as patients with IBD have an increased risk of gastro-intestinal infections.

Endoscopy is important to assess the appearance of bowel mucosa and also allows biopsies to be taken for histology. In the patient with acute colitis there is an increased risk of perforation. However, if the benefits are felt to outweigh the risks limited endoscopy may be appropriate. Once inflammation settles, colono-scopy will assess the sites and extent of the disease, which is important for future management.

(c) Markers of disease severity

Acute colitis is a life-threatening condition and the patient may need an urgent colectomy. Therefore it is crucial to monitor the patient's response to treat-ment using a combination of clinical features and laboratory results (see below).

Early assessment by both medical and surgical gastroenterologists is needed to formulate a clear management plan.

A severe attack of ulcerative colitis or Crohn's colitis would usually cause:

Stool frequency	>6 per day
Fever	>37.5°C
Tachycardia	>90 beats/min
Anaemia	Hb <10 g/dl
Albumin	<30 g/l
ESR	>30 mm/h
CRP	>10 µg/l.

Furthermore, simple observations can help predict the severity of disease. These include:

- stool chart
- weight chart.

Strict charting of stool frequency, consistency and presence or absence of blood is essential in assessing the severity of symptoms, and the response to treatment. Nocturnal defaecation is a particularly important sign in differentiating IBD from func-tional diarrhoea (see p. 183).

Inpatients should also be weighed regularly to assess their response to treatment. They should also be reviewed by a dietician, especially if nutritional supplements are needed.

(d) Differentiation of Crohn's colitis and ulcerative colitis

Remember that Crohn's disease can affect any part of the GI tract. This section focuses on colonic inflam-mation, and the features that will help differentiate Crohn's from ulcerative colitis. The features of Crohn's disease include:

- focal areas of inflammation/ulceration
- aphthoid ulcers
- skip lesions (separated by normal mucosa)
- 'cobblestone' appearance
- terminal ileal disease ('backwash ileitis' may occur in pancolitis but is uncommon)
- rectal sparing.

Histological features

- Granulomata present in 30% of patients
- Deep (transmural) inflammation
- Presence of goblet cells (depleted in UC)
- Absence of crypt abscesses

Radiological signs

- 'String-sign': presence of stricture
- 'Cobblestone' appearance
- Deep fissured 'rose-thorn' ulcers
- Skip lesion

> Use this opportunity to revise the struc-ture and function of the intestine wall. What are the important functions of the mucosa? What are the cells that achieve these functions? How do the findings in Crohn's disease relate to normal structure and function?

(e) Treatment of Crohn's disease

Before considering any specific therapy, ensure the patient is, and remains, well hydrated using intrave-nous fluids. 'Resting the gut' by keeping the patient 'nil by mouth' does not have any benefit apart from reducing the amount of diarrhoea. The colon nor-mally receives a significant volume of fluid from gastric, biliary, pancreatic and small bowel secretions, so normal water intake will not have any significant adverse effect.

Specific treatments include:

- 5-ASA-containing compound (e.g. mesalazine)
- steroids (initially intravenous if severe attack)
- bisphosphonate (e.g. alendronate 70 mg weekly) to prevent osteoporosis secondary to steroid treatment
- LMWH.

5-ASA (5-aminosalicylic acid) compounds such as mesalazine are used for their anti-inflammatory properties in mild to moderate inflammation. They have an added benefit in reducing 'flare-ups'; therefore they should be continued as maintenance treatment. Topical preparations are available in enema and suppository form, which are particularly useful if the inflammation is limited to the rectum. Oral 5-ASA compounds have different delivery systems to ensure the active component is delivered to the correct portion of the bowel. Some 5-ASA formulations are pH dependent and are released in the distal small bowel (more appropriate for use in Crohn's disease), whilst others are inactive until cleaved by large bowel flora (and hence suitable for colitis).

Ideally, steroids should only be used to treat an acute flare-up. The type of preparation will vary depending on the site and extent of the disease. If the patient is known to suffer from limited distal disease, steroid enemas can be used that limit side-effects, since there is limited systemic absorption. In contrast, intravenous steroids (e.g. hydrocortisone 100 mg qds) should be used in severe colitis, as oral steroids may be poorly absorbed due to rapid intestinal transit. Once symptoms are controlled, oral steroids can be substituted (e.g. prednisolone 40 mg od), reduced by 5 mg every 2 weeks (to zero if possible) provided the patient remains asymptomatic. A short course of steroids will not benefit patients with inflammatory bowel disease. A gradual reduction in steroid dose will maintain disease control, and prevent an Addisonian crisis.

> Use this opportunity to revise the physiological effects of corticosteroids. How do steroids work? What are the desirable therapeutic effects of steroids? What are the common side-effects, and how are they produced? What are the 'physiological' doses of both hydrocortisone, and prednisolone?

It is also beneficial to start patients on bone protection medication, as there is a risk of developing osteoporosis with recurrent or prolonged courses of steroids.

LMWH should be used to prevent venous thromboembolism. A high platelet count is a manifestation of the acute inflammatory response. This hypercoagulable state, combined with bed rest, increases the risk of DVT and PE (see p. 156).

Elemental diet can also be used to induce remission, particularly in patients with small bowel disease. Such diets improve nutrition, reduce the digestive burden on the bowel, and reduce the antigen load to the bowel mucosa. However, their precise mode of action is unknown. Unfortunately, many patients find these diets unpalatable and resort to a normal diet.

> Use this opportunity to familiarise yourself with the mechanism of action of the drugs used in the treatment of inflammatory bowel disease. What are the common side-effects?

(f) Erythema nodosum

Erythema nodosum can occur alone, or with other conditions including acute Crohn's disease. In this context, both conditions usually respond to steroids.

(g) Other extra-intestinal complications of Crohn's disease

- Pyoderma gangrenosum
- Uveitis
- Episcleritis
- Conjunctivitis
- Arthritis
- Ankylosing spondylitis
- Sacroiliitis
- Primary sclerosing cholangitis
- Amyloidosis (renal failure)
- Venous thromboembolism
- Gallstones (due to abnormal bile salt reabsorption)
- Renal stones

> How would these problems present? Familiarise yourself with the pathophysiology, clinical features, investigations and treatments for each of the above conditions. Which complications are related to disease activity?

(h) Azathioprine (complications and monitoring)

Azathioprine is an immunomodulator that is useful:

- to induce remission
- as a steroid-sparing agent
- in fistulating disease.

Azathioprine (1–2.5 mg/kg) is a derivative of thioguanine, a purine analogue. It is well absorbed from the gastrointestinal tract. Azathioprine is converted by glutathione in red blood cells to 6-mercaptopurine (6-MP) which is a purine nucleic acid antimetabolite that interferes with DNA synthesis.

Side-effects that are associated with azathioprine and 6-MP include:

- allergic reactions (high fever and/or rash and arthritis)
- leukopenia due to bone marrow suppression
- pancreatitis
- mild hepatitis.

Opportunistic infections can develop in patients on steroids and immunomodulators. Current recommendations are that the FBC should be checked weekly for the first four weeks after starting azathioprine, and then monthly for the duration of treatment. Bone marrow suppression and mild hepatitis are usually reversed by lowering the drug dose. Both 6-MP and azathioprine have also been rarely associated with severe cholestatic jaundice, which may progress to liver failure despite discontinuing therapy.

Other immunomodulators used in IBD include:

- methotrexate
- ciclosporin
- mycophenylate
- infliximab (anti-TNF receptor monoclonal antibody).

(i) Peri-anal fistulae

Perineal abscesses and fistulae occur in up to one-third of patients with Crohn's disease. Antibiotics are the first-line treatment especially in patients with draining fistulae and small abscesses that are not amenable to surgical drainage. Either metronidazole or ciprofloxacin are used. Before prescribing antibiotics it is important to take samples for microbiology. Unfortunately there is a high relapse rate when treatment is stopped.

If the perineal disease is resistant to antibiotic treatment, either treatment with immunomodulators or surgery should be considered.

> IBD is often diagnosed in the peak of childbearing years in women. What issues related to fertility, pregnancy, and breast feeding are important in treatment decisions?

(j) Other complications of Crohn's disease

- *Malabsorption* (depending on the site and extent of disease): terminal ileal disease (common) causes B_{12} deficiency and hence macrocytic anaemia. Proximal small bowel disease (rare) leads to deficiencies in iron, folate, calcium and magnesium, and electrolyte problems (*see* p. 201). Bile salt malabsorption can also occur following a right hemicolectomy, leading to gallstone formation and diarrhoea. If the patient has a significant small bowel resection, this can lead to 'short-

bowel syndrome', which causes malabsorption and diarrhoea owing to lack of absorptive surface area and shortened gut transit time.

- *Obstruction*: small bowel obstruction can occur in Crohn's disease, presenting with abdominal pain, swelling, vomiting and constipation (which may be absolute) (*see* p. 68). This may be due to adhesions, stricturing disease, or an inflammatory mass. An abdominal X-ray may show dilated small bowel loops proximal to the obstruction. Medical treatment with steroids may not be successful. In an attempt to preserve the length of the small bowel, a 'stricturoplasty' will open the narrowing and can prevent resection.
- *Fistulae*: can occur between the inflamed loop of bowel and any adjacent structure, e.g. other loops of bowel, bladder, vagina and skin. Symptoms will depend on the structures involved.
- *Intra-abdominal abscess*: abdominal pain, fever or rigors should alert you to the possibility of an abscess.
- *Perforation*: more common in cases of toxic megacolon (acute colitis) where there is gross swelling of the large bowel. Nevertheless, Crohn's disease affecting other parts of the gastrointestinal tract can perforate causing an acute abdomen (*see* p. 70).

> Remember that steroids can mask the symptoms and signs of intra-abdominal sepsis. What are the symptoms and signs of perforation and peritonitis? How might steroids mask these? (*see* p. 67).

- *Carcinoma*: both Crohn's disease and UC are associated with a higher rate of gastrointestinal malignancy. The disease extent and duration are important factors in determining the risk of developing adenocarcinoma of either the large bowel (UC and Crohn's) or the small bowel (Crohn's). For this reason patients with colonic Crohn's and UC should have surveillance colonoscopy (*see* BSG guidelines at www.bsg.org.uk).

(k) Indications for surgery in Crohn's disease

The main indication for surgery is the treatment of complications (e.g. stricture, stenosis, obstruction, fistula and bleeding). Resection is required in patients who do not respond to medical therapy.

(l) Prognosis after surgery

After surgery, the frequency of recurrence of Crohn's disease is high, usually at the site of the anastomosis. Approximately one-third of patients will have surgery again within 5 years, and the remainder within 15 years. Surgery is an important treatment option for Crohn's disease, but patients should be aware that it is not curative, and that disease recurrence after surgery is the rule.

Web resources

- British Society of Gastroenterology: www.bsg.org.uk
- National Association of Colitis and Crohn's Disease: www.nacc.org.uk
- NICE guidelines: www.nice.org.uk

Further reading

- Longmore M, Wilkinson I and Rajagopalan S (eds) (2004) *Oxford Handbook of Clinical Medicine* (6e). Oxford University Press, Oxford, pp. 244–7.
- Rampton DS (1999) Management of Crohn's disease. *British Medical Journal.* **319**: 1480.
- Forgacs I (1995) Clinical gastroenterology. *British Medical Journal.* **310**: 113.
- Kornbluth A and Sachar DB (2004) Ulcerative colitis practice guidelines in adults (update): American College of Gastroenterology, Practice Parameters Committee. *American Journal of Gastroenterology.* **99**: 1371.

A 40-year-old woman is admitted to the medical assessment unit. She has recently emigrated from Thailand and now works in a local supermarket. For the past 2 weeks, she has been feeling unwell, sweating, and has had a cough productive of blood-stained sputum. In addition she has been eating very little and has lost weight. On examination, she looks thin, her pulse is 90 beats/min and regular, her BP is 120/75 mmHg, and her respiratory rate is 18 breaths/min. Oxygen saturation is 98% on room air. She has a temperature of 37.5°C. On auscultation of her chest, there are a few inspiratory crackles at the right upper zone.

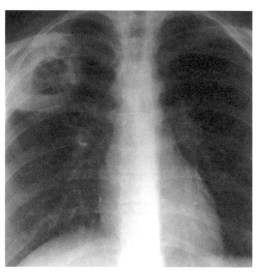

Figure 22.1 Chest X-ray from the patient.

(a) What are the differential diagnoses suggested by the history?

....
....
....

(b) What investigations would you order to confirm the diagnosis? Justify your answers.

....
....
....

Her chest X-ray is shown in Figure 22.1.

Later on, the laboratory technician telephones to confirm that the sputum sample is positive on auramine staining.

(c) What is your final diagnosis? What treatment is required?

....
....
....

(d) Do you think she requires any other tests before starting treatment? Explain your answer.

....
....
....

(e) What would you counsel her on before commencing treatment?

....
....
....

(f) Are there any public health issues that need to be addressed?

....

....

....

☞ She tolerates her treatment without any problems. After 5 days she still has a cough productive of green sputum. She wants to go home.

(g) Can she go home, and go back to work?

....

....

....

(h) Does she need any follow-up?

....

....

....

☞ Two days later, this patient's 17-year-old daughter is referred to the MAU with a strongly positive Mantoux test. She denies any respiratory symptoms and feels well. A chest X-ray arranged by her GP is reported as normal. She tells you she has never had any vaccinations.

(i) What is a Mantoux test?

....

....

....

(j) Does this patient have TB? Does she need any treatment?

....

....

....

☞ The Ward Clerk on the MAU tells you that her 11-year-old daughter is about to start at a private school. She asks you if she should arrange for her daughter to be vaccinated against TB.

(k) What advice would you give her?

....

....

....

Key cases

- Pneumonia
- Tuberculosis (TB)

Clinical context

The profile of infectious diseases has changed dramatically with the advent of air travel, immigration, and immunodeficiency/immunosuppression. Tuberculosis is a prime example that has many manifestations, of which pulmonary tuberculosis is the commonest. This condition is discussed in detail in the following scenario.

(a) Differential diagnoses

The possible diagnoses from this scenario include:

- *pneumonia*: patients may present with cough productive of purulent or blood-stained sputum. They may also be pyrexial and complain of breathlessness
- *pulmonary TB*: this should always be considered in an immigrant. Patients with pulmonary TB may present with a low-grade fever, a cough that may be productive of blood-stained sputum, and night sweats. Some patients may have minimal symptoms
- *malignancy* (*see* p. 128).

(b) Initial investigations

This patient has presented with a cough productive of sputum and a low-grade pyrexia. Initial investigations should include:

- blood cultures
- a chest X-ray, which may show the presence of infection or a tumour
- as pulmonary TB is suspected, sputum should be sent for direct smear microscopy. Sputum is smeared onto a slide and a stain e.g. auramine is applied. The stain is taken up by acid-fast bacilli (AFB) which are visible when the slide is examined under a microscope. A direct smear test will provide a faster result than sputum culture. Direct smear microscopy has a sensitivity of between 25% and 65%, and a specificity of more than 98%
- a sputum sample should be sent for microscopy and culture, including AFB. AFB cultures should be requested even if the direct smear test is negative
- if sputum cultures are repeatedly negative, an alternative would be to culture bronchial wash-

ings – obtained during bronchoscopy – for AFB. In the presence of a pleural effusion, pleural fluid can also be sent for culture of AFB, although the yield from this is low. Alternatively, a pleural biopsy can be done and tissue cultured for AFB
- in this scenario, TB is a differential diagnosis. An ECG is necessary to exclude TB pericarditis. It is an important diagnosis as active pericardial TB is an indication for high-dose corticosteroids.

> What is meant by the *sensitivity* and *specificity* of a test? What is the *predictive value* of a test?

(c) Diagnosis and treatment

The chest X-ray findings are consistent with pulmonary TB. The large irregular cavity in the right upper zone contains an air-fluid level. The direct smear test is positive for AFB. This patient requires treatment for TB. All pulmonary and extrapulmonary TB should be treated with 2 months of rifampicin, isoniazid, pyrazinamide and ethambutol. This should be followed by 4 months of rifampicin and isoniazid.

> Take this opportunity to revise the different ways in which antibiotics may work. What is the difference between *bacteriocidal* and *bacteriostatic*?

(d) Pretreatment precautions and testing

TB is an AIDS-defining illness. A patient with confirmed pulmonary or extrapulmonary TB is felt to be from an area or background with increased risk and should be tested for HIV.

Approximately 10% of patients treated will experience an adverse reaction to antituberculosis drugs. Some of these are summarised in Table 22.1.

Some pretreatment precautions and tests are recommended because of the risk of side-effects from antituberculosis therapy:

- ethambutol has a toxic effect on the eye. Although this is rare, visual acuity should be assessed using a Snellen chart before commencing treatment, and reassessed during the course of treatment to detect any deterioration as early as possible

Table 22.1 Adverse reactions to antituberculous drugs

Drug	Common	Uncommon	Rare
Isoniazid		Hepatitis	Optic neuritis
		Cutaneous hypersensitivity	Mental symptoms
		Peripheral neuropathy	Aplastic anaemia
			Haemolytic anaemia
			Agranulocytosis
Rifampicin		Hepatitis	Breathlessness
		Cutaneous reactions	Haemolytic anaemia
		Gastrointestinal disturbances	Acute renal failure
		Thrombocytopenic purpura	
		Flu-like symptoms	
Pyrazinamide	Nausea	Hepatitis	Gout
	Anorexia	Vomiting	Photosensitivity
	Flushing	Cutaneous reactions	
		Arthralgia	
		Hyperuricaemia	
Ethambutol		Retrobulbar neuritis	Hepatitis
		Arthralgia	Cutaneous hypersensitivity
			Peripheral neuropathy

Reproduced from: Joint Tuberculosis Committee of the British Thoracic Society (1998) Chemotherapy and management of TB in the UK: recommendations. *Thorax.* 53: 536–48.

- an uncommon side-effect of ethambutol is acute renal failure. Urea and electrolytes must be checked before starting treatment. It is also advisable to monitor renal function during antituberculosis treatment
- all antituberculosis drugs have the potential to cause hepatitis. Thus, patients should have liver function tests before treatment, and regularly throughout treatment.

(e) Counselling patients about to start antituberculosis therapy

- Patients should be told about the side-effects of antituberculosis drugs. If side-effects are experienced, patients should be encouraged to seek help.
- Rifampicin reduces the effect of the oral contraceptive pill. Female patients of childbearing age should be advised to use an additional or alternative form of contraception while receiving antituberculosis treatment.
- Rifampicin discolours urine and may also discolour contact lenses. Although not a serious side-effect, patients should be informed so as not to cause undue alarm.
- Compliance during antituberculosis chemotherapy is important. It is essential to ensure

complete resolution of TB, and to reduce the likelihood of relapse.

> Take this opportunity to read about directly observed therapy. How may it help with compliance with anti-TB chemotherapy?

(f) TB and public health

The management of TB is not confined to the patient in hospital, but extends into the community. As TB is highly infectious, anyone the patient has had recent close contact with must be traced and tested, as they are at risk of contracting the disease. This process is called contact tracing. Contact tracing is usually started once the diagnosis of TB has been confirmed.

Doctors in England and Wales have a statutory duty to notify a 'proper officer' of the local authority of suspected cases of certain infectious diseases. This includes cases of confirmed TB. The proper officers inform the Communicable Disease Surveillance Centre (CDSC) of the diseases notified on a weekly basis. The CDSC publishes these data weekly, in the form of local and national trends.

For the role of vaccination against TB, *see* the answer to (k), BCG vaccination.

> ☀ Which other infections diseases are classified as *notifiable*? You can revise this and read about the process of notifying infectious diseases in the CDSC publication at the Health Protection Agency website: www.hpa.org.uk/cdr/archives/CDRreview/1993/cdrr0293.pdf

(g) Returning to a normal life

Most patients with TB do not need admission to hospital. Treatment can be started and supervised as an outpatient. A patient who is HIV negative but who has sputum that is smear test-positive should be advised to remain at home for the first 2 weeks of treatment. A repeat sputum smear test is then performed. If this is negative for AFB, the patient may be allowed to continue with usual daily activities, including returning to work. Two weeks of chemotherapy are usually required before a patient is no longer infectious.

(h) Follow-up

Once TB therapy is completed, patients do not need regular follow-up with a chest physician unless they have had proven multi-drug-resistant TB (MDR TB). Patients should be informed of symptoms that may signify a relapse, and they should be advised to inform their GP if they occur. Patients who have had proven MDR TB should be followed up annually by a chest physician in the outpatient clinic.

(i) The Mantoux test

The Mantoux test is now the recommended standard method of tuberculin testing. It involves injecting 0.1 ml of 1 in 10,000 purified protein derivative (tuberculin) intradermally, producing a type IV hypersensitivity reaction. The result of the test is read after 48 to 72 hours. A positive reaction is the production of an erythematous induration of at least 10 mm in transverse diameter. A negative reaction is an induration of less than 5 mm. A positive Mantoux test implies previous exposure to tuberculin protein. This could be from BCG inoculation, active TB disease or TB disease that has been successfully treated in the past, or may indicate that the individual has been exposed to TB but does not have the disease. The Mantoux test is not used routinely to diagnose TB, because patients recently infected with TB or those that are immunocompromised may produce falsely negative results.

> ☀ The Mantoux test was named after the French physician Charles Mantoux, who developed the test in 1907 following the discovery of the *Tubercle* bacillus by Robert Koch in 1890.

(j) TB disease and TB infection

This person has a strongly positive tuberculin skin test, a normal chest X-ray and no other signs or any symptoms suggestive of TB. This is called TB infection or latent TB. Patients with latent TB do not need treatment for TB. However, patients identified with latent TB have an increased risk of developing TB, which may be prevented by chemoprophylaxis. This involves giving two anti-TB drugs for 3 months, or one anti-TB drug for 6 months. Anti-TB drugs have several potentially serious side-effects including hepatotoxicity, the risk of which increases with age (*see* p. 172). The evidence for the risks and benefits of chemoprophylaxis in latent TB are currently under review by NICE, which plans to issue guidelines in the near future.

> ☀ You can update yourself on the development of the tuberculosis NICE guidelines on the website www.nice.org.uk

(k) BCG vaccination

BCG stands for *bacillus of Calmette and Guérin* and is a vaccine against tuberculosis. It is prepared from a strain of the attenuated cow tuberculosis bacillus, *Mycobacterium bovis*.

> ☀ Take this opportunity to revise the difference between *live* and *killed* vaccines. Are attenuated vaccines live or killed? What are the benefits of a live vaccine?

Until recently, BCG vaccination was recommended for secondary school age children in the UK. Vaccination was also recommended for neonates born to new entrants to the UK from countries with high rates of TB. Since the introduction of these recommendations, the number of new cases of TB reported in the UK fell from 50,000 per year in the 1950s to 5800 in the late 1980s; most cases occurred in high-risk groups. These include people born abroad, the rate being higher in certain ethnic groups in the first few years after they enter the country, and their children, wherever they are born. They also include the homeless, those with HIV infection and contacts of known TB cases. As a result of the changing epidemiology of TB in the UK, the routine vaccination of secondary school age children is no longer recommended. The Joint Committee on Vaccination and Immunisation (JCVI) has advised BCG vaccination in the following groups:

- all infants living in areas where the incidence of TB is 40/100,000 or greater
- infants whose parents or grandparents were born in a country with a TB incidence of 40/100,000 or higher
- previously unvaccinated new immigrants from high-prevalence countries for TB.

Children who would otherwise have been offered BCG through the schools' programme will now be screened for risk factors, tested and only vaccinated if appropriate.

Individuals at risk due to their occupation, e.g. healthcare workers, should also be offered BCG vaccination.

The communication of these recommendations by the Chief Medical Officer (PL CMO (2005)3) can be found on the Department of Health website: www.dh.gov.uk/

Web resources

- British Thoracic Society: www.brit-thoracic.org.uk
- Department of Health: www.dh.gov.uk
- Health Protection Agency: www.hpa.org.uk
- National Institute for Health and Clinical Excellence: www.nice.org.uk
- World Health Organization: www.who.int/tb/en

Further reading

- Frieden TR (2002) Can tuberculosis be controlled? *International Journal of Epidemiology.* **31**: 894.
- Gamer P (1998) What makes DOT work? *Lancet.* **352**: 1326.
- Longmore M, Wilkinson I and Rajagopalan S (eds) (2004) *Oxford Handbook of Clinical Medicine* (6e). Oxford University Press, Oxford, pp. 564–5.
- Miller LG, Asch SM, Yu EI *et al.* (2000) A population-based survey of tuberculosis symptoms: how atypical are atypical presentations? *Clinical Infectious Diseases.* **30**: 293.
- Zumla A and Grange JM (1999) Doing something about tuberculosis. *British Medical Journal.* **318**: 956.

A 31-year-old woman presents to the GP complaining of feeling 'puffed' for the last few days. She has become breathless when walking upstairs at work, and is worried about it. Additionally she thinks she has experienced some palpitations. Furthermore, she has had trouble sleeping for a few months, and has been feeling anxious. She cannot point to any cause for her anxiety, since her work and home life have not changed recently. She works as a lawyer and was married last year.

(a) What further questions might the GP ask?

....

....

....

(b) What features on physical examination would the GP specifically seek to differentiate between the possible causes of this woman's symptoms?

....

....

....

On examination her pulse is found to be irregular and the GP does an ECG. A section of the rhythm strip is shown in Figure 23.1.

(c) Comment on the tracing. Which features define the diagnosis?

....

....

....

(d) What are the main concerns regarding this rhythm, and how might physical examination reveal whether they are important in this case?

....

....

....

The GP requests thyroid function tests.

(e) What would you expect to see on the laboratory report (use ↑↑, ↓↓, ↑, ↓, ↔ for highly/moderately raised/reduced or unchanged)?

	Patient's result	Normal range
Total T_3		1.1–2.8 nmol/l
Total T_4	200 nmol/l	60–135 nmol/l
TSH		0.5–5.5 mU/l

After receiving the result, her GP decides to refer her to an endocrinologist at the local hospital. Additionally, he decides to start treatment for her symptoms while waiting for the appointment.

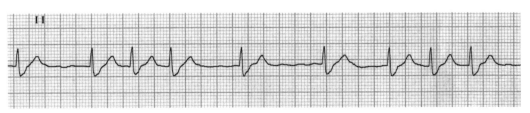

Figure 23.1 Rhythm strip from the ECG.

(f) What might he prescribe?

....

....

....

👉 She is referred to a consultant endocrinologist who discusses treatment options for her condition.

(g) What are the principal treatment options and what specific point would the consultant discuss with her?

....

....

....

👉 She is successfully treated, but 2 years later returns to her GP complaining that the lump in the front of her neck has become tight and has been making her cough. Her GP decides to refer her back to the endocrinologist. While waiting for her appointment she is rushed to hospital by ambulance, with dyspnoea and central cyanosis. She has a respiratory rate of 43 breaths/min, is sweating profusely and has audible stridor. After emergency intubation by an anaesthetist, she is rushed to theatre where a subtotal thyroidectomy is performed. The next day she is successfully extubated. Her voice is hoarse but her respiratory function is normal.

(h) What possible complications could develop in the immediate post-operative period and what are their causes?

....

....

....

(i) Which post-operative biochemical test is the most important and why?

....

....

....

(j) Which oral replacement therapies does this patient need?

....

....

....

👉 Post-operatively the patient makes rapid progress and her hoarseness improves. She is able to eat and drink easily and is discharged 7 days after surgery.

(k) What treatment/advice and reassurance would you give her about her voice?

....

....

....

(l) Which blood tests will her GP check regularly in the future?

....

....

....

Key cases

- Atrial fibrillation
- Hyperthyroidism

Clinical context

Breathlessness and palpitations, either separately or combined, are common symptoms. As always, an accurate history will provide clues to the final diagnosis, as exemplified by this scenario. Pay particular attention to the features that will help you discriminate between anxiety and those underlying conditions (especially endocrine ones) that have similar symptoms.

Thyrotoxicosis is a common cause of these symptoms, and in primary care is not always an easy diagnosis to make. It is much more common in women than in men. Hyperthyroidism has many clinical manifestations; however atrial fibrillation and anxiety are common. All cases should be referred to an endocrinologist in secondary care. It is often wise (with the patient's permission) to discuss the diagnosis with the patient's spouse and/or family members to ensure that they understand the time frame necessary to bring the disease and its symptoms under control.

(a) Anxiety as a symptom

Anxiety is a common presenting symptom. About 5% of all GP consultations are for anxiety-related symptoms.

Medical and psychiatric conditions can either mimic or precipitate anxiety, and anxiety states are amongst the most common psychological conditions of modern times. This situation arises because anxiety can provoke a host of symptoms such as palpitations, chest pain, hyperventilation, sweating and nausea, which only serve to make the patient more anxious.

Clearly this makes differentiating between physical and psychological causes extremely difficult on the basis of symptoms.

The symptoms described in this history could be attributed to many disease processes including free-floating anxiety disorder. However, breathlessness on exertion means that an underlying medical condition has to be excluded.

Specific points in the history that indicate an anxiety disorder include:

- *careful documentation of psychological symptoms*, including low mood, irritability, emotional lability, insomnia, and impaired concentration. It

may be helpful to talk to the patient's partner, or others they live with
- *physical symptoms* including hyperventilation (with hypocalcaemic symptoms (*see* p. 200)), poor appetite, sweating, preference for cold rooms, headaches, palpitations
- *situations that have precipitated the symptoms*: particular importance should be paid to the role of stress (it may be necessary to ask a family member if there have been any particular stresses)
- *a careful drug and alcohol history*: stimulants such as caffeine can produce anxiety, and both alcohol and alcohol withdrawal are common causes
- *symptoms of depression* (depression and anxiety frequently co-exist): these can be very difficult for the GP to manage.

Other aspects of the history should focus on other medical conditions that may either produce or mimic anxiety:

- *hyperthyroidism*: ask specifically about heat intolerance, weight loss, restlessness, muscle weakness, diarrhoea, increased appetite, family history
- *hypoglycaemia*: ask about symptoms of liver disease and alcohol use (*see* p. 60)
- *cardiac causes* (angina or arrhythmias): ask about risk factors (*see* p. 21), chest pain, shortness of breath, palpitations, dizziness, syncope
- *phaeochromocytoma*: ask about flushing, headaches, sweating, palpitations.

> Use this opportunity to look at the modes of presentation of anxiety disorders. You should be familiar with the differences between anxiety states, acute stress reaction, panic disorder and phobias. What are the main medical and non-medical treatments?

(b) Physical examination

Physical examination should help to exclude the medical conditions outlined above.

Useful clinical markers of hyperthyroidism include:

- goitre
- eye signs
- fine tremor
- proximal myopathy and wasting
- hyperdynamic circulation with warm peripheries

- cardiac examination may reveal a significant arrhythmia and/or heart failure.

> You should be familiar with signs of left and/or right ventricular failure. How are the cardinal signs produced by the underlying pathophysiology? What are the common causes of left and right ventricular failure?

Anxious patients may have:

- rapid respiratory rate
- tachycardia
- clammy hands
- tremor.

(c) (d) Atrial fibrillation (AF)

ECG interpretation

AF causes an irregularly irregular pulse that can be confirmed on clinical examination by demonstrating an apico-radial delay. However, normally the diagnosis of AF should be confirmed with an ECG. Multiple atrial or ventricular ectopic beats can produce an irregular pulse, and apico-radial delay may be difficult to detect.

The key ECG features are:

- discrete p waves are absent and are replaced by undulating fibrillation waves (which may not be obvious)
- the ventricular rate is irregularly irregular.

> Use this opportunity to revise ECG interpretation; you should be familiar with other common arrhythmias and their management.

AF is often talked about as being fast or slow. This is a common misconception. It is the ventricular response that is either fast or slow.

Atrial fibrillation

AF becomes more common with increasing age, affecting 0.5% of people aged 40–50 years, and 9% of those aged 80–90 years. The spectrum of presentations ranges from asymptomatic to haemodynamically compromised. Many patients experience a wide range of symptoms, including palpitations, dyspnoea, fatigue, dizziness, angina, and those of cardiac failure. In addition, AF can be associated with systemic and pulmonary emboli.

AF in the younger patient should prompt the following questions:

- is the patient hyperthyroid?
- is alcohol a factor?
- is illicit drug use a factor?
- could the patient have mitral valve disease?
- could the patient have cardiomyopathy?
- does the patient have an atrioseptal defect (ASD)?

> You should be aware of the differences in the pathophysiology, presentation and management of AF in young and old patients. What are the indications for anticoagulation and cardioversion respectively?

Consequences of AF

- Cardiac output can be compromised by the loss of atrial contractions and the irregular ventricular rate. This can lead to hypotension, heart failure, and ischaemia. People with pre-existing cardiac disease are particularly vulnerable.
- AF increases the risk of thromboembolism.

Physical examination

Examination should aim to determine the patient's risk from AF. High risk patients may need immediate cardioversion. A very fast ventricular rate (>150 bpm), heart failure, hypotension and poor perfusion are particular worries. On examination the following may be present:

- low BP
- raised JVP
- central cyanosis
- fine bi-basal crepitations consistent with pulmonary oedema
- a displaced apex beat
- third heart sound
- murmur (e.g. of mitral regurgitation or stenosis)
- ankle oedema
- ascites.

(e) Thyroid function tests

T_3, T_4 and TSH measurements are needed to diagnose and monitor patients with thyroid disorders.

Although T_3 is the form of the hormone that binds to intracellular receptors, the thyroid gland secretes much more T_4 than T_3. Around 20% of T_3 comes from direct thyroid secretion; the peripheral conversion of T_4 to T_3 accounts for the rest. Therefore T_3, T_4, and TSH should be tested in suspected thyroid disease. A more detailed analysis includes free T_4 and thyroid-binding globulin (TBG). Autoimmune thyroid disease (Graves' disease) can be confirmed by testing for thyroid peroxidase (TPO) antibodies.

Over 99% of cases of hyperthyroidism result from disorders primarily affecting the thyroid gland (pituitary causes are rare). TSH-secreting cells of the anterior pituitary are responsive to changes in the level of circulating thyroid hormones. If thyroid production of T_3 and T_4 is increased, pituitary production of TSH will be suppressed.

A characteristic feature of primary hyperthyroidism is a proportionately greater rise in serum concentrations of T_3 than of T_4.

Therefore the expected thyroid function test results would be:

	Patient's result	Normal range
Total T_3	↑↑	1.1–2.8 nmol/l
Total T_4	200 nmol/l	60–135 nmol/l
TSH	↓↓	0.5–5.5 mU/l

> ☀ You should be aware of the immunological, genetic and pathological principles underlying the pathogenesis of both autoimmune and non-autoimmune thyroid disease. How might HLA type influence the pathogenesis of Graves' disease?

(f) Initial management of hyperthyroidism

Definitive management should be instigated in secondary care. However since this patient is experiencing distressing symptoms, it would be wise to start her on a β-blocker, to provide symptomatic relief (slowing down her heart rate, reducing anxiety, and antagonising other sympathetic nervous system-driven physiological effects). β-blockers also reduce the peripheral conversion of T_4 to T_3.

Long-acting β-blockers (atenolol or nadalol) are often used as a once a day regime improves compliance.

> ☀ Use this opportunity to study the effects of thyroid hormones on different tissues. How do the hormones exert their effects at the cellular level?

(g) Management of hyperthyroidism

There are three treatments used by endocrinologists in the management of hyperthyroidism. They are all associated with similar improvements. The options are:

- antithyroid drugs such as carbimazole or propylthiouracil; 'block and replace' (the thyroid is prevented from secreting thyroxine and the hormone is replaced by levothyroxine tablets), or titration regime (the dose of antithyroid drug is slowly increased)

- radioactive iodine
- surgery (used in the minority of cases today).

There are benefits and risks associated with each approach, and the decision should rest with the properly informed patient.

One factor, which is important to establish in women of childbearing age, is *whether they are either pregnant or plan to get pregnant*, since both carbimazole and radioactive iodine are contraindicated in pregnancy. Additionally, it would be wise to discuss the use of different methods of contraception.

Other factors may determine which treatment is optimal. A rational approach might be a trial of 18 months of a 'block and replace' regimen to induce remission. If relapse occurs (50% of patients), initial management could be followed by either another attempt at a block and replace regimen or radioactive iodine treatment.

Indications for either surgery or radioactive iodine include:

- relapse after a course of antithyroid drugs
- large goitre
- toxic nodule or multinodular toxic goitre
- side-effects of antithyroid medication (particularly agranulocytosis)
- patient choice.

Indications for surgery alone include:

- hyperthyroidism complicating pregnancy, where drugs have failed
- patient preference
- suspected co-existent thyroid cancer (rare)
- tracheal/oesophageal compression.

Treatment is initially monitored by free T_4 level, since TSH suppression may persist for several months despite optimal treatment.

(h) (i) (j) Goitre and management

A large goitre can produce difficulty in breathing and dysphagia by compressing the trachea and oesophagus respectively. Multinodular goitre is the most common thyroid-related cause of either tracheal or oesophageal compression.

Stridor is a sign of extra-thoracic airway obstruction and is a medical emergency. If surgery is not immediately available, the patient should be anaesthetised, intubated and ventilated. Intubation becomes progressively more difficult as the trachea becomes oedematous, distorted and compressed.

Apart from in an emergency (as in this case), thyroidectomy should only be performed on patients who are euthyroid. Drug treatment should be stopped before surgery. A course of potassium iodide reduces the vascularity of the thyroid.

> Use this opportunity to revise the different types of goitre. What are common physiological causes of goitre? With a solitary nodular goitre what are the common investigations to exclude malignancy? What are the common forms of thyroid carcinoma?

Complications of thyroid surgery

- Damage to the recurrent laryngeal nerve causing transient hoarseness is common. Recurrent laryngeal nerve palsy occurs in only about 1%.
- Post-operative haemorrhage can cause compression of the trachea and hence respiratory distress. This is an emergency. Removal of the clips decompresses the area as blood escapes. Patients may also require intubation if the trachea has become oedematous.
- Wound infection.
- Transient hypocalcaemia occurs in up to 30% of patients due to removal of parathyroid gland tissue and hypoparathyroidism. However, permanent hypocalcaemia is rare, with a prevalence of about 2 per 100.

Post-operative recovery

- Calcium monitoring: since transient hypocalcaemia is so common, all patients should have their corrected calcium checked the day after surgery and daily until stable. Tests should be supplemented with documentation of hypocalcaemic symptoms (*see* p. 200).
- Calcium supplementation: calcium supplements should be started if the patient has a low corrected calcium level or complains of hypocalcaemic symptoms. Close monitoring is needed to prevent hypercalcaemia.

> What are the symptoms and signs of hypocalcaemia, and how do they arise? What is the correct calcium level?

Replacement therapy

- The patient may need thyroxine replacement. Regular monitoring of thyroid function will ensure the optimal dose of thyroxine if required. The incidence of hypothyroidism is proportional to the number of post-operative years.
- Immediately post-operatively, 30% of patients will require calcium supplementation. After 3 months only 2% require calcium.

(k) Voice dysfunction

Voice dysfunction may result from thyroid surgery if there is damage to the recurrent laryngeal or external laryngeal nerves. Some patients have a degree of hoarseness, and patients should be advised:

- not to strain their voices by excessive talking or shouting
- that their voices will gradually return to normal, but if the symptoms persist beyond 2 weeks after surgery, that they will be investigated by direct or indirect laryngoscopy.

> Use this opportunity to revise the innervation of the vocal cords. Why does surgery to the thyroid carry a significant risk of damage to these nerves?

(l) Follow-up

Follow-up of patients should involve routine assessment of symptoms and serum biochemistry. In particular this patient will need measurement of:

- T_4 and TSH
- serum calcium.

Patients may need monitoring for many years post-operatively since, as previously mentioned, hypothyroidism becomes progressively more common as time passes.

Web resources

- Management of AF: www.clinicalevidence.com
- Management of anxiety states: www.prodigy.nhs.uk
- Management of hyperthyroidism: www.prodigy.nhs.uk

Further reading

- Brent GA (1994) The molecular basis of thyroid hormone action. *New England Journal of Medicine.* **331**: 847.
- Hanna FW, Lazarus JH and Scanlon MF (1999) Controversial aspects of thyroid disease. *British Medical Journal.* **319**: 814.
- Longmore M, Wilkinson I and Rajagopalan S (eds) (2004) *Oxford Handbook of Clinical Medicine* (6e). Oxford University Press, Oxford, pp. 304–5, 130–1.
- Surks MI, Ortiz E, Daniels GH *et al.* (2004) Subclinical thyroid disease: scientific review and guidelines for diagnosis and management. *Journal of the American Medical Association.* **291**: 228.
- Woeber KA (1992) Thyrotoxicosis and the heart. *New England Journal of Medicine.* **327**: 94.

24 A lady with abdominal cramps

A 33-year-old lady is referred to clinic by her GP with a 4-month history of alternating diarrhoea and constipation, and cramping abdominal pain. When diarrhoea is the main feature she passes watery stool four to five times a day, mainly in the morning. In contrast, during the constipated phase, she defecates every 3 to 4 days, and her stools are like 'rabbit pellets'. Her pain is described as a 'cramp-like' sensation across her lower abdomen that is associated with a degree of urgency in needing to open her bowels. The pain eases once this has occurred.

She hasn't noticed any weight loss but tells you that her stomach seems to swell after food. This is associated with a 'bloated feeling'.

She works as a teacher, has recently started at a new school, and has found this change in work environment quite stressful.

There is no significant past medical history and she is not taking any medication at present.

On examination her abdomen is soft, non-tender and no masses are palpable. Bowel sounds and rectal examination are both normal.

(a) What is the differential diagnosis for this patient?

....

....

....

(b) What specific symptoms should be asked about to exclude organic disease?

....

....

....

(c) What symptoms in the above history might help confirm functional bowel disease?

....

....

....

(d) What initial investigations would you request?

....

....

....

You see the patient in clinic 3 months later. All her investigations are normal. A diagnosis of functional bowel disorder is made. She tells you that her symptoms are somewhat better now that she has settled into her job. Her main complaints at present are of cramping pain before defaecation and that she is more constipated than before.

(e) What pathophysiological processes are thought to be important in functional bowel disorder?

....

....

....

(f) What initial treatment would you consider given her current symptoms?

....

....

....

(g) What treatment would you suggest now?

....

....

....

You receive a letter from her GP a few months later telling you that her symptoms have deteriorated, and requesting a further clinic appointment. When she is seen she tells you that she is having increased cramping and bloating associated with more diarrhoea. At work she has had to take on extra duties owing to pending exams and again feels quite 'stressed-out'.

Key cases

- Chronic diarrhoea
- Functional bowel disorder (irritable bowel syndrome)

Clinical context

Diarrhoea and abdominal pain have been experienced, to varying extent, by virtually everyone. Often the symptoms are transient, possibly infective in origin, following a 'good night out'. On other occasions, these symptoms reflect pathology either in the intestine, or from an extra-alimentary site (*see* pp. 90, 163, 177 and 199). A carefully constructed, thorough, history will help you discriminate between the potential causes.

Functional bowel disorder (FBD), often referred to as 'irritable bowel syndrome' (IBS), is the most commonly diagnosed gastrointestinal condition affecting 10–15% of the population. It is characterised by altered bowel habit, either diarrhoea or constipation or a combination along with chronic abdominal pain, abdominal bloating and rectal hypersensitivity (without an organic cause). Although the actual numbers of people affected seem quite high (up to 20% of the population in some studies), only 15% of those seek medical advice. Furthermore, FBD still accounts for 25–50% of referrals to hospital gastroenterology clinics. It is also worth noting that FBD is second only to the common cold as a cause of absenteeism!

Organic causes of chronic diarrhoea have been discussed in other scenarios in this book. As the name implies, the cause of this extremely common disorder is still unknown. However as the pathophysiology of FBD is gradually deciphered contemporary management strategies emerge. Pharmacological treatment, lifestyle modification, and stress relief all have roles in the management of FBD, and their respective uses are discussed below.

(a) Differential diagnoses

- Functional bowel disorder
- Inflammatory bowel disease (*see* p. 163)
- Coeliac disease (*see* p. 199)
- Malignancy (*see* p. 90)

FBD can present with an array of symptoms that can mimic other, more sinister gastrointestinal problems, especially in patients over 45 years of age. Differentiating FBD from the conditions listed above can be challenging.

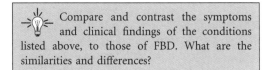

Compare and contrast the symptoms and clinical findings of the conditions listed above, to those of FBD. What are the similarities and differences?

(b) Features indicative of organic disease

Despite the frequency, timing and variation of symptoms in FBD some clinical features are not compatible with this diagnosis. Hence, prompt investigation for organic disease is needed if the patient's history includes:

- anorexia
- malnutrition
- weight loss
- pain, which is progressive, may either wake from, or prevent, sleep
- large-volume diarrhoea
- bloody stools
- nocturnal diarrhoea
- greasy stools (steatorrhoea).

(c) Features suggesting functional bowel disease

The Rome II criteria were developed to help diagnose functional bowel disorder without the need for further investigation. Patients should have the following recurrent symptoms for at least 3 months of a year:

- abdominal pain, the onset of which is associated with:
  - a change in stool frequency
  - a change in stool consistency
- supporting symptoms that include:
  - altered frequency of stool
  - altered form of stool
  - altered passage of stool
  - the presence of mucus
  - abdominal bloating
  - defecation relieves the pain.

The patient in the scenario has described all of these features, making the diagnosis of functional bowel disorder very likely.

(d) Initial investigations

- FBC
- U&E

- inflammatory markers (CRP/ESR)
- LFT
- TFT
- coeliac serology (transglutaminase antibody/endomysial antibody/IgA)
- colonoscopy (or flexible sigmoidoscopy and barium enema).

FBD mimics many common gastrointestinal conditions, and basic investigations should be aimed at excluding more sinister pathology, especially in the older patient. Anaemia would be a worrying finding as this could represent blood loss from inflammatory bowel disease, peptic ulcer disease, gastrointestinal malignancy, or malabsorption. If profuse diarrhoea is present, electrolytes may be deranged and the patient could be dehydrated. Elevation of inflammatory markers would not be expected in FBD and would point more toward a diagnosis of infection, inflammatory bowel disease or malignancy.

The clinical features of coeliac disease cover a wide spectrum from profuse diarrhoea with malabsorption and weight loss, to more vague symptoms such as bloating and cramping abdominal pain. Blood for serological markers of this disease (transglutaminase antibody, endomysial antibody, IgA) should be obtained. Biopsies from the distal duodenum taken during OGD are needed to give a definite diagnosis (see p. 201).

Colonoscopy is the investigation of choice to examine the mucosa of the colon and terminal ileum. Alternatively, flexible sigmoidoscopy will allow direct visualisation of large bowel mucosa, and the opportunity to obtain biopsies that will exclude left-sided colitis, while barium enema examination will exclude any mass lesions in the proximal colon. Subtle mucosal irregularities, however, are easily missed on barium examination.

Further investigations will depend on these initial tests, and patients' response to treatment. Small bowel Crohn's disease, for example, can present with intermittent diarrhoea and abdominal pain. A colonoscopy and small bowel barium studies will be needed to confirm the diagnosis. However, in contrast with FBD, Crohn's disease would also cause weight loss and raise inflammatory markers. Lactose intolerance and bacterial overgrowth could present with similar features to FBD, but diarrhoea is the predominant symptom (without alternating constipation). These diagnoses are confirmed using lactose-hydrogen and lactulose breath-testing respectively.

(e) Pathophysiological processes in functional bowel disorder

- Abnormal GI motility
- Abnormal sensory response: 'visceral afferent hypersensitivity'
- Post-infectious changes
- Stress: psychosocial dysfunction

The exact causes of functional bowel disorder remain unknown. They are likely to be heterogeneous given the complexity of the systems underlying the control of 'normal' gastrointestinal function. Intensive research centred on the areas outlined above has generated inconsistent and often conflicting findings.

Abnormal gastrointestinal motility

In FBD abnormalities in large and small bowel motility are inconsistent. Some studies have demonstrated a reduced rate of basal unstimulated colonic contractions whilst others have found basal motility to be increased.

Similarly the peristaltic response to stress, anger and infusions of cholecystokinin (CCK) is variable. Increased intestinal reactivity occurs in some patients with FBD, and also in healthy volunteer controls.

Other theories have suggested that motility may be increased by hypersensitivity of afferent pathways and changes in afferent-efferent reflexes.

> Use this opportunity to revise the control of peristalsis and mechanics of digestion in the GI tract. What are the gastroileal and gastrocolic reflexes? Which hormones regulate GI tract functions?

Visceral afferent hypersensitivity

A disproportionate response to visceral pain or discomfort in patients with FBD leads to the notion of visceral afferent hypersensitivity.

FBD patients often complain of 'bloating' or 'excess gas', however they have similar volumes to asymptomatic healthy people. Interestingly, rectal sensitivity is increased in patients with FBD. The pain threshold to rectal distension can be lowered even further by repeated stimulation of the sigmoid colon. This response also occurs in FBD patients who did not initially demonstrate afferent hypersensitivity. Although the sigmoid colon and rectum have been the most amenable sites for study, visceral hypersensitivity has also been demonstrated at other sites in the GI tract.

The higher perception of gastrointestinal pain relies on serial neural connections sometimes called the 'brain–gut axis'. Sensation in the gastrointestinal tract is controlled by various chemoreceptors and mechanoreceptors in the bowel wall. Sensory information is relayed through the nerves of the enteric plexuses to the nuclei in the dorsal horn of the spinal cord, and then via afferent nerves to the brain. Increases in the signal intensity at any point in this pathway could lead to the disproportionate response to bowel distension observed in FBD patients.

> Use this opportunity to revisit the enteric nervous system (ENS). What are the roles of the submucosal plexus and myenteric plexus? What are the effects of parasympathetic and sympathetic stimulation? Which neurotransmitters are important in ENS function?

Post-infectious changes

In this particular sub group of patients with FBD, diarrhoea is the predominant symptom and mucosal inflammation is present. The patient's history will provide the clues to this particular diagnosis. Jejunal biopsies taken from these patients have shown inflammatory infiltration of the myenteric plexus and associated degeneration of the nerves. Similar immunohistological changes have been observed in patients with gastroenteritis. The link between FBD and infection is made stronger by the observation that persistent FBD symptoms occur in a proportion of patients following an acute episode of bacterial gastroenteritis.

This could be part of the pathogenesis of FBD in some – but not all – patients.

Psychosocial dysfunction

Anxiety, depression, phobias and somatisation disorders are common in patients with FBD who present to their GP or hospital for medical attention. These psychological disorders are not usually present in patients with FBD who don't seek medical attention. Therefore it appears that psychological distress might influence the perception that patients have of their symptoms, but is probably not the cause of the symptoms.

> What are the methods of screening for a psychological disorder? What key questions should be asked to assess the presence of anxiety or depression? What are the forms of formal psychological testing available? Who usually performs these tests?

Other observations suggest that 'stress' may be causal. Stressful tasks can alter gastrointestinal motility and increase the perception of pain to colonic balloon distension in healthy controls.

Most doctors will have experienced patients with FBD who present with intolerable symptoms during times of stress. The symptoms often improve when the psychosocial stressors are removed.

Anxiety management can often help with the symptoms of FBD. Forming a therapeutic relationship and giving appropriate reassurance can reduce patients' anxiety surrounding their symptoms.

(f) Initial treatment in functional bowel disorder
- Development of a 'therapeutic relationship' with the patient
- Reassurance
- Dietary modification
- Increase fibre
- Anti-spasmodics (e.g. mebeverine/hyoscine)

> What are the components involved in the development of a therapeutic relationship? How do they help in a patient's acceptance of a psychosocial component to their disease?

Reassuring patients that no sinister problems have been identified despite thorough planned assessment can alleviate anxiety that could potentially increase their symptoms, without re-inforcing the 'ill role'. Helping them to understand the possible processes underlying the condition (*see* above) can also be beneficial.

Vegetables such as beans, broccoli, brussel sprouts and cabbage rely on commensal gut flora in the colon for their digestion. The production of gas during digestion can lead to uncomfortable distension in FBD sufferers with visceral hypersensitivity. Consequently, a trial of a modified diet with reduced leguminous or cruciferous vegetable content may help.

Increasing dietary fibre or adding fibre supplements may help in patients with constipation- or diarrhoea- predominant FBD. Fibre can facilitate the transit of stool and may improve its consistency. Increasing fibre may worsen patients' symptoms so, if supplements are used, they should be increased gradually over a period of time.

As well as lifestyle modification, a sensible starting point for this patient would be to prescribe a course of an antispasmodic. Mebeverine (135 mg up to 3 times/day) or hyoscine butylbromide (10 mg up to 3 times/day) could be of potential benefit. Hyoscine (buscopan), an antimuscarinic (anticholinergic) drug, reduces intestinal motility, while mebeverine is thought to have a direct relaxant effect on intestinal smooth muscle.

(g) Further treatment
- Loperamide
- Amitriptyline
- Anxiety management/referral to psychologist

The management of FBD has been likened to a triangle or pyramid, in that most patients – the base – will respond to reassurance. The next 'level' will require antispasmodic treatment with or without fibre supplements. The apex represents the minority of patients who will require specialist psychological assessment.

Anti-diarrhoeal drugs such as loperamide (Imodium) may be useful in patients who experience uncomfortable or frequent diarrhoea. They should be used sparingly since they can cause significant constipation.

Antidepressants have been shown to have useful analgesic effects in FBD. Despite the links between anxiety, depression and FBD, the pain relieving effect of antidepressants is unrelated to a reduction in depressive symptoms and much lower doses are used than in the treatment of depression. Tricyclic antidepressants such as amitryptiline are often used. They have the added benefit of reducing gastrointestinal motility, which may help patients with diarrhoea. Up to a month of treatment may be required for tricyclics to have a therapeutic effect. If patients are clinically anxious or depressed a trial of a selective serotonin reuptake inhibitor (SSRI) is worthwhile.

As previously described, psychosocial stressors can worsen the abdominal pain associated with FBD. There are many approaches to reducing stress and anxiety. Relaxation techniques, exercise or support groups can help some patients. Others with more severe symptoms may benefit from formal counselling or cognitive behavioural therapy (CBT). If anxiety is acute and related to stressful life events, a short course of benzodiazepines (e.g. diazepam) may be warranted.

Web resources
- Guidelines for FBD management: www.bsg.org. uk
- Information on FBD: www.gpnotebook.co.uk

Further reading
- Drossman DA, Creed FH, Olden KW *et al.* (1999) Psychosocial aspects of the functional gastrointestinal disorders. *Gut.* **45** Suppl 2: II25–II30.
- Mertz HR (2003) Irritable bowel syndrome. *New England Journal of Medicine.* **349**: 2136.

25 An unsteady pensioner

Patrick is an 88-year-old retired dentist. He has been referred to the medical assessment unit by his GP with a one-week history of increasing confusion, urinary incontinence and frequent falls.

He lives with his son and daughter-in-law who accompany him to the hospital. They tell you that before this week, he was a normal, fit and independent man, and all his other medical problems were well controlled! The son says that he is 'very concerned about how fast his father has deteriorated', and despite considerable efforts to care for him over the past week, he is only safe with hospital care.

(a) Acute confusion in the elderly is a common presenting complaint. What are likely causes for Patrick's confusion?

....

....

....

(b) What formal assessment can be used to monitor a patient's level of confusion?

....

....

....

(c) What investigations might help you diagnose a cause for his confusion?

....

....

....

Patrick has a past medical history of congestive heart failure, and osteoarthritis. He has suffered from depression and insomnia since his wife died 2 years ago. His regular medications are:

- bendrofluazide 2.5 mg mane
- ramipril 5 mg mane
- nitrazepam 5 mg nocte
- paroxetine 30 mg mane
- paracetamol 1g qds
- diclofenac 50 mg tds
- omeprazole 20 mg od.

(d) Which risk factors for falling should be assessed in the history?

....

....

....

During Patrick's hospital stay, the healthcare team caries out a falls assessment. They identify several potential areas for intervention to reduce his risk of further falls.

(e) What should be specifically addressed in a falls assessment?

....

....

....

(f) Which interventions might reduce the risk of further falls?

....

....

....

(g) Discuss the psychosocial impact of having a fall in an elderly patient, and how this might lead to increased morbidity.

....

....

....

Following the results of initial investigations, Patrick has a 7-day course of levofloxacin for a urinary tract infection, and left lower lobe pneumonia. He is transferred to a care of the elderly ward. His condition improves, and after 4 days he is orientated in time and place. During his stay on the ward Patrick receives daily physiotherapy.

During one of his physiotherapy sessions, the physiotherapist identifies a gait abnormality but is unsure what it represents.

(h) What common gait abnormalities may be found in elderly patients, and what are their causes?

....

....

....

After a successful period of rehabilitation, Patrick is seen by the discharge liaison team, who organise an appropriate package of care involving a period of 'intermediate care'. Two days before he is due to be discharged he develops acute malodorous diarrhoea in the night. A stool sample confirms *Clostridium difficile* toxin. He is transferred to a side room and started on appropriate antibiotic treatment.

(i) How can the transmission of hospital-acquired infections be reduced?

....

....

....

(j) Discuss the causes, consequences, and treatment of *Clostridium difficile* diarrhoea.

....

....

....

After 7 days of treatment Patrick has formed stool. Unfortunately the intermediate care bed that had been arranged for him is no longer available. On the ward round the consultant discusses the problems that prolonged hospital admissions can have for elderly patients.

(k) What common complications can occur in elderly patients after hospital admission?

....

....

....

Key cases

- Acute confusion (delirium)
- Falls in the elderly
- Acute infectious diarrhoea

Clinical context

Over the last half century, life expectancy has increased on average by 15 years. The elderly now comprise a quarter of the western world's population. We must learn to appreciate the physiology of ageing, and complex multisystem pathology.

Elderly patients are often defined by the frequent presence of multiple pathologies, and the atypical presentation of illness. Additionally the presentation of a social problem may obscure an underlying disease or complicate its management. Acute myocardial infarction, pneumonia, urinary tract infection, and anaemia (to mention a few) can present with confusion, falls, and loss of either mobility or day-to-day functioning. Specific symptoms and signs may not be present. Furthermore there is often an acceptance that ill health is normal in old age, and patients often present late – a common cause for patients' poor prognoses!

Understanding the atypical nature of illness in the elderly is important. What affects one patient will not affect the next. Ageing affects organ function, leading to a reduced reserve capacity. Thus when an elderly patient has a minor illness, or when a new drug is introduced, the balance can be tipped, causing either a new problem or exacerbating a chronic problem.

> ⚐ Use this opportunity to reflect on the importance of the 'geriatric giants'. The symptoms of falls, incontinence, confusion, and immobility are common to a number of diseases of old age.

(a) Causes of acute confusion (delirium)

'Delirium' is a term often used interchangeably with phrases such as 'acute confusional state', 'acute organic brain syndrome', and 'toxic confusional state'. Delirium is usually reversible. The onset may be relatively sudden, however symptoms may progress over hours or days. It typically fluctuates in severity, is usually worse at night, and can affect the young and old alike. Elderly patients may become delirious following any 'balance-tipping' insult.

Infection at any site, particularly the urinary tract, is a common precipitant.

A patient with an acute confusional state may have the following features:

- *mild global impairment of cognitive processes*: associated with reduced awareness of the environment (i.e. a reduced level of consciousness)
- *disorientation*: time, place, and person
- *memory loss*: after recovery there is little or no memory for events during the period of confusion
- *mood disturbance*: lability, agitation, anxiety or depression
- *behavioural changes*, including inactivity, hyperactivity, or irritability
- *perceptual disturbance*: delusions, or perceptual misperceptions (illusions) and hallucinations
- *disturbance of the sleep–wake cycle*: this is referred to as '*sundowning*'.

Nurses often inform junior doctors that a patient was confused and agitated overnight. However, when the patient is assessed during the working day there can be little to suggest that this was the case, i.e. no obvious signs of delirium. This is what is known as 'sundowning', where there is increased agitation and activity late in the day, and through the evening and night.

It is important to understand that delirium is often differentiated from dementia, depression and schizophrenia by the acute and fluctuating character of patients' symptoms. Nevertheless, the boundaries are often blurred, especially when there is co-existing illness. This is particularly true of a prolonged delirious state, or dementia with Lewy bodies (a type of dementia that has a fluctuating course, and symptoms that can frequently include psychosis). Furthermore, following the treatment of the underlying condition (e.g. infection), there may be a lag period in which the delirious symptoms resolve slowly.

Common causes of acute confusion include:

- Infection:
  - **urinary tract infection**
  - **chest infection**
  - meningitis, encephalitis
  - septicaemia
- Metabolic encephalopathies:
  - **hypo/hypernatraemia**
  - **hypo/hyperglycaemia**
  - **hypo/hypercalcaemia**
  - **renal failure: uraemia**

- hypothermia
- hepatic failure – encephalopathy
- Wernicke's encephalopathy and other vitamin B deficiencies
- hypo/hyperthyroidism
- Cushing's disease, Addison's disease
- Hypoxaemia:
  - **pneumonia**
  - **exacerbation of COPD (hypoxaemia +/− hypercapnia)**
  - pulmonary oedema
  - pulmonary embolism
- Cerebral pathology:
  - **stroke/TIA**
  - **subdural haematoma**
  - raised intracranial pressure, hydrocephalus
  - subarachnoid haemorrhage
  - malignancy (primary or secondary)
  - epilepsy, i.e. post-ictal states and non-convulsive status
  - cerebral abscess
  - trauma
- Cardiovascular:
  - **acute myocardial infarction**
  - **anaemia (chronic/acute)**
- Drugs:
  - **drug intoxification: anticholinergic agents, benzodiazepines, narcotics, tricyclic antidepressants**
  - drug and alcohol withdrawal syndromes
- Gastrointestinal:
  - constipation/ diarrhoea.

This patient's acute confusion is likely to be due to multiple causes. Given the history, all the above that are in bold are likely, and therefore should be excluded.

This, in theory, is easy to do. In practice, however, the patient with a confusional state can be very challenging to assess and treat. Often no reliable history is available, and information from relatives/ friends can be very valuable. This can save time and fruitless investigations.

> Use this opportunity to think about what other sources of information about a patient are available. Who should you contact if unsure about the history given?

(b) Formal assessment of confusion

The abbreviated mental test was developed by Hodkinson in 1972 as a tool to aid the diagnosis of dementia. It is commonly used in confusion and is the most appropriate initial test to rapidly assess and monitor a patient's cognition. The maximum score achievable is 10 (*see* below). Score: 8–10 probably normal, 7 probably abnormal, 0–6 abnormal. It is a brief measure of cognitive impairment in adults:

1 *age*: must be correct
2 *time*: correct to the nearest hour
3 *'42 West Street'*: give this and ask for it to be repeated to ensure it has been heard correctly. Ask for it again at the end of the test
4 *month or year*
5 *place* (name of hospital)
6 *date of birth*
7 *recognition of two people*
8 *year of the start of the Second (or First) World War*
9 *name of the present monarch*
10 *count backwards from 20 to 1.*

Serial scores can be a very useful way of monitoring improvement. You must ensure that the same questions are used, and do not correct the patient if a wrong answer is given. Repeated corrections, especially of the same answer may produce a learned response.

The mini-mental state examination (MMSE) assesses five areas of cognitive function: orientation, registration, attention and calculation, recall and language. The maximum score achievable is 30. A score of 23 or below indicates cognitive impairment. It is used to screen for, and establish, the severity of cognitive impairment. It is useful for monitoring changes in cognition using sequential assessments, e.g. for assessing the progression of dementia. Dementia is a syndrome of global impairment of cognition in clear consciousness. Compare this with the definition of acute confusional state/delirium.

> What is the definition of consciousness? How is this different from cognition? How is consciousness assessed?

(c) Investigations for a patient with acute confusion

The following initial investigations should be done on patients presenting with acute confusion with no obvious cause:

- plasma glucose
- FBC
- U&E
- markers of myocardial injury
- LFTs and bone profile (Ca^{2+}, HPO_4^{2-}, ALP)
- CRP
- ECG
- CXR
- dipstick of urine (and if required microscopy, culture and sensitivity)

- ABG (only if low SpO_2, or abnormal venous HCO_3^-).

> How do the investigations above relate to the common causes of confusion? For example, what consequences of acute or chronic anaemia might cause an acute confusional state?

Further investigations may be ordered after the interpretation of the initial investigations, combined clues from specific symptoms and/or signs, and collateral history. Below are some common examples:

- thyroid function tests
- clotting screen
- blood cultures
- vitamin B_{12} and folate levels
- urine and serum osmolality
- ultrasound of the liver/kidneys
- CT of the brain
- lumbar puncture
- electroencephalogram (EEG).

Falls in the elderly

Falls are a common problem causing considerable mortality, morbidity, reduced function and premature nursing home admission. They have major effects on patients, their relatives, and NHS resources.

- Approximately 33% of the elderly population (>65 years) fall at least once a year in the community. This increases to 50% when in hospital or nursing home environments.
- Women generally fall 2–3 times more frequently than men.
- Falls are the leading cause of death from injury among people over the age of 75 years.
- 3–10% of falls in the elderly result in serious injury.
- Only 1% of falls result in hip fractures; however approximately 30% of patients with a fractured neck of femur are dead within 12 months (*see* p. 104).
- Falls account for 10% of emergency admissions.
- Patients who are unable to get up after a fall have significant risks of further morbidity (*see* pp. 104–9).

> What are the older people's National Service Framework (NSF) standards? How do they relate to problems affecting the elderly, such as stroke, falls, and mental health?

(d) Causes and risk factors for falls

Falls have multiple precipitating causes and predisposing risk factors. It is important to establish whether a potentially treatable medical cause, environmental factors, or a combination are responsible. Most falls are multifactorial in origin e.g. tripping over a rug, precipitated by an abnormal gait and poor vision. Common causes and risk factors include:

- *impairment in hearing, vision, and balance*
- *environmental factors*: inadequate lighting, ill-fitting shoes/slippers, slippery floors, loose rugs, and inadequate handholds
- *poly-pharmacy*: use of four or more drugs, particularly benzodiazepines, SSRIs, neuroleptic agents, antihypertensives and anticonvulsants. This may be particularly important if a new drug has recently been introduced
- *hypotension*: postural, drug-induced, post-prandial
- *syncope*: cough, micturition, defaecation
- *arrhythmia*
- *intermittent delirium*: *see* causes above
- *dementia, depressive symptoms*
- *unstable knee due to quadriceps weakness*
- *previous stroke*
- *arthritis*
- *Parkinson's disease.*

(e) Falls risk assessment

The National Institute for Health and Clinical Excellence (NICE) provides guidance for the healthcare team to identify and assess falls in the elderly. NICE set out three key areas in Guideline 21 (2004):

1 case/risk identification
2 multifactorial risk assessment
3 multifactorial interventions.

All health professionals who care for elderly patients should ask about falls in the past year, and their frequency, context, and characteristics.

Patients at high risk of falling need further assessment to identify underlying problems. They should be referred for a multifactorial falls risk assessment with appropriate intervention including:

Physical factors

- Neurological examination including gait, balance, mobility, muscle weakness and visual impairment
- Urinary incontinence
- Cardiovascular examination
- Osteoporosis risk
- Medication review

Psychological factors

- Cognitive impairment
- Perceived functional abilities and anxiety surrounding falling

Home assessment

- Home hazards
- Falls history

Assessment of each area in the above list may be complex and should be done by trained members of a multidisciplinary team. Often hospitals will have a proforma used to document the findings in each area. An example of a postural stability assessment is shown in Figure 25.1a and b.

> Use this opportunity to think about members of the healthcare team who may be involved in falls assessments. What forms of assessment does your hospital use? What is the role of occupational therapy in the hospital, and in the community?

(f) Interventions to reduce the likelihood of further falls

After assessing and treating both acute and chronic co-morbidities, and assessing risk factors, a successful management plan should include the following components (NICE Guideline 21, 2004):

- strength and balance training with walking aid provision
- OT assessment of home hazards with appropriate intervention
- vision assessment and referral
- a review of medication aiming to minimise poly-pharmacy
- promoting patients' independence by addressing their overall physical and psychological wellbeing.

A review of medication is crucially important in preventing further falls. Many elderly patients have several chronic conditions requiring poly-pharmacy. Often, new drugs will be added without considering either ageing physiology, altered drug metabolism, interactions, or the cumulative effect. However, with the perceived benefit of each drug comes the most common adverse effect – increased risk of a fall. A risk–benefit assessment of each medication is required.

(g) Psychosocial impact of falls in the elderly

Despite many falls in the elderly having an underlying cause (e.g. UTI, atrial fibrillation, heart failure, anaemia, pneumonia, etc), the fall itself often has the greatest effect on the patient's lifestyle. Falling, especially when patients are unable to get up unaided, is an extremely unpleasant experience, and the fear of further falls tends to lead to a vicious cycle (i.e. the fear itself leading to deteriorating mobility).

Following a fall, elderly patients often enter a vicious cycle of anxiety caused by:

- lost confidence in mobility, and fear of falling
- a reminder that their general health is poor
- loss of independence and a need to rely on others.

Depression may follow as patients become:

- housebound and fail to continue with their hobbies and interests
- detached from social circles.

In addition, as a result of reduced mobility, elderly patients are at greater risk of:

- constipation
- infections: chest and urinary tract
- deep vein thrombosis or pulmonary embolus
- muscle atrophy: precipitating more falls
- accelerated osteoporosis: increasing the risk of fracture on the next fall
- orthostatic postural hypotension: precipitating more falls.

Additionally, there are many other factors that can influence a patient's quality of life after a fall. These must be investigated with individualised intervention aimed at improving physical and psychological function.

(h) Gait abnormalities

Watching someone walk can provide valuable clinical information. A gait abnormality is an uncontrollable problem with walking. Abnormalities include:

- *waddling gait*: broad-based: 'duck-like' waddle resulting from proximal muscle weakness (e.g. proximal myopathy)
- *scissor gait*: characterised by leg flexion at the hips and knees. Patients appear as if crouching; the knees and thighs hit or cross in a scissors-like movement (e.g. spastic paraplegia)
- *antalgic gait*: someone trying to minimise pain in a limb. The patient leans to the side of the painful hip and takes a rapid, heavy step, followed by a slower step on the unaffected side (e.g. osteoarthritis)
- *parkinsonian gait*: hesitation in starting walking, accompanied by small, shuffling and hurried steps (festination), and lack of normal arm swing (e.g. Parkinson's disease/antidopaminergic drugs)
- *sensory ataxic gait*: (spinal) posterior column damage leads to a loss of proprioception resulting in a stamping, broad-based gait. Patients tend to look at their feet throughout the process of walking and are worse in poor light. This gait is also seen in patients with peripheral neuropathy

Name . . . . Hosp No . . . . . .

Forenames . . . .

Mr / Mrs / Miss / Ms . . . . M / F DoB . . . /. . /. .

NHS

POSTURAL STABILITY

FALLS in the elderly are usually <u>multifactorial</u> and are <u>rarely simple</u>. The provoking factor may be trivial but for those with postural instability it is a potent catalyst, which launches a chain reaction leading to a fall.

- Do not accept a fall as mechanical until postural stability has been considered systematically.
- Multiple factors are the norm.

FALLS(S)	✓		✓		✓		✓		✓
Single	☐	Multiple	☐	Indoors	☐	Outdoors	☐	Day	☐
Fracture(s)	☐	Frail	☐	Nutrition poor	☐	BMI <19	☐	Night	☐
Dehydration	☐	Hypothermia	☐	Pressure Sore	☐	Length of lie		......hours	

Witness account

Previous injuries

PROVOKING FACTORS	✓	**Synopsis**
(Pre)-Syncope	☐	
Postural hypotension	☐	
TIA	☐	
Vertigo/dizziness	☐	
Chronic illness, Epilepsy	☐	
Acute illness	☐	
Other		

SUSPECT MEDICATIONS, ALCOHOL	**ACTION**
1	•
2	•
3	•
4	•
5	•
6	•

PHYSICAL FINDINGS		BP Lying
		BP Sitting
		BP Standing 0'
Current injuries		BP Standing 2'
Gait		
Romberg's test		
Timed up and go	Seconds	Time to rise from an armed chair, walk 3 metres, return and sit down. N ≤ 15 sec
Misc:		

Figure 25.1 Postural stability assessment. (Reprinted with permission from the Countess of Chester NHS Foundation Trust.)

An unsteady pensioner

Which components of POSTURAL STABILITY are compromised?

DETECTION	✓	Finding	Eg
P' Neuropathy	☐		Spinothalamic and posterior column functions
Myelopathy	☐		Spinal disease, motor/sensory level, sphincters?
Visual	☐		Cataracts, Macular degeneration, ..
Labyrinthine	☐		Vertigo, nystagmus, cf cerebellum
Other	☐		
COMPUTATION	✓		
Stroke	☐		Lateralising, focal signs
Medication/alcohol	☐		Suspicion, history, cogeners, Abnormal LFTs, ..
Confusion, acute	☐		AMT and Folstein score
Dementia	☐		AMT and Folstein score
Other	☐		
CORRECTION	✓		
Neurological	☐		Cerebellar signs, dyspraxia, gait characteristics
Parkinsons/ism	☐		Extrapyramidal signs, gait characteristics
Muscular	☐		Myopathy, wasting, fasciculation, ..
Skeletal	☐		Deformity, fracture,
Other	☐		

INVESTIGATIONS			(Indicated investigations, ✓ and order)	
Basic	ECG	☐	Routine bloods	☐
Supplementary	24 hour Halter Monitor	☐	Echocardiogram	☐
Special, consultant	Carotid sinus massage	☐	Tilt table test	☐

MANAGEMENT

-
-
-
-
-
-

Dr . . . . Signature . . . . Bleep . . . . . Date . . . / . . / . .

THERAPIES	✓	
Environment	☐	
Feet/shoes	☐	
Walking aids	☐	
Home visit	☐	
Visual acuity	☐	R /6 L /6

MET Visual contrast acuity	24 V Good ☐	20-23 Good ☐	16-19 Fair ☐	1-15 Poor ☐

Recommendations

PT/OT . . . . Signature . . . . Date . . . / . . . / . . .

- *hemiplegic gait (or spastic gait)*: the affected leg is weak and spastic, with dorsiflexion and weakness of the foot resulting in the leg being swung in an arc-like fashion (e.g. following a stroke)
- *steppage gait*: also known as foot drop. The foot hangs down causing the toes to scrape the ground whilst walking (e.g. common peroneal nerve palsy).

> Use this opportunity to revise the control of walking. What features on physical examination might suggest cerebellar, cortical, spinal, and sensory disorders?

(i) Hospital-acquired infections

Hospital-acquired (or nosocomial) infections are common in elderly patients with frequent admissions to hospital. Other risk factors include:

- immunosuppression due to drugs or disease
- surgical and intensive care patients
- patients with catheters and other indwelling devices (e.g. peripheral and central cannulae).

Hand washing is the most effective way of reducing patient-to-patient spread of infection in hospitals. Unfortunately, this can be suboptimal due to the length of time suggested for adequate washing, allergies to antiseptic cleaners, and a high ratio between patients and staff. Other measures used in hospitals in an attempt to reduce the spread of infection include the following:

- gloves, masks, gowns
- isolation of infectious, or potentially infectious, patients
- barrier or reverse barrier nursing
- regular cleaning of the hospital environment
- closing infected wards/bays on a ward
- avoiding insertion of unnecessary cannulae and removing them when not required. Most trusts have specific policies regarding indwelling devices
- removing other indwelling devices if not required, e.g. central lines and catheters
- clean uniforms
- hand washing by relatives
- using sterile equipment.

(j) *Clostridium difficile*

Clostridium difficile is a major nosocomial infection associated predominantly with antibiotic use. It is an anaerobic, spore forming, Gram-positive bacterium. The normal bowel flora in some way inhibits the overgrowth of *C. difficile* in the large intestine (natural, native resistance). However, when this mechanism is disrupted, *C. difficile* proliferates.

Some strains of *C. difficile* secrete two exotoxins: exotoxins A and B. Both A and B bind to receptors on epithelial cells resulting in fluid secretion and mucosal damage. Exotoxin B is used for the diagnosis, based on its response during culture.

Antibiotics (particularly cephalosporins and clindamycin) are known to reduce natural bowel flora, allowing *C. difficile* to proliferate.

The colonisation rate in normal members of the public is less than 5%. Spores are found on the hands of patients and staff, as well as beds and floors. It is highly contagious, and barrier nursing is required.

Clinically there is a spectrum of disease from asymptomatic carriers to fulminant colitis exhibiting symptoms of malodorous diarrhoea, crampy abdominal pain, fever and vomiting. Complications of *C. difficile* include toxic megacolon, perforation, electrolyte disturbances, and hypoalbuminaemia.

In the treatment of acute infectious diarrhoea it is important to:

- isolate from other patients, particularly those receiving antibiotics
- take a full history and examine, particularly for abdominal tenderness and hydration status (*see* p. 105)
- stop the likely culprit (i.e. antibiotic)
- ensure the patient is well hydrated
- investigate (abdominal X-ray for toxic megacolon; blood biochemistry and haematology (particularly U&E, FBC, albumin, and CRP))
- treat with oral or intravenous metronidazole, or oral vancomycin as a second-line agent (after consulting your hospital's policy).

> 'Superbug' stories are common in the media. How does antibiotic resistance arise? Which organisms have become particularly problematic in hospital patients? What is your hospital's policy regarding MRSA treatment? Which organisms are predicted to become problematic in the near future?

(k) Common complications following admission to hospital

Elderly patients have a fear of admission to hospital. It is common to hear 'I don't want to go to hospital because I might catch something'. Hospital admission-associated complications (e.g. hospital-acquired infections) are extremely important to consider before admitting any patient to hospital. Every admission should have the risks and benefits carefully balanced.

Common complications of admission to hospital include:

- *hospital-acquired infections*: LRTI, gastro-enteritis (diarrhoea and vomiting), UTI, MRSA-colonisation, septicaemia, cellulitis (from venflon site)
- *constipation*: resulting from immobility, poor diet, lack of appetite, associated with depression
- *depression*
- *deep vein thrombosis* (+/− pulmonary embolus)
- *a reduction of level in activities of daily living*
- *worsening of mobility*
- *increased dependency.*

Web resources

- Falls – NICE (2004) *Guideline 21: The Assessment and Prevention of Falls in Older People*: www. nice.org.uk
- J Starr (2005) *Clostridium difficile*-associated diarrhoea: diagnosis and treatment. BMJ Learning. www.bmjlearning.com

Further reading

- Brown TM and Boyle MF (2002) ABC of psychological medicine: delirium. *British Medical Journal*. **325**: 644.
- Chang JT, Morton SC, Rubenstein LZ *et al.* (2004) Interventions for the prevention of falls in older adults: systematic review and meta-analysis of randomised clinical trials. *British Medical Journal*. **328**: 680.
- Feder G, Cryer C, Donovan S and Carter Y (2000) Guidelines for the prevention of falls in people over 65. The Guidelines' Development Group. *British Medical Journal*. **321**: 1007.
- Horan MA (1998) Presentation of disease in old age. Chapter 14. In: R Tallis and H Fillit (eds) *Brocklehurst's Textbook of Geriatric Medicine and Gerontology* (5e). Churchill Livingstone, Edinburgh, pp. 201-05.
- Meagher DJ (2001) Delirium: optimising management. *British Medical Journal*. **322**: 144.
- Woolf AD and Akesson K (2003) Preventing fractures in elderly people. *British Medical Journal*. **327**: 89.

26 A diabetic with diarrhoea

Dianne is a 32-year-old insulin-dependent diabetic. She normally has good glycaemic control, regularly attends her review clinics, and has not suffered any significant complications from the disease.

She visits her GP complaining that she has been feeling weak and tired recently, and has been having intermittent bouts of diarrhoea. She says that she thinks she has lost some weight over the last month.

(a) What further questions would the GP ask Dianne?

....

....

....

(b) Which symptoms indicate the need for further investigation?

....

....

....

(c) Which disease processes could be responsible for Dianne's symptoms?

....

....

....

She additionally complains of stiffness in her fingers and a tingling sensation in her fingers, toes and around her lips.

(d) List two possible metabolic explanations for the tingling sensation in her fingers, toes and lips.

....

....

....

On examination she is found to have superficial bruising and proximal muscle weakness.

(e) Which two vitamin deficiencies could account for this?

....

....

....

Initial investigations included a full blood count, which showed a low Hb and raised MCV. Additionally the requested blood film showed the presence of both macrocytes and microcytes.

(f) Account for these findings.

....

....

....

(g) What overall diagnosis is most likely?

....

....

....

(h) Which diagnostic tests should now be done?

....

....

....

Initial biochemistry results showed increased ALP.

(i) Give an explanation for this. What are the other causes of a raised ALP level?

....

....

....

(j) Which investigations could confirm the initial suspicion?

....

....

....

(k) Which other healthcare professionals should now be involved in her care?

....

....

....

(l) The GP suggests that Dianne should have regular follow-up for her condition. What would he check during her review?

....

....

....

She does not attend her reviews and 15 years later presents with weight loss and central abdominal pain. A small bowel barium meal shows strictures in the distal duodenum.

(m) Which possible complications of the disease could cause this?

....

....

....

(n) How could she have prevented this sequel of her disease?

....

....

....

✓ Answers and teaching notes

Key cases

- Chronic diarrhoea
- Coeliac disease
- Diabetes mellitus

Clinical context

Acute diarrhoea is a symptom that nearly everybody has experienced. Thankfully most diarrhoeal illnesses are self-limiting, and most sufferers do not seek medical advice. In contrast, chronic diarrhoea is associated with significant morbidity. There are many underlying causes and sequelae. This scenario shows how the patient's history will define the cause, direct relevant investigations, and predict/identify potential associations and complications.

Chronic diarrhoea

Chronic diarrhoea is an extremely common reason for patients to visit their GP. It is defined as the frequent passage of abnormally liquid stool, and is chronic if it lasts for more than a month. Patients who present with 'diarrhoea' may just mean frequent stools. Clarifying the history is vital.

(a) History

The history should include:

- blood or mucus in stool
- nature of stools (consistency and other features e.g. floating/pale/foul-smelling – steatorrhoea)
- frequency of the stool
- abdominal pain including the nature of the pain (e.g. colicky?)
- vomiting
- length of time
- return from a foreign country
- occupation
- drug history
- sexual history
- family history.

Other important points to consider include:

- the patient's age is important in deciding between possible causes
- weight loss in chronic diarrhoea is suspicious and should be investigated
- nocturnal diarrhoea is always pathological (i.e. wakes from sleep)
- in chronic diarrhoea it is important to exclude a rectal lesion, and a rectal examination must be done. However, there is a high false-negative rate with the untrained finger
- dehydration in either an infant or elderly person with diarrhoea necessitates admission to hospital.

A differential diagnosis for chronic diarrhoea includes conditions shown in Table 26.1.

> 🔅 Use this opportunity to revise the mechanisms of diarrhoea. You should be familiar with the concepts of osmotic, secretory and inflammatory diarrhoea, in addition to problems affecting gut motility. How do these concepts apply to the causes of diarrhoea listed below?

(b) Associated symptoms

The key features that would be particularly worrying in this patient are:

- weight loss
- symptoms of anaemia
- chronicity (over a month).

Chronic diarrhoea always needs investigation. Whether the large and/or small bowel is investigated would depend on the history.

Table 26.1 Differential diagnosis of chronic diarrhoea

Common	Less common	Rare
Functional bowel disorder	Bowel carcinoma	Thyrotoxicosis
Diverticular disease	Inflammatory bowel disease	Chronic pancreatitis
Antibiotic use	Excess alcohol	Diabetes (autonomic nephropathy)
Overflow in constipation	Malabsorbtion (e.g. coeliac disease)	Laxative use
Lactose intolerance	Bacterial overgrowth	

(c) Disease processes

The differential diagnoses listed above are not exhaustive. The key features in this case are the patient's age, history of chronic fatigue, weight loss and ongoing GI upset, in combination with a history of autoimmune diabetes.

Clinical suspicion would therefore include:

- malabsorbtion (coeliac disease)
- diabetic autonomic neuropathy
- thyrotoxicosis
- inflammatory bowel disease
- bacterial overgrowth.

A diagnosis of carcinoma is unlikely.

The presence of autoimmune disease should always lead to the clinical suspicion of other associated autoimmune diseases. These include Graves' disease, Hashimoto's thyroiditis, vitiligo, Addison's disease, coeliac disease, pernicious anaemia, primary ovarian failure, and myasthenia gravis.

(d) Symptoms and signs of hypocalcaemia

Hypocalcaemia is characterised by sensory symptoms consisting of paresthesiae of the lips, tongue, fingers and feet, and motor symptoms and signs including carpopedal spasm, generalised muscle aching and spasms of facial muscles (tetany).

- tetany results from a severe degree of hypocalcaemia
- it also results from a reduction in ionised plasma calcium. This occurs in severe alkalosis due to increased calcium binding to albumin.

A reduction in extracellular calcium lowers action potential thresholds and increases tissue excitability causing continuous muscular contractions.

Chovstek's (tapping the facial nerve over the zygomatic arch to produce twitching of the facial muscles), and Trousseau's signs (inflating a cuff over the brachial artery to produce carpal spasm) can be used to assess for tetany.

> How does hypocalcaemia cause the symptoms of tetany? What are the effects of hypocalcaemia on the resting membrane potential and gated sodium channels? How does alkalosis produce the same effect?

(e) Vitamin deficiency

- Bruising can be a sign of abnormal clotting, and in this case vitamin K deficiency.
- Proximal muscle weakness is a sign of vitamin D deficiency.

Vitamins are either water soluble (B-complex and C) or fat soluble (A, D, E and K). Water-soluble vitamins are more rapidly turned over, and are less readily stored than fat-soluble vitamins, which are stored in the liver and fatty tissues.

Vitamin A (retinol)

Vitamin A has many functions. In addition to its critical role in photoreceptor function, it is important in bone growth, cell division and gene expression.

Vitamin D (cholecalciferol)

Vitamin D regulates calcium and phosphate. In its active form (1,25-dihydroxycholecalciferol) it increases calcium absorbtion from the small intestine, and increases both bone calcification and resorption.

Vitamin D deficiency in growing children causes rickets. Vitamin D deficiency in adults results in osteomalacia, and muscular weakness.

> You should be familiar with regulation of calcium homeostasis by vitamin D, parathyroid hormone, and calcitonin. What are the roles of the skin, liver and kidneys in vitamin D metabolism?

Vitamin E (various tocopherols)

Vitamin E is an important antioxidant, it protects vitamins A and C, erythrocytes and fatty acids from oxidative damage and destruction.

Vitamin K (phylloquinone (K_1) and menaquinone (K_2))

Vitamin K_2 is naturally produced by commensal bacteria in the GI tract. It is a co-factor required for the synthesis of factors II, VII, IX, and X, and proteins C and S. Additionally osteoblasts contain vitamin K-dependent proteins such as osteocalcin.

Patients taking antibiotics may lack vitamin K because intestinal flora are destroyed. Additionally, people with chronic diarrhoea may have problems absorbing sufficient amounts of vitamin K.

> Use this opportunity to revise the intrinsic and extrinsic coagulation pathways. Which pathway would vitamin K deficiency primarily affect? What would be the effect on the PT and APTT?

(f) Mixed or bimodal anaemia

A blood film should always be ordered in the investigation of anaemia. Although automated counts provide a rapid estimate of the Hb and MCV, they do not provide information on cell morphology, which may provide a definitive diagnosis.

A systematic approach to understanding anaemia is important. A raised MCV is usually due to Vitamin B_{12} or folate deficiency, chronic alcohol consumption or hypothyroidism. Microcytosis is usually due to iron deficiency or blood loss. In this scenario, the presence of both macrocytes and microcytes should alert to the possibility of B_{12} and/or folate deficiency, and iron deficiency (*see* p. 228).

(g) Coeliac disease (gluten-sensitive enteropathy)

The key points outlined in the scenario include a history of weight loss, diarrhoea, and malabsorption of fat-soluble vitamins, folate, and iron. Taken together with the patient's known type 1 diabetes, the most likely diagnosis would be coeliac disease.

Coeliac disease is a relatively common, lifelong inflammatory disease predominantly affecting the upper small intestine due to gluten in the diet of genetically susceptible patients. The disease may be as prevalent as 1 in 100, and consequently there are a large number of patients with undiagnosed coeliac disease.

T-cell-mediated immune response to gluten is the major cause of mucosal damage. A series of inflammatory processes results in damage to the mucosa of the proximal small bowel. The mucosal damage is a spectrum with the classical change being subtotal villous atrophy. Damage leads to poor absorption of nutrients including iron, folic acid and fat-soluble vitamins (all the F's – Fe^{2+}, folate, fat-soluble vitamins).

Clinically this manifests as:

- symptoms of anaemia: iron, folate and rarely B_{12} deficiency
- weight loss due to malabsorption
- ongoing GI upset: diarrhoea, abdominal pain, indigestion, bloating, wind.

Other features of iron or folate deficiency include angular stomatitis and mouth ulcers respectively, which are frequently found in coeliac disease. Rarer complications such as tetany and osteomalacia can result from more severe malabsorbtion (as in this scenario).

(h) Diagnosis of coeliac disease

Tests include:

- endomysial and transglutaminase (IgA) antibodies
- distal duodenal or oblique jejunal biopsy.

The definitive method for diagnosing coeliac disease is still a biopsy of the small intestine. A specimen is taken from the distal end of the duodenum via upper GI endoscopy for microscopic analysis.

Endomysial (EMA) and transglutaminase antibody (TGA) tests may suggest a diagnosis of coeliac disease, but the bowel must still be biopsied for confirmation.

False negatives for EMA/TGA include:

- IgA deficiency (2% of coeliac patients are IgA deficient)
- gluten-free diet
- infancy (EMA/TGA are not consistently positive until > 4 years).

(i) (j) Osteomalacia

Alkaline phosphatase (ALP)

Alkaline phosphatase is present in all body tissues. However high concentrations are found in osteoblasts, hepatocytes, canalicular epithelial cells and placental tissue. Different cells produce different isoenzymes and these may aid diagnosis. ALP levels rise considerably when bones are growing, liver cells are damaged, or biliary obstruction occurs.

Possible causes of increased levels of plasma ALP include:

- *hepatobiliary disease* including:
  - cholestasis: increased synthesis of hepatocyte ALP and increased secretion into plasma (*see* p. 61)
  - hepatocellular disease, including all causes of hepatitis (moderate elevations in ALP)
- *bone disease* – bone isoenzyme, reflecting increased osteoblastic activity, may be raised in:
  - osteomalacia and rickets
  - renal osteodystrophy
  - bone metastases (or rarely a primary bone tumour)
  - recent fracture
  - a growing child – especially at puberty
  - Paget's disease
- *pregnancy*: the placenta secretes its own isoenzyme, which raises ALP concentration
- *malignancy*.

Osteomalacia

Osteomalacia is caused by vitamin D deficiency. Failure of calcium absorbtion leads to low serum calcium. PTH is secreted to try and compensate, leading to increased osteoclastic and osteoblastic activity and overall loss of bone mineral content. Key investigations include:

- *biochemistry*: low or normal Ca^{2+}, low HPO_4^{2-}, secondary to renal PTH effects
- *radiology* shows osteopenic bone and decalcification of bone, particularly of any concave surfaces.

(k) (l) Follow-up

Education is important in the management of patients with coeliac disease and chronic malabsorbtion. Patients require vitamin replacement, calcium supplements, and bisphosphonates to treat osteoporosis. The only definitive treatment is the strict adherence to a gluten-free diet, which may prove difficult. Many patients benefit from attending a local coeliac support group. Other healthcare professionals essential to the management of coeliac patients include:

- dieticians
- nurses
- gastroenterologists
- clinical biochemists.

> Adherence to a gluten-free diet may prove difficult. What are the reasons for intentional and non-intentional non-adherence? How might psychological aspects of chronic disease be related to these?

Long-term follow-up is essential to monitor disease control and complications. Review may be carried out by dieticians, nurses, GPs or gastroenterologists, and may be in primary or secondary care. Regular review involves:

- *monitoring the disease status*:
  - asking about symptoms
  - height, weight, BMI, hip/waist ratio
  - FBC
  - LFTs
  - bone profile (Ca^{2+}/HPO_4^{2-}/ALP)
  - serum folate/ferritin/B_{12}
- *preventing disease complications*:
  - osteoporosis risk assessment and treatment includes dual emission X-ray absorptiometry (DEXA) scans for all patients. Menopausal women should be scanned every 3 years. Lifestyle advice should be given, including exercise, smoking and alcohol advice. Calcium and vitamin D_3 supplements should be prescribed if patients are poorly mobile, and bisphosphonates used if patients have osteoporosis
  - a significant proportion of coeliac patients have some degree of splenic atrophy, therefore they should be vaccinated against haemophilus influenza B and streptococcal pneumonia
- *patient awareness and self-care*:
  - compliance with a gluten-free diet should be discussed
  - gluten-free food and drink directories are available through the Coeliac Society (*see* web resources), and many supermarkets now have sections containing gluten-free products
  - dieticians may be able to help with advice on weight, and both dietary and supplemental sources of calcium, vitamin D and iron
- *other issues*:
  - patients may want to consider screening of first-degree relatives
  - the genetic link to type 1 diabetes may warrant random or fasting plasma glucose testing.

(m) Coeliac complications

Complications of coeliac disease include the sequelae of dietary deficiencies discussed above. Other complications and associations include:

- osteoporosis (even in treated cases)
- an increased risk of small bowel adenocarcinoma
- an increased risk of oesophageal and oropharyngeal squamous cell carcinoma (*see* p. 135)
- intestinal T-cell lymphoma
- primary biliary cirrhosis
- neurological conditions (epilepsy, ataxia and neuropathy).

Strictures in the distal duodenum could represent adenocarcinoma or intestinal T-cell lymphoma.

(n) Prevention

The only way to reduce the sequelae of coeliac disease is strict adherence to a gluten-free diet.

Web resources

- British Society of Gastroenterology: www.bsg.org.uk
- Coeliac disease information: www.patient.co.uk
- The Coeliac Society: www.coeliac.co.uk

Further reading

- Fasana A (2003) Celiac disease – how to handle a clinical chameleon. *New England Journal of Medicine*. **348**: 2068.
- McManus R and Kelleher D (2003) Celiac disease – the villain unmasked. *New England Journal of Medicine*. **348**: 2573.

27 A builder with back pain

During your clinical attachment in general practice you see John, a 42-year-old builder who is complaining of lower back pain. He is well known to the practice and frequently presents with similar complaints, requesting a sick note.

He says 'I was carrying a wardrobe down the stairs with my son and suddenly I had this intense pain in my back. It's more on the left and moves into my bottom. Occasionally I also get a severe shooting pain down my left leg'. On examination John is reluctant to move his back and there is visible and palpable muscle spasm with diffuse tenderness. Straight leg raising test of his left leg is positive at 40 degrees. There are no 'red flags'.

(a) List 'red flags' (symptoms and signs suggestive of serious spinal pathology) you should assess in all patients presenting with back pain.

....
....
....

(b) What is the most likely diagnosis in this case, and how do the features described support this?

....
....
....

(c) How should this be managed, and what information should you give John about his condition?

....
....
....

Later that day you go with the GP to visit Jack, a 78-year-old retired gentleman with hypertension. Jack had called the practice early that morning complaining of a 'bad back' and 'problems with his water works'. The GP informs you Jack rarely visits the practice. He has only met Jack once before when visiting his wife who died 2 years ago from heart failure. The GP takes a history from him and learns that he has had a 'bad back' for approximately 2 months, but the pain has been much worse this week. He also enquires further about the problems with Jack's waterworks.

(d) From one part of the physical examination the GP confirms his suspicion as to the diagnosis. What is that part?

....
....
....

Jack is sent to the local hospital's surgical assessment unit. He is seen by an SHO who quite reasonably orders some imaging which proves informative.

(e) What imaging would be requested regarding the back pain, and why is it likely to have been informative?

....

....

....

(f) What further investigations should or could be done and why?

....

....

....

Jack is admitted to the urology ward. When the SHO gets there, he checks the fluid chart and there is no record of Jack having passed urine. His bladder is palpably grossly enlarged but is not tender.

(g) The SHO is worried that this may be due to spinal cord compression. What features in either the history or on examination could confirm his suspicions?

....

....

....

(h) The SHO's worries prove to be justified. What urgent treatment should now be given?

....

....

....

(i) How should the cancer be treated?

....

....

....

His 55-year-old son asks to see you. He says that he is beginning to experience similar symptoms to his father. He is concerned that he may have prostate cancer.

(j) What ethicolegal principle prevents open discussion with the son?

....

....

....

(k) Before starting investigations to detect prostate cancer what should the patient receive?

....

....

....

(l) What steps are required to detect early prostate cancer?

....

....

....

(m) The tests prove positive – what are the potential treatments?

....

....

....

(n) Treatment with curative intent is only possible in early prostate cancer. In view of this fact, should this man have already been screened?

....

....

....

Key cases

- Back pain
- Disc prolapse
- Cauda equina syndrome
- Prostatic cancer

Clinical context

Back pain is one of the most common reasons for patients to present to their GP, and accounts for a majority of chronic disability and incapacity from work. In the UK up to 50 million working days are lost each year. Nearly half a million people receive a long-term state incapacity benefit because of back pain. The cost of this to the UK economy is estimated at £5 billion/year (Department for Work and Pensions). To address this impact on society, the Government White Paper (1998) commenced the healthy workplace initiative 'Back in work'.

Back pain is a regrettably common result of our evolutionarily recent adaptation to an upright posture. Both benign and malignant causes are discussed here, using a slipped disc and metastatic prostate cancer as common examples. The need to prevent, or to treat with great urgency, incipient paraplegia is stressed. There are many links with other aspects of medicine, which are mentioned in the text and in text boxes. Finally the opportunity is taken to cover early, as opposed to late prostate cancer, and the role of screening.

Spectrum of back pain

The causes of back pain are extensive. Developing a good understanding is essential. At one end of the spectrum there is simple backache (caused by ligamentous or muscle strain) and lumbar disc prolapse, both self-limiting conditions. In contrast, at the other end of the spectrum, malignancy and cauda equina syndrome are potentially fatal and disabling. The prognoses of these conditions are dependent on timely diagnosis and treatment. In the middle of the spectrum there are the systemic and inflammatory conditions that are neither self-limiting nor fatal, requiring further investigations for diagnosis. In reality, common things occur commonly and around 90% of conditions are self-limiting and secondary to simple strain. Nevertheless, a thorough history and examination are needed each time to rule out any sinister pathology.

> ☀ To aid a comprehensive understanding of back pain, review the anatomy of the lumbar spine while studying the causes of back pain.
>
> What are the symptoms and signs of lumbar nerve root entrapment at each level from L2 to S1?

(a) 'Red flags' in back pain

- Structural deformity
- Weight loss
- Night pain (wakes from sleep)
- Past medical history of carcinoma
- Medication: e.g., systemic steroids
- Genitourinary symptoms: difficulty with micturition
- Gastrointestinal symptoms: constipation or diarrhoea
- Saddle anaesthesia
- Leg weakness/gait disturbance
- Patient systemically unwell
- Marked morning stiffness

> ☀ It is essential to develop your own personal formulae for assessing and managing common complaints. Identifying 'red flags' in the history and examination helps confirm or exclude serious pathology. Such a system should be developed for assessing back pain.

(b) Diagnosis

In this patient the likely underlying pathology is an acute lumbar disc prolapse. This is suggested by:

- acute lower back pain
- history of heavy lifting
- restricted spinal movements
- radiating leg pain
- a positive straight leg test.

These symptoms often follow a disc injury produced by sudden straining of the spine. There is acute low back pain, and when the nerve roots have been compressed, there may be radiating pain, paresthesiae, and motor weakness.

Examination commonly reveals pain and spasm of the paraspinal muscles, with restricted spinal movements. Patients may lean away from the side of any leg pain, in an effort to reduce the pain.

The straight leg raising test stretches the sciatic nerve, and pain associated with L5 and S1 roots gets worse.

(c) Management of simple back pain, and information given to patients

- Reassure the patient that you do not think there is a sinister cause for the back pain.
- Explain the cause of the pain.
- Inform the patient you expect a full recovery.
- Advice: a short period of rest (2–3 days at most) until pain settles slightly. Long-term rest is contraindicated; the best advice is to stay active within the limits of pain.
- Prescribe analgesia and an anti-inflammatory drug: e.g. regular paracetamol and an NSAID (e.g. naproxen (if no contraindications)).
- Prescribe a short-term muscle relaxant (<2/52): e.g. diazepam.

Prostate cancer with spinal metastases

Prostate cancer is the most common cancer in UK males. In 2000 there were 27,149 reported new cases of prostate cancer in the UK. Prostate cancer is predominantly a disease of elderly men, with almost half of all registered cases in patients aged over 75 years (Toms, 2004).

In the absence of screening (*see* later in this question), a common problem of prostate cancer is late presentation with metastatic bone disease. Often this involves the lumbosacral spine. Patients' first symptoms of the disease may include backache. The 'red flags' to assess in patients aged over 55 years old with back pain are that the pain is:

- constant
- progressive
- non-mechanical
- localised: worse at night or pain 'wakes from sleep'
- severe, with a sudden onset, e.g. following cough – pathological fracture
- associated with significant weight loss
- associated with past medical history of carcinoma.

Other common malignancies that metastasise to bone arise from the bronchus, breast, thyroid, kidney and oesophagus.

Extensive para-aortic lymph node metastases can cause similar back pain. Clinically, there is a remarkable sign of such metastases: patients sit bending forward or lie on their side curled up. This is because flexing their lumbar spine takes some of the tension off the unstretchable plaque of nodes. Conversely, asking the patient to extend their lumbar spine acutely exacerbates the pain.

> Think about how you would investigate such a patient who you suspect has presented with para-aortic lymph node metastases.

> Use this opportunity to revise the 'red flags' and appropriate investigations for the cancers listed above. Depending on the stage of the disease it is also important to understand the different definitive and palliative treatments offered to patients.

(d) Digital rectal examination

Yet again, the importance of rectal examination cannot be overemphasised. In this case, it is very likely that the GP will feel an extensive carcinoma as a craggy fixed mass, which cannot be distinguished from the prostate. The history of lower urinary tract symptoms (*see* p. 95) is why the rectal examination is essential.

(e) Investigations in suspected bone metastases

The investigations needed are:

- chest X-ray
- abdominal X-ray
- pelvic X-ray
- spinal X-ray
- myeloma screen.

Bone metastases from most types of cancer are usually lytic but, in the case of prostate cancer, they are usually sclerotic and therefore visible as dense deposits in bones on a plain X-ray. Interestingly, not all are initially sclerotic but may 'appear' on a follow-up X-ray after starting treatment in hormone-responsive cases. This is a sign of bone healing (recalcification). Therefore this should not be interpreted as evidence of progression of the bony metastatic disease without other evidence. To get a full picture of bone metastases, an isotope bone scan is useful.

> What is a bone scan? How would you limit the number of bone scans for prostate cancer to cases in which the result will affect treatment? What are the general indications for a bone scan? What other urological abnormalities can incidentally be revealed by a bone scan and why? What is a 'superscan'?

As prostate cancer-related bone metastases tend to be sclerotic, pathological fractures are relatively less common. Lytic metastases are much more likely to cause fractures.

> What is the approach of orthopaedic surgeons to pathological fractures of the femur and to their prophylaxis?

(f) Further investigations

- *U&E*: to exclude uraemia, which is quite likely in this case, and which could also cause anaemia.
- *FBC*: the patient could have anaemia from haematuria but also from bone marrow replacement (*see* p. 227).
- *Prostate-specific antigen* (PSA): the chance of this *not* being prostate cancer with bone metastases is very slim, but a raised PSA would confirm the diagnosis. It is also a tumour marker and, as with all other such markers, is therefore very useful in assessing response to treatment.

> Take this opportunity to consider which tumour markers are useful in monitoring the progression or response to treatment of which tumours. How can such markers lose their value in such monitoring over time?

- *ALP*: this is a marker of bone healing rather than bone destruction. It is also likely to be raised and is another marker of metastases in bones (in this case) and the liver (*see* p. 201).
- *Serum calcium*: hypercalcaemia can occur in any advanced malignancy. It is not a marker for bone metastases.

> What are the clinical characteristics of hypercalcaemia? How do the symptoms arise? What are the indications for treatment as opposed to letting nature take its course? What treatment is available?

- *Prostate biopsy* is easy to do but unnecessary if the PSA is raised. There are times when tests and invasive investigations are done which don't *need* to be done.
- *Bone scan – see* (e).
- *Ultrasound of the kidneys and bladder.*

(g) Retention of neurogenic cause (i.e. the cauda equina syndrome)

If the metastases are causing problems below L1, this will be due to compression of the cauda equina, leading to lower motor neurone damage, causing anaesthesia and/or paralysis. Compression of either the spinal cord or the cauda equina is more common in patients with spinal metastases, but you must be aware that prolapsed discs can also do the same at any level.

The function of the sacral nerves is most at risk in cases of compression (UMN or LMN lesion). Function can be lost by local damage (LMN lesion) or damage to the spinal cord at any higher level (UMN lesion).

History

- *Bladder symptoms*: has not passed urine, or just dribbles from overflow incontinence. The bladder is often not painful but this is not invariably the case.
- *Bowel*: the first symptom is the subtle one of inability to distinguish between faeces and flatus. This precedes the onset of faecal soiling or incontinence.
- *Sensation*: 'saddle' anaesthesia.

Examination

- Full neurological examination: for sensory level, including specific examination of the perineum for loss of sensation.
- Abdominal examination: including palpation for an enlarged bladder and rectal examination for altered sensation and/or sphincter tone. The tone is decreased in LMN lesions and increased in UMN lesions.

> Take this opportunity to revise the neurological examination of the parts of the body supplied by the lumbar and sacral nerves.

It is all too easy to miss urinary retention of neurological cause in patients who are more likely to develop retention from bladder outflow obstruction.

Cauda equina syndrome is a condition with a specific window of opportunity for treatment (48 hours from the onset of urinary/bowel dysfunction). Failure to treat promptly may leave the patient with permanent disabilities, and often the clinician facing potential allegations of negligence.

The Medical Defence Union (www.the-mdu.com) produces educational material on the diagnosis, delay and litigation risk of common conditions. These are informative articles regarding real-life reports of incidents where doctors have failed to manage a patient's complaint correctly, leading to an adverse event in care.

It is better to learn from other people's mistakes rather than from your own.

(h) Treatment of cord and cauda equina compression

There is no simple answer which is applicable to all cases. However, one or more of the following may be effective:

- dexamethasone 4 mg tds as a short-term treatment to try to relieve any oedema-related compression from inflammation while other treatments start to work
- treatment of the tumour itself, if this has not already been given. This would be appropriate in this patient's case (*see* (i) below)
- radiotherapy is also appropriate in this case because prostate cancer is usually radiosensitive
- surgical decompression. This is quite an undertaking in cases with bone metastases but may be the only option. It is the obvious option when the compression is from a prolapsed disc.

(i) Palliative prostate cancer treatment

Obviously the only treatment possible will be palliative, in other words, the treatment of symptoms and delaying the onset of further symptoms. Such treatments include:

- hormone manipulation
- treatment of outflow obstructive symptoms
- treatment of pain
- specific treatments for bone metastases. These include radiotherapy and, in fit patients, radioactive strontium (which is expensive).

Hormone treatment depends on the fact that, being a sex gland, the prostate is sensitive to circulating levels of testosterone. Removing testosterone from the circulation causes the regression of prostate cancer cells. Such manipulation started with either bilateral orchidectomy or stilboestrol. Since then, many further forms of hormone manipulation have been developed. The essence of treatment is to maximise the benefits, which have altered little since the introduction of the initial methods of hormone manipulation, while minimising side-effects. Such treatment is often given in primary care with the advice of a urologist. An important point to remember is that the LHRH analogues (Zoladex) cause an initial increase in testosterone levels, which could briefly exacerbate symptoms. Therefore, in this case cyproterone acetate (Casodex) should be given for the first 2–3 weeks in addition to any such treatment.

(j) Ethicolegal considerations: confidentiality

A relative's consent is required before detailed information may be shared with a patient about that relative's past medical history. In certain situations a doctor may be required to break confidentiality (*see* p. 142).

 Why is the principle of confidentiality of paramount importance in the doctor–patient relationship? When can, or should, a doctor break confidentiality?

(k) Counselling regarding implications of investigations

When a patient is about to have a test that might have profound implications on their life, and the lives of those close to them, they should undergo a degree of counselling.

This may consist of information regarding the implications of both positive and negative test results given by the doctor, or referral to specialist counselling services. Who to counsel is also important. In this case, either patients who are requesting to be 'screened' for prostate cancer with a view to possible treatment with curative intent, or patients in whom *you* think it is necessary to make a diagnosis, so that you can give treatment, may be eligible. It is unethical to test the PSA level in old, or unfit, asymptomatic men, except for specific reasons.

(l) Investigation of prostate cancer

- PSA.
- Rectal examination.
- TRUS (transrectal U/S-guided) biopsies of the prostate.

Rectal examination and PSA often suggest that the diagnosis is quite possible, but only histological analysis of biopsied prostate tissue can give a definitive diagnosis. Remember that a normal biopsy result does not exclude the possibility of prostate cancer (since the disease is often focal). In these circumstances, the decision to repeat a biopsy is highly specialised.

Another problem is setting the level of PSA (which is also age related) to optimise the indications for prostatic biopsy, particularly if one is seeking to cure early prostatic cancer. If the level is set too high, many patients will only be diagnosed when the cancer is too locally extensive, or has metastasised, so that it is too late to give curative treatment. If the level is set too low, too many patients will be subjected to prostatic biopsy – which has its own morbidity and mortality – resulting in benign histology. The setting of the parameters for any method of screening is always problematical, and it is important to be aware of this.

(m) Treatment

Options for treatment are tailored to the individual patient. They include:

- prostatectomy
- radiotherapy/brachytherapy
- hormone manipulation
- observation.

There is no best treatment. The type of treatment depends on the stage of the cancer. Possible treatments are: open or laparoscopic radical prostatectomy, radical radiotherapy, brachytherapy, hormone manipulation (probably in combination with one of the other treatments), and 'watchful waiting' (i.e. no immediate active treatment). So you can legitimately argue that the one the patient chooses after discussion with the urologist is the 'best' treatment. The point is that there are no properly conducted (controlled) trials that have established the best treatment.

(n) Screening

- This man should not have already been screened.

Asymptomatic males are not routinely screened in Britain. PSA is an inadequate mass screening tool for many reasons. When considering mass screening, the Wilson and Junger criteria are often consulted. Mass screening has unacceptable false-positive rates and inclusion of benign disease that may never have otherwise affected the patient. A European trial by Schroder (in Rotterdam) in evaluating screening confers survival benefit when suitable patients are treated with curative intent. The question of choosing the parameters in screening has already been discussed. There are exceptions to the rule not to screen routinely. A good example is men who are at increased risk because of a positive family history.

Web resources

- Clinical guidelines for the management of acute back pain: www.rcgp.org.uk
- Medical Defence Union – case presentations: www.the-mdu.com
- NICE guidance on cancer services: www.nice.org.uk
- Prostate cancer risk management: www.cancerscreening.nhs.uk/prostate

Further reading

- Crawford ED (2005) PSA testing: what is the use? *Lancet.* **365**: 1447.
- Collier J, Longmore M and Scally P (eds) (2003) *Oxford Handbook of Clinical Specialities* (6e). Oxford University Press, Oxford, pp. 618–26.
- Longmore M, Wilkinson I and Rajagopalan S (eds) (2004) *Oxford Handbook of Clinical Medicine* (6e). Oxford University Press, Oxford, p. 410.
- Shekelle PG and Delitto AM (2005) Treating low back pain. *Lancet.* **365**: 1987.
- Speed C (2004) Low back pain. *British Medical Journal.* **328**: 1119.
- Toms JR (ed) (2004) *Cancer Stats Monograph 2004.* Chapter 8: Prostate cancer. Cancer Research UK, London, p. 55.
- Wilson JMG and Junger G (1968) *Principles and Practice of Screening for Disease.* World Health Organization, Geneva.
- Van Tulder M and Koes B (2003) Low back pain and sciatica. *Clinical Evidence.* **Issue 10**: 1343.

A 71-year-old lady is admitted to the medical assessment unit following a 2-day history of increasing shortness of breath. She is extremely fatigued, denies any chest pain but has been complaining of a worsening cough with sputum production. She has a medical background of chronic disease that includes chronic bronchitis and emphysema (on home oxygen), ischaemic heart disease, hypertension and heart failure with multiple past hospital admissions. On examination her pulse is 102 beats/min and regular, she has a BP of 151/78 mmHg, and her respiratory rate is 28 breaths/min. On auscultation of her chest there are early inspiratory crackles, which are worse on the right. Diffuse wheeze with prolonged expiration can be heard throughout the remainder of her chest.

(a) Comment on the disease processes and how they may be contributing to her symptoms.

....

....

....

(b) What symptoms or signs could help distinguish between the possible causes of this patient's breathlessness?

....

....

....

(c) What further investigations would you order and why?

....

....

....

The poorly positioned chest X-ray is shown in Figure 28.1.

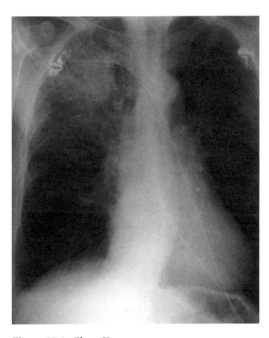

Figure 28.1 Chest X-ray.

(d) What treatment would you now initiate?

....

....

....

(e) How would you monitor the response to treatment?

....

....

....

☞ She initially responds to treatment but then starts to deteriorate. Eight days later she is seen by the on-call team at 2 am, distressed and finding it difficult to breathe. She is given 2.5 mg diamorphine and nebulised salbutamol. When you arrive in the morning she is cyanosed, with a respiratory rate of 13 breaths/min. Her oxygen saturation is 81% on 28% O_2 via face mask. She tells you that she doesn't think she's going to make it, and that she doesn't want to have her heart restarted if it stops.

(f) Is this the correct amount of oxygen?

....

....

....

(g) What further treatment options are available?

....

....

....

(h) When is it generally acceptable to consider issuing a 'do not attempt resuscitation' (DNAR) order?

....

....

....

(i) What issues would the consultant want to clarify before issuing a DNAR order in this case?

....

....

....

☞ Her family are called and are at her bedside during the morning ward round. They ask to see a doctor in private.

(j) What would you discuss with them?

....

....

....

☞ During the discussion the daughter comments that all of this is due to smoking, and tells you how they have tried to tell their mother to give up for many years. She asks for advice on how to give up smoking herself.

(k) What help is available through the NHS?

....

....

....

(l) Describe the government's health promotion strategies regarding smoking cessation.

....

....

....

Key cases
- Chronic obstructive pulmonary disease (COPD)
- Congestive cardiac failure (CCF)
- Left ventricular failure (LVF)

Clinical context

The patient with acute on chronic breathlessness can be a difficult diagnostic dilemma, especially – as in this case – where there is a background history of COPD and heart failure. Both conditions frequently co-exist, and a deterioration in one can trigger an exacerbation of the other. The main problem will be identified by a well-taken history combined with an accurate physical examination. This scenario provides the essential features that will help you to discriminate between COPD and LVF, and to manage a patient with an infective exacerbation of COPD. It also tackles some of the difficult issues that have to be considered in the dying patient, in particular 'resuscitation, yes or no?'

(a) Symptoms

An acute increase in breathlessness in COPD is usually due to a bacterial or viral chest infection, while in heart disease it is often due to pulmonary oedema, perhaps precipitated by either an MI or an arrhythmia.

The three key symptoms of COPD – dyspnoea, cough and sputum – are also signs of pulmonary oedema, with both conditions also potentially causing severe fatigue:

- *acute increase in dyspnoea*: infection in COPD, or acute pulmonary oedema in cardiac disease
- *cough*: attempt to clear sputum or fluid in COPD, or LVF respectively
- *sputum*: infection, secretions or pulmonary oedema
- *fatigue*: chronic disease, respiratory failure in COPD, poor perfusion, low output, and low SpO_2 in CCF.

> Take this opportunity to revise the causes of breathlessness. What is the difference between breathlessness and dyspnoea?

The main pathophysiological features causing irreversible airflow limitation in COPD are:

- narrowing of the small airways due to inflammation, smooth muscle hypertrophy, and fibrosis

- alveolar destruction leading to a loss of lung framework, elasticity and recoil
- reduced patency of small airways from loss of alveolar support
- increased mucus production.

COPD is a mixture of emphysema and bronchitis that often overlap. The airway obstruction and alveolar destruction lead to air trapping and hyper-inflation of the lungs. This leads to decreased inspiratory capacity and increased accessory muscle use. The laboured use of accessory muscles to move very little air into the lungs gives rise to the distressing sensation of dyspnoea in COPD.

In left-sided cardiac failure, the sensation of dyspnoea is caused by back pressure in the pulmonary circulation. Increased hydrostatic pressure leads to pulmonary venous congestion and fluid transudation, which builds up in the interstitium and eventually affects the alveoli. The result is heavy, stiff lungs and consequently difficulty in breathing.

In both COPD and LVF, chronic dyspnoea worsens as the disease progresses. Eventually the patient will feel breathless at rest.

> Use this opportunity to revise the management of 'stable' COPD. What are the mainstays of treatment? What are respiratory function tests? What are the FEV_1, FVC and FEV_1/FVC ratio? What are the indications for home oxygen therapy?

(b) Key differentiating symptoms and signs

- Sputum characteristics
- Orthopnoea or paroxysmal nocturnal dyspnoea (PND)
- Gallop rhythm or third heart sound on cardiac auscultation (caution, *see* notes below)
- Late fine inspiratory crackles at the bases that do not clear on coughing are suggestive of pulmonary oedema. Early coarse inspiratory crackles are more suggestive of infection or viscous secretions.

The nature of the sputum is a key differentiating feature; pink frothy sputum may indicate pulmonary oedema, whereas thick mucoid or purulent sputum probably indicates an infective exacerbation of COPD.

Dyspnoea that occurs soon after the patient lies down and improves on sitting up (orthopnoea) would suggest LVF. Orthopnoea occurs because when lying flat there is an increase in venous return to the right atrium and ventricle. This increases the blood flow to the lungs and the pressure in the pulmonary vessels, leading to further fluid transudation.

COPD can also produce an increase in breathlessness on lying flat, but the accumulation of secretions takes longer than in pulmonary oedema. When COPD is responsible, nocturnal breathlessness is usually caused by accumulation of secretions, coupled with a gravity-induced decrease in lung volume. Patients wake with a productive cough, but the breathlessness resolves as the secretions clear.

An S3 gallop rhythm associated with a decrease in ventricular compliance may suggest LVF. However the same can occur with RVF (cor pulmonale) secondary to the prolonged pulmonary hypertension of COPD. Additionally, emphysema may muffle the heart sounds.

Patients with LVF have characteristic crepitations that are characterised as fine late inspiratory crackles. The sounds are gravity dependent, so they are first heard at the bases.

> You should be familiar with the regulation of both ventilation and perfusion in the lung. How does the pathophysiology of COPD cause pulmonary hypertension?

(c) Investigations

In all patients with an exacerbation of COPD the following investigations should be ordered:

- *chest X-ray*: findings of COPD are hyperinflation of the lung fields, flattened diaphragm, narrow cardiac silhouette ('tube heart'), and decreased peripheral vascular markings. Consolidation may point to an infective exacerbation of COPD (*see* X-ray in Figure 28.1). These findings are quite distinct from those of LVF. Dilatation of pulmonary veins is often the first X-ray finding in LVF; bilateral pleural effusions are a later feature. X-rays may show cardiomegaly, Kerley B lines, interstitial oedema, or upper lobe diversion
- *arterial blood gases*: provide a good measure of the acuteness and severity of an exacerbation. The degree of hypoxaemia and carbon dioxide retention are important when deciding on optimal O_2 therapy. When measuring ABGs it is important to note the FiO_2, the patient's Hb level, and temperature

- *pulse oximetry*: not as reliable as ABG measurement, but when combined with clinical observation, can be a powerful tool for instant feedback on the degree of hypoxaemia
- *an ECG to exclude co-morbidities*: this patient has known cardiac disease, and hypoxaemia can precipitate myocardial ischaemia
- *a full blood count*: should be performed to check for any anaemia, which may add to the sensation of breathlessness
- *U&E*: should be measured since the patient may be dehydrated or have an infection. Additionally COPD patients tend to retain sodium, and use of the common bronchodilators can lead to hypokalaemia
- *if the sputum is purulent, a sample should be sent for microscopy and culture*: this can help confirm the diagnosis and will give information on antibiotic sensitivities
- *blood cultures*: should be taken if the patient is pyrexial.

(d) Management

The chest X-ray shows chronic changes of COPD with right upper lobe consolidation and a small right pleural effusion. This points to an acute exacerbation of COPD. There are no obvious features of LVF.

The management of an acute exacerbation of COPD is to treat hypoxaemia and any precipitating/concurrent infection. Infection worsens the already chronic bronchitis, and this is often further exacerbated by airways hyper-reactivity.

- A combination of nebulised bronchodilators, steroids and theophylline may be required to reverse bronchospasm and keep the small airways patent.
- Additional steroids should be given. If the patient has been on long-term corticosteroids, the added stress of an acute exacerbation can provoke an Addisonian crisis. Therefore a double dose is often given.
- Oxygen is given at a concentration determined by the results of serial ABG measurements. Treatment should aim to keep the SpO_2 above 90% and minimise the amount of CO_2 retention.
- Bacteria are isolated in about 40–60% of acute exacerbations of COPD. The common bacteria found in patients' sputum are *Haemophilus influenzae*, *Streptococcus pneumoniae* and *Moraxella cattarhalis*. Antibiotic treatment follows the local microbiology guidelines.
- Appropriate analgesia must be provided to ensure patient comfort. One of the common reasons for deterioration is physical exhaustion due to the increased effort of respiration.
- Intravenous fluids should be given since these

patients may be dehydrated due to infection and increased insensible losses.
(NICE Guideline 12, 2004)

> Use this opportunity to revise the pharmacology of commonly used bronchodilators. How do these drugs act? Can you predict their side-effects from their actions?

(e) Monitoring

The purpose of monitoring is to assess respiratory function and to give early warning of any deterioration. As such, monitoring and documentation of clinical features, hypoxaemia and markers of infection are important.

- Patients can be monitored by regular clinical assessment.
- Pulse oximetry should be continuous.
- Intermittent ABG measurements should be used to monitor patients with respiratory failure who are retaining CO_2, until they are stable.
- Temperature and clinical features are the best measures of the success of antibiotic therapy. Serial CRP and FBC measurement may also be useful.

> You should be familiar with interpreting ABG measurements. What is the difference between type 1 and type 2 respiratory failure? How can the bicarbonate level tell you whether the problem is chronic?

(f) Oxygen therapy

- There is no correct answer. Oxygen should be given to ensure that SpO_2 is above 90%. If, despite increasing FiO_2, this is not possible, or the patient is retaining CO_2, or is becoming tired, then ventilatory support is needed.

Hypoxaemia can kill quickly. Adequate oxygen should always be given to relieve hypoxaemia. Aim for a saturation level of above 90%. Care should be exercised since too much oxygen can cause respiratory depression in some patients who chronically retain CO_2.

Large increases in $PaCO_2$ can lead to deterioration of mental function and narcosis. If respiratory drive is severely inhibited by high $PaCO_2$, then decreasing O_2 leads only to worsening hypoxaemia. Immediate positive pressure ventilation (either invasive (IPPV) or non-invasive (NIPPV)) is necessary.

> Use this opportunity to revisit the control of respiration. Where are the main receptors? How do the central and peripheral chemoreceptors differ in their sensitivities?

(g) Further treatment

Once patients suffer from severe muscle fatigue, they may be unable to make sufficient respiratory effort to enable effective air movement into the lungs. This rapidly leads to worsening hypoxaemia, carbon dioxide retention and severe respiratory acidosis. These patients need to be either ventilated, or given sufficient pain relief and/or sedation for palliation of their distressing dyspnoeic symptoms.

The treatment options are therefore:

- use of a respiratory stimulant such as doxapram
- NIPPV
- symptomatic relief with morphine (with careful dose titration), oxygen, saline nebulisers and fluids if indicated
- transfer to ITU for invasive ventilation (after discussion with intensivists).

(h) DNAR orders

The decision to institute a DNAR order is the responsibility of the consultant in charge, or in emergencies with the most senior member of the team. It is important to ensure that a valid directive is in the patient's notes if resuscitation is considered inappropriate.

DNAR orders are generally considered acceptable in the following circumstances:

- where a competent patient has indicated that they do not want CPR
- where the patient's condition indicates that CPR is unlikely to be successful
- where successful CPR is likely to be followed by a length and quality of life that would be unacceptable to the patient.

(i) Issues

As with the general circumstances relating to issuing a DNAR order, the issues that need to be considered relate to the patient's wishes, and the likely clinical outcome.

Issues specific to this case that would need to be clarified include:

- *the patient's wishes*: what does she mean by 'restarting her heart'? Does this mean further aggressive treatment?
- *that the patient is competent to make the decision*
- *the likely clinical outcome*: in general, during exacerbations of COPD, functional status, BMI,

requirement for oxygen when stable, co-morbidities and previous admissions to intensive care units should be considered, in addition to age and FEV_1
- *that there is consensus* with other members of the healthcare team looking after the patient, and with the patient's family.

(j) Involving relatives

People close to patients often feel that they are not sufficiently involved in decisions that are made about their relatives in hospital. Even though their views have no legal status in terms of actual decision making, they should be involved if the patient wants them to be (i.e. if the patient consents).

- The family should be informed that the patient has decided that she doesn't want CPR.
- They should be informed that her condition is serious and that giving CPR would probably prove to be futile.
- They should be asked for their opinions about what they think the patient wants.
- Their agreement should be sought, but the patient's decision is final.

(k) Smoking cessation

The aims of smoking cessation programmes in the UK are threefold:

- to encourage smokers to stop smoking
- to reduce their chances of relapse
- to reduce the amount of tobacco smoked if people cannot stop.

The help that is currently available in the UK through primary care includes:

- face-to-face behavioural support including counselling and advice, teaching coping skills training, and group support
- nicotine replacement therapy in the form of chewing gum, patches or inhalators
- bupropion (Zyban): there is evidence that it reduces the severity of withdrawal symptoms and facilitates stopping smoking
- self-help literature.

(l) Public health policy

The Tannahill model is a useful way of thinking about public health promotion (Downie *et al.*, 1996). Health promotion is stylised as three overlapping areas: health education, health protection and disease prevention:

- *health education*: preventing ill health by influencing the knowledge, beliefs, attitudes and behaviour of the community
- *health protection*: refers to the policies and codes of practice preventing ill health, e.g. no smoking in public places
- *disease prevention*: refers to both the initial occurrence of disease (primary prevention) and also to the progress (secondary prevention), and subsequently the final outcome (tertiary prevention).

Regarding public health policy on smoking these are:

- *health education*: education, advertising dangers (TV/billboard advertising), warnings on packets etc. Additionally, brief advice (up to 5 minutes) from a GP given to all smokers to encourage them to make an attempt to stop is effective in promoting smoking cessation
- *health protection*: taxation, age restriction, advertising bans, a ban on smoking in public places is pending
- *disease prevention*: help with stopping as above.

Web resources

- COPD guidelines (SIGN Guideline 59): www.sign.ac.uk
- DNAR orders: www.resus.org.uk
- Ethics of DNAR orders: www.ethics-network.org.uk
- Global initiative for chronic obstructive lung disease: www.goldcopd.com
- Health and social care on tobacco: www.dh.gov.uk
- Smoking cessation: www.prodigy.nhs.uk

Suggested reading

- Chinn S, Jarvis D, Melotti R *et al.* (2005) Smoking cessation, lung function, and weight gain: a follow-up study. *Lancet.* 365: 1629.
- Downie R, Tannahill A and Tannahill C (1996) *Health Promotion.* Oxford University Press, Oxford.
- Murphy R, Driscoll P and O'Driscoll R (2001) Emergency oxygen therapy for the COPD patient. *Emergency Medicine Journal.* 18: 333.
- National Institute for Clinical Excellence (2004) *Guideline 12: Chronic Obstructive Pulmonary Disease – management of chronic obstructive pulmonary disease in adults in primary care and secondary care.* NICE, London.

29 A patient with high blood pressure

Mr Jones, a 50-year-old man, attends his GP for a routine assessment. He is a smoker and has a BMI of 35 but is otherwise well. The GP measures his BP and notes that it is 178/88 mmHg. He is advised to return in a week to see the practice nurse. On repeat measurement his BP is 184/94 mmHg. The nurse asks for him to return again the following week at which time his BP remains elevated at 176/86 mmHg.

(a) What is the patient suffering from?

....

....

....

(b) Why is it important to control blood pressure?

....

....

....

(c) What are the risk factors for high blood pressure?

....

....

....

Mr Jones returns to visit his GP following his BP measurement. The GP explains to him that he is likely to have primary hypertension.

(d) What is primary hypertension and why is it likely that he has this?

....

....

....

(e) What pathophysiological factors might maintain high blood pressure in primary hypertension?

....

....

....

(f) What are the important causes of secondary hypertension?

....

....

....

(g) What blood tests would be arranged for Mr Jones, and why are they important?

....

....

....

The GP examines Mr Jones' fundi and detects nothing abnormal. Additionally, Mr Jones does not complain of any visual problems. The ECG is shown in Figure 29.1.

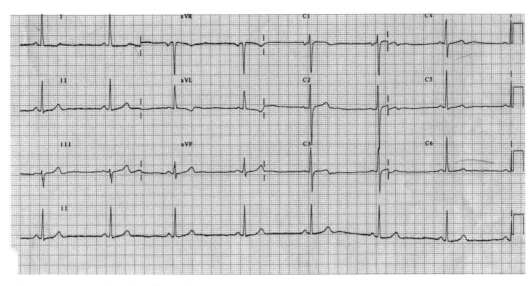

Figure 29.1 ECG taken from the patient.

(h) Comment on the tracing. What other ECG abnormalities are associated with hypertension?

....

....

....

(i) What lifestyle changes would the GP advise his patient to make?

....

....

....

(j) What antihypertensive drugs might the GP consider using to treat this patient?

....

....

....

The GP prescribes his patient an anti-hypertensive, and asks him to return in 4 weeks. However he does not return to the practice and avoids attempts to reassess his condition.

The patient presents to the A&E department at the local hospital 2 years later. He is complaining of intermittent exercise-induced chest pain, left arm pain and breathlessness, he also describes a 3-day history of orthopnoea and a 1-month history of peripheral oedema. He is also experiencing altered vision and a headache. He has a BP of 230/120 mmHg.

(k) What is the patient suffering from?

....

....

....

(l) The SHO in A&E performs fundoscopy. How is hypertensive retinopathy graded, and what are the changes?

....

....

....

(m) His ECG shows some ST segment depression and T wave inversion, and he has proteinuria on the urine dipstick test. What actions would the SHO take?

....

....

....

(n) What are the dangers of reducing this patient's blood pressure too rapidly?

....

....

....

Key cases

- Primary hypertension
- Malignant hypertension
- Angina pectoris

Clinical context

Blood pressure is often not taken by medical students as they use the readings from the patient's observation chart. This is not good enough. You must ensure you know the theory and practice of blood pressure measurement. It is one quick and easy bedside skill that can significantly influence a patient's health.

Hypertension is common, and if left untreated is a major cause of morbidity and mortality. This scenario will take you through the assessment, diagnosis, causes and management of hypertension.

Current guidelines quote normal blood pressure as <140/90 mmHg. However blood pressure should be measured regularly, even in those patients with normal values (*see* Table 29.1).

Table 29.1 Blood pressure measurements

BP (mmHg)	
< 120/75	Normal
120–130/75–85	Normal range, BP should be checked annually
130–139/85–89	Upper range of normal, recheck BP in 2 months and give lifestyle advice
140–159/90–99	Mild hypertension
160–179/ 100–109	Moderate hypertension, two further measurements should be taken at weekly intervals to confirm the diagnosis
> 180/110	Severe hypertension, requires immediate confirmation within one day, and BP repeated within one week depending on the clinical situation

(a) Isolated systolic hypertension (ISH)

The sequential measurements show:

- borderline ISH: 140–159/ <90 mmHg
- established ISH: > 160/< 90 mmHg.

ISH is currently defined as a systolic blood pressure (SBP) >140 mmHg, with a diastolic blood pressure (DBP) < 90 mmHg. It was once thought to be relatively benign. However it is now recognised that systolic hypertension, even without diastolic hypertension, is a significant risk factor which, if left untreated, increases morbidity and mortality. It is the most common and the most difficult type of hypertension to treat. The prevalence of ISH increases with age, occurring in 50% of those aged 60 years and over, rising to 75% in those 75 years and over.

> What are the guidelines for the management of hypertension in 'special circumstances'. You should be familiar with the target values for BP in diabetic patients, patients with renal disease, and pregnancy-induced hypertension.

(b) Consequences of hypertension

- Increased risk of stroke
- Increased risk of heart disease
- Increased risk of renal failure

Hypertension is usually symptomless (often called the 'silent killer'), but it should be treated to reduce the risk of developing complications. The prevalence and risk of developing complications of hypertension increase with age. It is important to realise that hypertension is *the* major cardiovascular risk factor that is amenable to intervention and prevention.

There is strong evidence that hypertension is a significant risk factor for stroke, coronary heart disease, peripheral vascular disease, and renal disease. Much of this evidence has come from The Framingham Heart Study and other large epidemiological studies like the Multiple Risk Factor Intervention Trial.

> What is the difference between population-based health intervention, and individual, or high-risk-based intervention? You should be able to think of examples of both. What is the concept of 'shifting the curve to the right'?

(c) Risk factors for hypertension

The risk factors for hypertension are similar to those for heart disease. Black populations in North America have been shown to have higher BPs than their white counterparts, but this relationship is less convincing in the UK and Europe. An inverse relationship exists between educational achievement and BP in both black and white people. Social factors affect these measurements.

As such, the key risk factors are:

- age
- ethnicity
- family history
- obesity, sedentary lifestyle
- dyslipidaemia
- pharmacological, including alcohol, NSAIDs, and the OCP
- others, including a high salt intake and 'stress'.

(d) Primary hypertension

- This is hypertension of non-defined origin (idiopathic/essential).
- Approximately 90–95% of cases of hypertension are defined as 'primary'.

Primary (essential) hypertension, as the name implies, has no known cause. However, as mentioned, heredity is a predisposing factor. Environmental factors seem to have a more pronounced effect on blood pressure in genetically susceptible individuals.

(e) Pathophysiological factors in primary hypertension

Multiple factors sustain elevated BP. Many normally adaptive physiological mechanisms are prone to positive feedback in the hypertensive state, leading to worsening hypertension. Factors which maintain an elevated BP include:

- atherosclerosis
- salt and water retention
- activation of the renin–angiotensin–aldosterone system
- raised sympathetic tone.

The pathophysiology of hypertension is believed to be due to progressive stiffening of the small and large vessels of the arterial tree, due to ageing. This results in a continuous rise in systolic blood pressure, which in turn causes thickening of the arterial medial and intimal layers, further stiffening the arteries, accelerating artherosclerosis and exacerbating hypertension.

In the kidneys, damage to the microvasculature can reduce renal function by impairing glomerular filtration. This causes sodium and water retention, secondary hyperaldosteronism, and further hypertension.

Use this opportunity to revisit the renin–angiotensin–aldosterone system. What are the stimuli for release of renin from the juxtaglomerular apparatus? How might microvascular damage and impaired glomerular perfusion lead to salt and water retention?

High sympathetic tone disproportionately raises BP in hypertensive patients, or those who will develop hypertension compared with normotensive patients. A high resting pulse rate can be a manifestation of increased sympathetic activity, and is an accepted predictor of subsequent hypertension.

The increased resistance of the arterial tree results in an increase in the workload of the left ventricle, resulting in left ventricular hypertrophy (see Figure 29.1). DBP often remains normal or even decreases with age, resulting in widened pulse pressure. Decreased DBP can result in reduced coronary blood flow, and therefore increase the risk of developing myocardial ischaemia.

Remember that:

blood pressure = cardiac output × peripheral vascular resistance

and that:

cardiac output = stroke volume × pulse rate

How do the factors outlined above relate to these parameters?

(f) Causes of secondary hypertension

Secondary causes account for approximately 10% of cases of hypertension. The secondary causes follow from the pathophysiological mechanisms outlined above. It is important to at least consider these causes, since correct treatment may cure hypertension.

Common causes therefore include:

- *intrinsic renal or renovascular disease*: e.g. due to diabetes, or renal artery stenosis
- *endocrine disorders*: including hyperthyroidism, phaechromocytoma (catecholamine excess), Conn's syndrome (primary aldosterone excess), Cushing's syndrome (corticosteroid excess) and acromegaly (growth hormone excess)
- *cardiovascular disorders*: including coarctation of the aorta
- *iatrogenic*: NSAIDs, oral contraceptives, steroids.

(g) Investigations in hypertension

Investigations in hypertension are used to detect any end-organ damage, and to exclude a cause of secondary hypertension.

Such investigations include:

- urinalysis
- serum U&E
- 24-hour creatinine clearance
- CXR
- ECG
- renal U/S
- echocardiography
- serum glucose and lipids.

The urine should be tested for evidence of primary renal disease or hypertensive nephropathy. Urine should be examined for dysmorphic red cells, casts, and cultured. If there is proteinuria or evidence of renal disease, a 24-hour urine sample is needed.

Serum U&E will detect renal impairment, and may suggest Conn's syndrome or Cushing's disease.

A CXR will help in the assessment of cardiomegaly or pulmonary oedema (LVF), and can be used to detect the presence of rib notching, which is suggestive of coarctation of the aorta (rare).

The echocardiogram is more sensitive than either the ECG or CXR in determining left ventricular hypertrophy and failure. This is not always done in day-to-day practice, but is advocated by many as a key investigation for all hypertensive patients.

The need for renal ultrasound depends on the clinical history, physical examination, and urinalysis result.

Diabetes mellitus and hyperlipidaemia are associated with hypertension and increase the likely risk of cardiovascular disease. It is important to measure both glucose and a lipid profile in a fasting blood sample.

(h) ECG changes

The ECG shows left ventricular hypertrophy (LVH). There are many criteria for diagnosing LVH on an ECG. One way to determine this is to measure the height of the S wave in V1 and the R wave in V5 or V6 (Soklow and Lyon). If the two waves add up to more than 35 small squares, then the left ventricle is hypertrophied. This is because large voltages are recorded in the leads over the thickened muscle.

In general, on the ECG, it is important to look for signs of LVH and strain or ischaemic heart disease, both of which constitute target organ damage. In addition, atrial fibrillation (AF), premature ventricular contractions, ventricular arrhythmias, and sudden cardiac death are observed more often in patients with LVH than in those without LVH.

(i) Lifestyle modification

Lifestyle modification is the first step in the treatment of primary hypertension. The key changes that need to be made include:

- weight loss
- smoking cessation
- dietary modification, low-salt diet, five portions of fruit/vegetables per day
- reduction in alcohol intake (<3 units/day for men and <2 units/day for women)
- regular exercise.

Central obesity is measured by the waist-to-hip circumference ratio. This shows a stronger correlation to BP than the overall body mass. Intervention trials have demonstrated that weight loss is associated with a reduction in blood pressure.

Smoking causes cardiovascular disease and stimulates the sympathetic nervous system.

The relationship between alcohol intake and blood pressure is causal. Reduction in alcohol intake in heavy drinkers results in lowering of blood pressure.

Vegetarians have lower blood pressure than non-vegetarians. Increased intake of fruit and vegetables has been shown to lower blood pressure in hypertensive patients who were predominantly meat eaters.

There is conflicting evidence regarding the role of exercise in the prevention and treatment of hypertension.

(j) Pharmacological management of hypertension

In a 50-year-old Caucasian man, the drugs that should be considered for the initial treatment of hypertension are:

- *ACE inhibitors*: ramipril, enalopril
- *Calcium channel antagonists*: amlodipine, felodipine, nifedipine
- *Thiazide diuretics*: bendrofluazide.

ACE inhibitors reduce the formation of angiotensin II and hence reduce peripheral vascular resistance. It is important to note that these drugs may cause a sharp fall in BP with the first dose. Some patients are intolerant of the side-effects of ACE inhibitors and therefore an angiotensin II receptor agonist (e.g. losartan or valsartan) may be used.

Selective calcium channel antagonists bind to calcium channel receptors, blocking the entry of calcium into the cell, and hence causing relaxation of the arteriolar smooth muscle.

Thiazide diuretics reduce salt and water reabsorption in the distal convoluted tubule. Consequently, initial falls in BP are thought to occur due to a reduction in total blood volume, venous return and cardiac output. Cardiac output does return to normal, but the antihypertensive effect persists as the peripheral resistance has decreased.

If BP control proves difficult, other drugs to be considered include loop diuretics, potassium sparing diuretics, α-blockers, β-blockers, angiotensin II receptor antagonists or centrally acting antihypertensives.

> ☀️💡 Use this opportunity to revise the common side-effects of antihypertensive drugs. What are the absolute contraindications to ACEi or β-blocker use?
>
> What side-effects of calcium channel antagonists do elderly patients frequently complain about?

Combination therapy has yielded significant improvements in the control of hypertension. The treatment algorithm suggested by the Royal College of Physicians (RCP) is shown in Figure 29.2.

(k) Malignant hypertension

This patient is suffering from:

- malignant hypertension
- angina.

Malignant hypertension is rare. Visual disturbance, headache and breathlessness may occur when the diastolic pressure is greater than 130 mmHg, and systolic pressure is greater than 220 mmHg. Fundoscopy may reveal retinal changes and papilloedema, and patients may have overt signs of cardiac failure (*see* pp. 178 and 213). Patients may present with decreased consciousness, focal neurological signs, fits (hypertensive encephalopathy), and stroke.

(l) Hypertensive retinopathy

The changes that may be visible in the retina of a hypertensive patient include:

- narrowed arterial lumen (grade 1)
- 'nipping' (where thickened arteries cross veins) (grade 2)

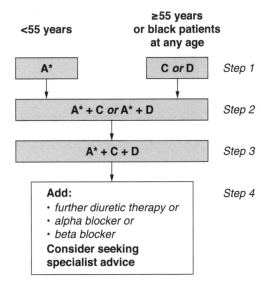

A = ACE inhibitor (* or ARB if ACEi-intolerant); C = calcium-channel blocker; D = thiazide-type diuretic. Beta-blockers are not a preferred initial therapy for hypertension but are an alternative to A in patients <55 years in whom A is not tolerated, or contraindicated (includes women of child-bearing potential). Black patients are only those of African or Caribbean descent. In the absence of evidence, all other patients should be treated according to the algorithm as non-black.

Figure 29.2 RCP algorithm for the treatment of hypertension in primary care. Copyright © 2006 Royal College of Physicians. Reproduced by permission. Full text available online at www.rcplondon.ac.uk/pubs/books/HT/HypertensionGuide.pdf

- flame-shaped haemorrhages and cotton wool spots (grade 3)
- papilloedema (grade 4).

Hypertensive retinopathy is graded 1 to 4 as shown above. In this case you would expect a hypertensive retinopathy of 3–4.

(m) (n) Management of malignant hypertension

The 1-year mortality of untreated malignant hypertension is approximately 90%. Malignant hypertension occurs in 1% of patients with primary hypertension.

The aim of treatment in a hypertensive emergency is immediate action to bring about a gradual, controlled reduction of blood pressure. A good rule of thumb is to aim for a reduction of approximately 25% of mean arterial pressure or reduce diastolic pressure to 100–110 mmHg over 24 hours.

- This is an emergency, therefore ABCDE should be assessed and treated appropriately.
- Treatment is with intravenous antihypertensives. Labetolol is the first line in the absence of

pulmonary oedema or other contraindications to β-blocker treatment. Nitroprusside, hydralazine, and nitrates are alternatives.

- Regular cardiovascular and neurological observations are critical. For this reason, patients should ideally be admitted to HDU/ITU. This is an emergency.
- Patients should have an arterial line +/– central line.
- Scrupulous fluid balance is essential, and patients should be catheterised and urine output monitored.

The reason for these measures is that a rapid reduction in blood pressure can result in end-organ hypoperfusion, potentially causing ischaemia and/or infarction. If a patient complains of cardiac symptoms (e.g. development/worsening of chest pain), has a dramatically reduced urine output (renal hypoperfusion) or develops neurological symptoms and/or signs during the reduction of blood pressure, then the rate of drug infusion should be slowed or stopped.

Web resources

- British Hypertension Society: www.bhsoc.org
- Guidelines on hypertension management: www.sign.ac.uk
- The Merck Manual of Diagnosis and Therapy: www.merck.com

Further reading

- Adamczak M, Zeier M, Dikow R and Ritz E (2002) Kidney and hypertension. *Kidney International*. **61** Suppl 80: 62.
- Brown MJ, Cruickshank JK, Dominiczak AF *et al.* (2003) Better blood pressure control: how to combine drugs. *Journal of Human Hypertension*. **17**: 81.
- Luft FC (2004) Geneticism of essential hypertension. *Hypertension*. **43**: 1155.
- National Collaborating Centre for Chronic Conditions (2006) *Management of Hypertension in Adults in Primary Care: partial update*. Royal College of Physicians, London.
- National Institute for Clinical Excellence (2004) *Guideline 18: Management of Hypertension in Adults in Primary Care*. NICE, London.
- O'Brien E, Beavers D and Marshall H (eds) (1995) *ABC of Hypertension* (4e). BMJ Publishing, London.
- Vaughan CJ and Delanty N (2000) Hypertensive emergencies. *Lancet*. **356**: 411.
- Williams B, Poulter NR, Brown MJ *et al.* (2004) British Hypertension Society guidelines for hypertension management 2004 (BHS-IV): summary. *BMJ*. **328**: 634.

(30) A tired old lady

Beryl is a 72-year-old woman, who presents to her GP feeling tired all the time. She was last seen in the surgery 1 month ago when she was diagnosed as having a viral illness, with symptoms of a dry cough, sore throat and headache. She says that the symptoms have not really improved, and over the last few days her cough has got worse and is now productive. She lives with her sister, who commented that she was looking pale, and urged her to go back to the GP. Her GP thinks that she looks anaemic. He tells her that he needs to ask her some questions and examine her, and then she needs to see the practice nurse to have some blood tests.

(a) What features of the history would her GP concentrate on?

....

....

....

(b) What specific features would the GP be looking for on clinical examination?

....

....

....

The GP does a thorough physical examination and finds nothing remarkable, apart from the fact that she looks very pale. He says he will call her with the results of the blood tests.

Two days later the GP receives the blood results, which show a severe anaemia with a haemoglobin of 7.0 g/dl and an MCV of 97 fl. Additionally, her white cell count is 1.2×10^9/l and platelets are 80×10^9/l. The GP tells Beryl that her blood tests are abnormal, and that she needs to be admitted to hospital for further investigations.

(c) What conditions could cause the abnormalities seen on her full blood count?

....

....

....

She is sent to the haematology day ward for further investigation.

(d) How will she be investigated?

....

....

....

The SHO on the day ward says that Beryl needs a blood transfusion because her Hb is less than 8.0 g/dl.

(e) What general points should be considered before giving a blood transfusion?

....

....

....

(f) What complications should you be wary of when transfusing blood?

....

....

....

She is successfully transfused 3 units of blood without significant complications and is sent home with an appointment to come back to the haematology clinic in a week's time for review of the results.

Her results are reviewed at the haematology meeting and she is shown to have a form of acute myeloid leukaemia (AML). The team discusses the treatment options in an elderly patient.

(g) What are the principal treatment options available?

....

....

....

(h) What factors should be considered when deciding the best option?

....

....

....

At her follow-up appointment the consultant breaks the bad news to Beryl and her sister. He explains the possible treatment options and their risks and benefits. He says that there isn't any particular evidence that one treatment is superior to another; there are clinical trials in which different treatment regimes are being tested. The consultant says that the unit's policy is to enrol patients who want to try chemotherapy on the AML 14 trial, which is a clinical trial specifically aimed at finding out the best treatment for patients over 60 years old.

(i) Discuss the ethical issues involved in clinical trials.

....

....

....

Beryl decides to opt for chemotherapy. She is admitted to hospital during her consolidation phase and is found to have a neutrophil count of 0.2×10^9/l. The registrar is concerned about the possibility of her getting infected.

(j) What specific measures can reduce the chances of neutropenic sepsis?

....

....

....

Beryl recovers from the first course of chemotherapy and the consultant says that there is a good chance of her having a complete remission.

(k) What is her long-term prognosis?

....

....

....

Key cases

- Anaemia
- Myelodysplasia (MDS)
- Acute myeloid leukaemia (AML)

Clinical context

The definition of anaemia is a reduction in the Hb concentration of the blood. The Hb concentration must be more than two standard deviations below the mean for a population of healthy people of the same age and sex. This represents a level of less than 13.5 g/dl for men, and less than 11.5 g/dl for women.

Anaemia is extremely common, and globally constitutes an enormous health problem. The most common causes in the developing world are malnutrition, increased circulatory demands (i.e. pregnancy), hookworm infection, and malaria. Although these causes must also be considered in the West, it is important to establish an index of clinical suspicion when considering the causes of suspected anaemia. Anaemia in the West is most commonly due to blood loss. The most common causes are menorrhagia in premenopausal women, and gastrointestinal bleeding in postmenopausal women and in men. Other causes to be considered include malabsorbtion (e.g. coeliac disease), anaemia of chronic disease, renal disease, haemolytic anaemia, myelodysplasia, haematological malignancy, alcohol use, liver disease and pernicious anaemia. A further detailed history will be guided by the results of the laboratory investigations.

The most important lesson from this scenario is that anaemia is a symptom of an underlying condition, and not a diagnosis. In your future career you will see many examples of anaemic patients being treated empirically, usually with iron, and not being investigated. The underlying cause must be sought. A comprehensive history and thorough examination will often provide the answer when combined with appropriate investigations. This scenario uses the example of AML in an elderly patient to illustrate salient information regarding anaemia, pancytopenia, blood transfusion, and chemotherapy complicated by neutropenic sepsis.

(a) History in suspected anaemia

The history should concentrate on the general symptoms of anaemia, and symptoms that might suggest an underlying cause.

Symptoms of anaemia include:

- shortness of breath (particularly on exercise)
- headaches
- palpitations and anginal pain
- intermittent claudication
- lethargy and weakness.

Symptoms that might suggest an underlying cause should be broken down into systems:

Symptoms suggestive of a GI cause

- Rectal bleeding or melaena (*see* p. 90)
- Haematemesis (*see* p. 122)
- Dyspepsia (*see* p. 122)
- Abdominal pain (*see* p. 70)
- Change in bowel habit (diarrhoea or constipation) (*see* p. 90)
- Symptoms of chronic bowel disease (*see* p. 163)

Symptoms suggestive of a GU cause

- Vaginal bleeding (full menstrual/gynaecological history)
- Haematuria (*see* p. 40)
- Urinary symptoms
- Symptoms of renal disease (*see* p. 97)

Symptoms suggestive of a haematological cause (which should be qualified, e.g. when/where)

- Bruising
- Bleeding
- Recurrent infections
- Weight loss, fevers, sweats, pruritus

Symptoms of chronic disease

- Rheumatological, pulmonary (especially important in this case), cardiac symptoms (*see* p. 178)
- Weight loss
- Anorexia
- Fevers
- Sweats

Additionally, a general history should be taken which should include:

- Previous medical history (chronic disease)
- Drug history (particularly aspirin, NSAID and steroid use)
- Family history (sickle-cell, thalassaemia)
- Social and dietary history
- Alcohol history.

(b) Clinical examination in anaemia

Systematic examination is important when considering both the severity and the cause of anaemia. Signs of anaemia can be divided into general and specific signs. When assessing the general signs it is important to examine for any features of 'organ' decompensation. This is particularly true in elderly patients who are prone to cardiac failure precipitated by the higher output needed to maintain tissue perfusion.

When assessing potential causes of anaemia it is important to exclude the common causes first. This includes systematic assessment of potential sources of blood loss from the gastrointestinal and genitourinary systems. Additionally, there are many specific signs that may indicate an underlying cause.

General signs of anaemia

- Pallor of the eyelids, tongue, nail beds and palms (Hb of less than 9 or 10 g/dl).
- Tachycardia, bounding pulse and cardiomegaly are associated with a hyperdynamic circulation (reflects an attempt to increase oxygen delivery to the peripheral tissues).
- Decompensation may be demonstrated by hypotension, tachycardia, dyspnoea, or, in severe cases, by features of congestive cardiac failure.

Specific signs of anaemia

- Angular stomatitis, painless glossitis and very rarely spoon-shaped nails (koilonychia) in iron deficiency anaemia.
- Painful glossitis and angular stomatitis in megaloblastic anaemias.
- Bruising combined with features of infection might suggest marrow failure (malignancy, myelodysplasia).
- Mild jaundice is associated with haemolytic anaemias, or may be a sign of liver disease.
- Stigmata of alcoholism.
- Abdominal examination.
- Features of GI malignancy (see p. 90).
- Features of liver disease (see p. 63).
- Splenomegaly may indicate haematological malignancy and can also cause haemolysis, and sequestration of blood cells.
- Palpable kidneys may indicate polycystic kidney disease causing chronic renal failure and its associated features (see p. 97).

(c) Pancytopenia

Pancytopenia is a reduction in the peripheral circulation of red cells, white cells, and platelets. Generally pancytopenia is caused by decreased cell production in the marrow, or increased cell destruction by an enlarged spleen. When a reduction in all cell lines is observed, the main diseases that need to be excluded are:

- acute leukaemia (AML or ALL)
- myelodysplasia (MDS)
- myeloma
- marrow infiltration by lymphoma or solid tumours
- aplastic anaemia (idiopathic, or secondary to drugs, infection, or radiation exposure)
- splenomegaly.

Thus patients may present with symptoms and signs of anaemia, and are prone to infection and bleeding.

(d) Haematological investigation

- Repeat FBC
- Haematinics (see p. 91)
- Peripheral blood film
- Bone marrow aspirate and trephine biopsy

Anaemia always requires further investigation, particularly within the context of pancytopenia. An FBC should be repeated to confirm the degree of pancytopenia, and provide a baseline measurement for treatment. Additionally, red cell indices from the

FBC, combined with haematinics can help define the type of anaemia.

The peripheral blood film is important in the investigation of anaemia and other cytopenias. Microscopic examination of the blood is used to assess abnormalities in the number and morphology of red blood cells, white blood cells and platelets. Additionally, the peripheral blood film can detect the presence and number of other cells such as reticulocytes and myeloid or lymphoid blast cells.

> Use this opportunity to revise normal and commonly abnormal morphology. What important information can be gained from a blood film? You should be familiar with some of the more common variations in size and shape of the cells commonly seen using light microscopy.

Examination of the bone marrow is one of the most valuable diagnostic tests in the evaluation of haematological disorders. Bone marrow is usually extracted from the iliac crest using either aspiration or trephine biopsy. The aspirate is then spread onto a slide and stained for microscopy. A trephine biopsy is a solid cylinder of bone, which is fixed, decalcified and sectioned. The aspirate is useful for examination of single marrow-derived cells, whereas trephine biopsy provides architectural information. Marrow samples can be analysed for immunological and cytochemical markers, which are assuming greater importance in the diagnosis of haematological disorders.

> Use this opportunity to revise the common myeloid and lymphoid cell lines. How are growth and differentiation controlled? How is the marrow architecture and microenvironment involved in effective haematopoiesis? What are the important extramedullary sites of haematopoiesis?

(e) Blood transfusion

The BCSH guidelines on blood transfusion (2001) highlight the importance of factors including 'the cause of the anaemia, its severity and chronicity, the patient's ability to compensate for anaemia, the likelihood of further blood loss, and the need to provide some reserve before the onset of tissue hypoxaemia'.

In general:

- blood should only be given if absolutely necessary
- treat the patient, not the number. There is no universal haemoglobin concentration below

which red cell transfusions should be given. Clinical judgement plays a role in the decision to transfuse red cells
- the cause of anaemia should be found. Transfusions should be avoided when there are alternatives, e.g. treatment of iron, B_{12} or folate deficiency, anaemia of chronic renal failure or autoimmune haemolytic anaemia
- blood tests aimed at finding the cause of anaemia should always be done before transfusion
- patients should be properly informed about the benefits, risks and alternatives to blood transfusion. Remember that they have the right to refuse transfusion.

(BCSH, 2001)

> People differ in their response to anaemia. Use this opportunity to revise the way in which the body compensates for anaemia. Which factors determine oxygen delivery and consumption? What are the physiological adaptations and haemodynamic mechanisms that determine patients' ability to tolerate anaemia? How do these change over time?

(f) Complications of blood transfusion

Most acute haemolytic reactions due to ABO incompatibility can be avoided by appropriate testing before transfusion, and use of procedures to prevent errors.

> What procedures do most hospitals use to prevent errors in blood transfusion? How are the forms different from normal blood investigation forms? What checks are carried out in the laboratory?

In addition to acute haemolysis, several complications may be fatal: delayed haemolysis, anaphylaxis, transfusion-related acute lung injury (similar to ARDS, see p. 124), and graft-versus-host disease.

Other more common transfusion problems which patients should be told about include:

- febrile reactions caused by HLA antibodies
- allergic reactions caused by donor plasma proteins
- post-transfusion circulatory overload
- bacterial transmission
- viral transmission
- other infections.

Although patients have to be told about the possibility of infection from blood products, this is rare. It is important to realise that there have been no cases of transfusion-transmitted (new) variant Creuzfeldt–Jakob disease (vCJD).

Major transfusion reactions are rare. However, monitor the patient for pain, fever, flushing, rash, shortness of breath, wheeze, vomiting or hypotension. If any symptoms occur, the transfusion should be stopped and appropriate management commenced.

>  Use this opportunity to revise blood groups, rhesus and other antigen systems. What are the alternatives to donor blood transfusion? How do patients' religious beliefs differ relating to transfusion? What is the local protocol for blood transfusion in your hospital? What are the financial costs of the commonly used blood products?

(g) (h) Treatment of AML in the elderly

The symptoms of AML are caused by the clonal expansion of malignant myeloid precursor cells in the marrow and blood, causing bone marrow failure and infiltration of other organs. AML is classified according to the morphology of the most common blast cells found on examination of the marrow.

The largest proportion of AML cases occur in the elderly. In contrast to younger patients with AML, AML in the elderly is often highly resistant to chemotherapy due to differences in cell biology, cytogenetics and drug resistance. Furthermore, co-existing medical problems make elderly patients less tolerant of the cardiotoxic and nephrotoxic side-effects of conventional chemotherapy regimes.

The decision to give intensive chemotherapy in the elderly may prove difficult. Treatment-related mortality can be as high as 30%, and often these patients can be maintained on blood transfusions and platelet support for many months. Quality of life issues may be more important than the duration of survival.

The main treatment options for elderly patients are:

● supportive treatment with blood and platelet transfusions
● conventional combination chemotherapy
● low-dose, or single-agent chemotherapy
● immunotherapy (using anti-CD33 mononoclonal antibody complexed with anti-tumour antibiotic, gemtuzumab ozogamicin (Mylotarg)).

> Use this opportunity to revisit the common haematological malignancies. Which myeloid precursors are commonly affected in AML? What are the general phases of chemotherapy? What are the different types of stem cell transplantation?

In general, the factors that should be used when deciding a management plan are:

● age and general fitness
● severity of disease
● co-morbidities
● prognostic factors
● personal preference.

(i) Clinical trials

The ethics of clinical trials are complex and have seen considerable change over the last century. Just because something can be done does not mean it should be done. The Declaration of Helsinki (1964) contains recommendations guiding biomedical research involving humans, and was revised in 2000:

● *Article 2*: the potential benefits, hazards and discomforts of a new method should be weighed against the advantages of the best current diagnostic and therapeutic methods
● *Article 5*: in medical research on human subjects, considerations related to the well-being of the participants should take precedence over the interests of science and society
● *Article 9*: no clinical trial can commence until an appropriate ethics committee approves the protocol.

In practice this means that any research must have been approved by the local research and ethics committee (LREC). Department of Health guidance to ethics committees requires the committee to look at the protocols on the basis of three different approaches:

● *patient welfare*: duty based
● *patient dignity*: rights based
● *scientific validity*: goals based.

In general the factors that make a clinical trial ethical include:

● social or scientific value
● scientific validity and independent review
● risk–benefit ratio
● unbiased subject selection
● informed consent
● respect for potential and enrolled subjects.

> Use this opportunity to revisit the principles of duty-based, rights-based and goals-based ethical principles. What are the similarities and differences of these approaches?

> Use this opportunity to revise the components of a standard septic screen. Which additional samples would be requested in a patient with febrile neutropenia?

(j) Neutropenic sepsis

Neutropenia can result from both AML and more commonly, the treatments used. Neutrophils are the most common phagocytic cells involved in the normal immune response, and depletion places patients at enormous risk of bacterial, viral, fungal and protozoal infection. Many of these infections arise from patients' own commensal bacterial flora, and normally non-pathogenic organisms may cause severe life-threatening infection.

When there is severe depletion of neutrophils there may be no pus formation, and pyrexia may be the only sign of infection. Cultures should be taken from all suspected sites of infection and empirical antibiotic treatment started – according to local protocols.

Although prompt recognition of any infection is vital, prophylaxis of infection is more important. Haematology units will all have protocols in place, and it is important to be familiar with these. The general measures used include:

- isolation facilities with air filtration and positive pressure ventilation
- attention to hygiene by all staff members, with careful handwashing before and after patient contact
- barrier nursing
- freshly cooked thoroughly heated meals. Avoidance of unpasteurised dairy foods, pepper and herbs that might contain fungi
- oral antimicrobial treatment to reduce gut flora
- oral antifungals
- topical antiseptics for bathing and mouthwashing
- regular cultures from the mouth, skin, stool to document a patient's bacterial flora and their sensitivities.

(k) Long-term prognosis

Although the initial response to treatment is a major predictor of prognosis, the chance of a long-term remission in elderly patients remains poor. Only 5% of patients older than 65 years can expect to remain disease free.

Web resources

- Blood transfusion guidelines: www.bcshguidelines.com
- Clinical trials in leukaemia: www.cancerbackup.org.uk
- Information on anaemia: www.prodigy.nhs.uk

Further reading

- BCSH (2001) Guidelines for the clinical use of red cell transfusions. *British Journal of Haematology.* 113(1): 24.
- Fitzsimons EJ and Brock JH (2001) The anaemia of chronic disease. *British Medical Journal.* 322: 81.
- Greer JP, Foerster J, Lukens JN *et al.* (2003) *Wintrobe's Clinical Haematology* (11e). Lippincott Williams and Wilkins, Philadelphia.
- Hoffbrand AV, Pettit JE and Moss PAH (2001) *Essential Haematology* (4e). Blackwell Publishing, Oxford.
- Nardone DA, Roth KM, Mazur DJ *et al.* (1990) Usefulness of physical examination in detecting the presence or absence of anemia. *Archives of Internal Medicine.* 150: 201.
- Oscier DG (1997) ABC of clinical haematology. The myelodysplastic syndromes. *British Medical Journal.* 314: 883.

Quick symptom reference guide

Main index